10th edition – Part B: Exotic Pets

Editor-in-Chief:

Joanna Hedley BVM&S DZooMed(Reptilian) DipECZM(Herpetology) MRCVS
Beaumont Sainsbury Animal Hospital, Royal Veterinary College,
Royal College Street, London NW1 0TU

Published by:
British Small Animal Veterinary Association
Woodrow House, 1 Telford Way, Waterwells Business Park,
Quedgeley, Gloucester GL2 2AB

A Company Limited by Guarantee in England.
Registered Company No. 2837793.
Registered as a Charity.

Copyright © 2020 BSAVA

Small Animal Formulary
First edition 1994
Second edition 1997
Third edition 1999
Fourth edition 2002
Fifth edition 2005
Sixth edition 2008
Seventh edition 2011
Eighth edition 2014
Small Animal Formulary – Part A: Canine and Feline
Ninth edition 2017
Tenth edition 2020
Small Animal Formulary – Part B: Exotic Pets
Ninth edition 2015
Tenth edition 2020

All rights reserved. No part of this publication may be reproduced, stored in a retrieval system, or transmitted, in form or by any means, electronic, mechanical, photocopying, recording or otherwise without prior written permission of the copyright holder.

A catalogue record for this book is available from the British Library.

ISBN 978-1-910443-71-2

The publishers, editors and contributors cannot take responsibility for information provided on dosages and methods of application of drugs mentioned or referred to in this publication. Details of this kind must be verified in each case by individual users from up to date literature published by the manufacturers or suppliers of those drugs. Veterinary surgeons are reminded that in each case they must follow all appropriate national legislation and regulations (for example, in the United Kingdom, the prescribing cascade) from time to time in force.

Printed in the UK by Cambrian Printers, Aberystwyth SY23 3TN
Printed on ECF paper made from sustainable forests.   10010PUBS20

Contents

Editorial Panel

Preface

Welcome to Part B of the 10th edition of the *BSAVA Small Animal Formulary*, covering those drugs used in exotic pets. Treatment of exotic pets can be challenging due to the wide variety of species and conditions that may be encountered, in addition to the many anatomical and physiological differences between the different species groups. Although our knowledge is progressing all the time, unfortunately there is still a lack of pharmacological studies and clinical efficacy trials for many commonly used drugs in these species. Consequently, many drug dosages are extrapolated from those used in other species or have been derived from anecdotal recommendations based on apparent clinical efficacy. As in the previous edition, primary references indicate where information is available, but for most drugs it is important to be aware that evidence is limited. Additional references are provided in the online version of the Formulary and we look forward to expanding this resource in the future.

Since the last edition, various new drugs have become available and information on other drugs has increased with some modifications to recommended dosages or treatment protocols. Some drugs have been deleted if they are no longer available or their use is no longer recommended. The majority of drugs listed are still not licensed for use in these species, so need to be prescribed via the cascade with informed client consent.

I would like to thank all the Editorial Panel members for their hard work reviewing each monograph and ensuring that dosages and evidence are as up-to-date as possible. I would also like to thank the BSAVA Publishing team at Woodrow House for all their editorial and administrative assistance, without which this Formulary would not have been possible.

Joanna Hedley
January 2020

Foreword

The *BSAVA Small Animal Formulary: Part B – Exotic Pets* has developed over the last few years from an appendix in the cat and dog Formulary to a standalone resource and is a reflection of the increasing popularity of the non-traditional pets. Busy small animal clinicians in both primary care and referral practice will find this evidence-based resource an invaluable help with immediate prescribing advice, especially for some of the more unusual exotic pets they can be presented with.

This new edition of the Formulary sees Joanna Hedley take up the editorial reins from Anna Meredith. Joanna has assembled a knowledgeable and experienced group of subject experts to review the Formulary, which has been completely updated. This comprehensive resource covers small mammals (including primates, sugar gliders and hedgehogs in addition to rodents, rabbits and ferrets), birds, reptiles, fish and amphibians, and contains twelve new drug monographs.

Joanna and her team are to be congratulated on bringing out this new and updated small animal exotic Formulary.

Sue Paterson MA VetMB DVD DipECVD FRCVS
BSAVA President 2019–2020

Introduction

Notes on the monographs

- **Name.** The rINN generic name is used where this has been agreed. When a choice of names is available the more commonly used in the UK has been provided. The list of trade names is not necessarily comprehensive, and the mention or exclusion of any particular commercial product is not a recommendation or otherwise as to its value. Any omission of a product that is authorized for a particular small animal indication is purely accidental. All monographs were updated in the period March–September 2019. Products that are not authorized for veterinary use by the Veterinary Medicines Directorate are marked with an asterisk. Products that are authorized for use in one or more of the exotic species listed in a monograph are marked by bold text. Note that an indication that a product is authorized does not necessarily mean that it is authorized for all species and indications listed in the monograph; users should check individual data sheets. You may also wish to refer to the VMD's Product Information Database (www.vmd.defra.gov.uk/ProductInformationDatabase/).

- **Formulations.** Only medicines and formulations that are available in the UK have been included – many others are available outside the UK and some medicines in different formulations. Common trade names of human medicines are provided. In many cases they are available as generic formulations and may be cheaper. However, be careful of assuming that the bioavailability of one brand is the same as that of another. Avoid switching between brands unnecessarily.

- **Action** and **Use**. Veterinary surgeons using this publication are warned that **many of the drugs and doses listed are not currently authorized** by the Veterinary Medicines Directorate (VMD) or the European Agency for the Evaluation of Medicinal Products (EMEA) (either at all or for a particular species), or manufacturers' recommendations may be limited to particular indications. **The decision, and therefore the responsibility, for prescribing any drug for an animal lies solely with the veterinary surgeon.** Expert assistance should be obtained when necessary. The 'cascade' and its implications are discussed below.

- **Safety and handling.** This section only outlines specific risks and precautions for a particular drug that are in addition to the general advice given below in the 'Health and safety in dispensing' section.

- **Contraindications** and **Adverse reactions.** The list of adverse reactions is not intended to be comprehensive and is limited to those effects that may be of clinical significance. The information for both of these sections is taken from published veterinary and human references and not just from product literature.

- **Drug interactions.** A listing of those interactions which may be of clinical significance.

- **Doses.** These are based on those recommended by the manufacturers in their data sheets and package inserts, or are based on those given in published articles or textbooks, or are based on clinical experience. These recommendations should be used only as guidelines and should not be considered appropriate for every case. Clinical judgement must take precedence. Where possible, doses have been given for individual species; however, sometimes generalizations are used. 'Mammals' includes ferrets, lagomorphs and rodents. Doses for small primates and other exotic mammals, such as African pygmy hedgehogs and sugar gliders, are given on a species basis only. 'Birds' includes psittacines, raptors, pigeons and others. 'Reptiles' includes chelonians, lizards and snakes. Amphibians and pet fish are also included. Except where indicated, all doses given for reptiles assume that the animal is kept within its Selected Temperature Range (Ts). Animals that are maintained at different temperatures may have different rates of metabolism and therefore the dose (and especially the frequency) that is required may require alteration.
- **References.** Primary references are given to support doses where available and are denoted by a letter. Such primary references describe a pharmacokinetic or clinical efficacy trial in that species or species group (not case reports). Primary references are generally not given where doses are considered very well established in the scientific literature, particularly for rabbits and rodents (e.g. from studies on laboratory mammals), or where the product is authorized in that species or species group. For some drugs, non-primary references are also given and are denoted by a number. These generally refer to sources of information such as textbooks where no other primary information can be found and the reference is deemed a useful resource in itself. All other doses can be assumed to be taken from other non-primary sources such as other formularies, book chapters or reviews, or are anecdotal.

Distribution categories

Authorized small animal medicines now fall within the first four categories below and all packaging supplied by drug manufacturers and distributors was changed in 2008. Medical products not authorized for veterinary use retain their former classification (e.g. P, POM). Some nutritional supplements (nutraceuticals) are not considered medicinal products and therefore are not classified. Where a product does not have a marketing authorization it is designated 'general sale'.

AVM-GSL: Authorized veterinary medicine – general sales list (formerly GSL). This may be sold by anyone.

NFA-VPS: Non-food animal medicine – veterinarian, pharmacist, Suitably Qualified Person (SQP) (formerly PML companion animal products and a few P products). These medicines for companion animals must be supplied by a veterinary surgeon, pharmacist or

SQP. An SQP has to be registered with the Animal Medicines Training Regulatory Authority (AMTRA). Veterinary nurses can become SQPs but it is not automatic.

POM-VPS: Prescription-only medicine – veterinarian, pharmacist, SQP (formerly PML livestock products, MFSX products and a few P products). These medicines for food-producing animals (including horses) can only be supplied on an oral or written veterinary prescription from a veterinary surgeon, pharmacist or SQP and can only be supplied by one of those groups of people in accordance with the prescription.

POM-V: Prescription-only medicine – veterinarian (formerly POM products and a few P products). These medicines can only be supplied against a veterinary prescription that has been prepared (either orally or in writing) by a veterinary surgeon to animals under their care following a clinical assessment, and can only be supplied by a veterinary surgeon or pharmacist in accordance with the prescription.

Exemptions for Small Pet Animals (ESPA): Schedule 6 of the Veterinary Medicine Regulations 2013 (unofficially known as the Small Animal Exemption Scheme) allows for the use of medicines in certain pet species (aquarium fish, cage birds, ferrets, homing pigeons, rabbits, small rodents and terrarium animals) the active ingredient of which has been declared by the Secretary of State as not requiring veterinary control. These medicines are exempt from the requirement for a marketing authorization and are not therefore required to prove safety, quality or efficacy, but must be manufactured to the same standards as authorized medicines and are subject to pharmacovigilance reporting.

CD: Controlled Drug. A substance controlled by the Misuse of Drugs Act 1971 and Regulations. The CD is followed by (Schedule 1), (Schedule 2), (Schedule 3), (Schedule 4) or (Schedule 5) depending on the Schedule to The Misuse of Drugs Regulations 2001 (as amended) in which the preparation is included. You could be prosecuted for failure to comply with this act. Prescribers are reminded that there are additional requirements relating to the prescribing of Controlled Drugs. For more information see the *BSAVA Guide to the Use of Veterinary Medicines* at www.bsavalibrary.com.

Schedule 1: Includes LSD, cannabis, lysergide and other drugs that are not used medicinally. Possession and supply are prohibited except in accordance with Home Office Authority.

Schedule 2: Includes etorphine, morphine, papaveretum, pethidine, diamorphine (heroin), cocaine and amphetamine. Record all purchases and each individual supply (within 24 hours). Registers must be kept for 2 calendar years after the last entry. Drugs must be kept under safe custody (locked secure cabinet), except secobarbital. Drugs may not be destroyed except in the presence of a person authorized by the Secretary of State.

Schedule 3: Includes buprenorphine, pentazocine, the barbiturates (e.g. pentobarbital and phenobarbital but not secobarbital – which is Schedule 2), tramadol, gabapentin and others. Buprenorphine, diethylpropion and temazepam must be kept under safe custody (locked secure cabinet); it is advisable that all Schedule 3 drugs are locked away. Retention of invoices for 2 years is necessary.

Schedule 4: Includes most of the benzodiazepines (temazepam is now in Schedule 3), and androgenic and anabolic steroids (e.g. clenbuterol). Exempted from control when used in normal veterinary practice.

Schedule 5: Includes preparations (such as several codeine products) which, because of their strength, are exempt from virtually all Controlled Drug requirements other than the retention of invoices for 2 years.

The prescribing cascade

Veterinary medicinal products (VMPs) must be administered in accordance with the prescribing cascade, as set out in The Veterinary Medicines Regulations 2013. These Regulations provide that when no authorized VMP exists for a condition in a particular species, veterinary surgeons exercising their clinical judgement may, in particular to avoid unacceptable suffering, prescribe for one or a small number of animals under their care other suitable medications in accordance with the following sequence:

1   A VMP authorized in the UK for use in another species with the same condition, or for a different condition in the same species.
2   A medicine authorized in the UK for human use or a VMP authorized in another EU member state for use in any species under the Special Import Scheme.
3   A VMP prepared extemporaneously by a properly authorized person as prescribed by the veterinary surgeon.

'Off-label' use of medicines

'Off-label' use is the use of medicines outside the terms of their marketing authorization. It may include medicines authorized outside the UK that are used in accordance with an import certificate issued by the VMD. A veterinary surgeon, with detailed knowledge of the medical history and clinical status of a patient, may reasonably prescribe a medicine 'off-label' in accordance with the prescribing cascade. Authorized medicines have been scientifically assessed against statutory criteria of safety, quality and efficacy when used in accordance with the authorized recommendations on the product literature. Use of an unauthorized medicine provides none of these safeguards and may, therefore, pose potential risks that the authorization process seeks to minimize. Note that the use of an ESPA medicine not in accordance with the product's labelling would be classed as use under the cascade and considered an extemporaneous preparation.

Medicines may be used 'off-label' for a variety of reasons including:

- No authorized product is suitable for the condition or specific subpopulation being treated
- Need to alter the duration of therapy, dosage, route of administration, etc., to treat the specific condition presented
- An authorized product has proved ineffective in the circumstances of a particular case (all cases of suspected lack of efficacy of authorized veterinary medicines should be reported to the VMD).

Responsibility for the use of a medicine 'off-label' lies solely with the prescribing veterinary surgeon. He or she should inform the owner of the reason why a medicine is to be used 'off-label' and record this reason in the patient's clinical notes. When electing to use a medicine 'off-label' always:

- Discuss all therapeutic options with the owner
- Use the cascade to determine your choice of medicine
- Obtain signed informed consent if an unauthorized product is to be used, ensuring that all potential problems are explained to the client
- Administer unauthorized medicines against a patient-specific prescription. Do not administer to a group of animals if at all possible.

An 'off-label' medicine must show a comparative clinical advantage to the authorized product in the specific circumstances presented (where applicable). Medicines may be used 'off-label' in the following ways (this is not an exhaustive list):

- Authorized product at an unauthorized dose
- Authorized product for an unauthorized indication
- Authorized product used outwith the authorized age range
- Authorized product administered by an unauthorized route
- Authorized product used to treat an animal in an unauthorized physiological state, e.g. pregnancy (i.e. an unauthorized indication)
- Product authorized for use in humans or a different animal species to that being treated.

Adverse effects may or may not be specific for a species, and idiosyncratic reactions are always a possibility. If no adverse effects are listed, consider data from different species. When using novel or unfamiliar drugs, consider pharmaceutical and pharmacological interactions. In some species, and with some diseases, the ability to metabolize/excrete a drug may be impaired/enhanced. Use the lowest dose that might be effective and the safest route of administration. Ensure that you are aware of the clinical signs that may suggest toxicity.

Information on 'off-label' use may be available from a wide variety of sources (**see Further reading and useful websites**).

Drug storage and dispensing

For further information on the storage and dispensing of medicines see the *BSAVA Guide to the Use of Veterinary Medicines* available at www.bsavalibrary.com. Note that veterinary surgeons may only supply a veterinary medicine from practice premises that are registered with the RCVS and that these premises must be inspected. It is recommended that, in general, medications are kept in and dispensed in the manufacturer's original packaging. Medicines can be adversely affected by adverse temperatures, excessive light, humidity and rough handling. Loose tablets or capsules that are repackaged from bulk containers should be dispensed in child-resistant containers and supplied with a package insert (if one exists). Tablets and capsules in foil strips should be sold in their original packaging or in a similar cardboard box for smaller quantities. Preparations for external application should be dispensed in coloured fluted bottles. Oral liquids should be dispensed in plain glass bottles with child-resistant closures.

All medicines should be labelled. The label should include:

- The owner's name and address
- Identification of the animal
- Date of supply (and, if applicable, the expiry date)
- Product name (and strength)
- Total quantity of the product supplied in the container
- Instructions for dosage
- Practice name and address
- The name of the veterinary surgeon who prescribed the medication (if not an authorized use)
- Any specific pharmacy precautions (including storage, disposal, handling)
- The wording 'Keep out of reach of children' and 'For animal treatment only'
- Withdrawal period, if relevant
- Any other necessary warnings.

The words 'For external use only' should be included on labels for products for topical use. All labels should be typed. If this information will not fit on a single label then it is permissible to include the information on a separate sheet.

For medicines that are not authorized for veterinary use, and even for some that are, it is useful to add to the label or on a separate information sheet the likely adverse effects, drug interactions and the action to be taken in the event of inadvertent mis-dosing or incorrect administration written in plain English.

In order to comply with the current Veterinary Medicines Regulations, records of all products supplied on prescription must be kept for 5 years. When a batch is brought into use in a practice, the batch number and date should be recorded. It is not necessary to record the batch number of each medication used for a given animal.

Health and safety in dispensing

All drugs are potentially poisonous to humans as well as animals. Toxicity may be mild or severe and includes carcinogenic and teratogenic effects. Warnings are given in the monographs.

However, risks to humans dispensing medicines are not always well characterized and idiosyncratic reactions may occur. **It is good practice for everyone to wear protective clothing (including gloves) when directly handling medicines, not to eat or drink (or store food or drink) near medicines**, and to wash their hands frequently when working with medicines. Gloves, masks and safety glasses should be worn if handling potentially toxic liquids, powders or broken tablets. Do not break tablets of antineoplastic cytotoxic drugs, and use laminar flow cabinets for the preparation and dispensing of these medications. **See Appendix** for more information.

Many prescribers and users of medicines are not aware of the carcinogenic potential of the drugs they are handling. Below are lists of medicines included in the *BSAVA Formulary* that are known or potential carcinogens or teratogens. The lists are not all-inclusive: they include only those substances that have been evaluated. Most of the drugs are connected only with certain kinds of cancer. The relative carcinogenicity of the agents varies considerably and some do not cause cancer at all times or under all circumstances. Some may only be carcinogenic or teratogenic if a person is exposed in a certain way (for example, ingesting as opposed to touching the drug). For more detailed information refer to the International Agency for Research on Cancer (IARC) or the National Toxicology Program (NTP) (information is available on their respective websites).

Examples of drugs known or suspected to be human carcinogens (c) or teratogens (t):

- ACE inhibitors (t), e.g. benazepril, enalapril
- Androgenic (anabolic) steroids (t, c)
- Antibiotics (c), e.g. metronidazole, chloramphenicol
- Antibiotics (t) e.g. aminoglycosides, doxycycline, trimethoprim, sulphonamides
- Antifungals (c), e.g. fluconazole, itraconazole
- Antineoplastic drugs (c, t) – all
- Antithyroid drugs (t), e.g. carbimazole/methimazole
- Beta-blockers (t)
- Deferoxamine (t)
- Diltiazem (t)
- Finasteride (t)
- Immunosuppressives (c), e.g. azathioprine, ciclosporin
- Methotrexate (t)
- Misoprostol (t)
- NSAIDs (t)
- Penicillamine (t)
- Phenoxybenzamine (c)
- Progesterone (c) and some oestrogens (c)
- Vitamin A (t)

Note that most carcinogens are also likely to be teratogens.

Acepromazine (ACP)
(ACP) **POM-V**

Formulations: Injectable: 2 mg/ml solution. Oral: 10 mg, 25 mg tablets.

Action: Phenothiazine with depressant effect on the CNS, thereby causing sedation and a reduction in spontaneous activity.

Use: Sedation or pre-anaesthetic medication in small mammals and other exotic species. ACP raises the threshold for cardiac arrhythmias and has antiemetic properties. Sedation is unreliable when ACP is used alone; combining ACP with an opioid drug improves sedation (neuroleptanalgesia) and the opioid provides analgesia. The depth of sedation is dose-dependent up to a plateau (0.1–5 mg/kg dependant on species and size). Increasing the dose above this does little to improve the predictability of achieving adequate sedation but increases the risk of incurring adverse effects, the severity of adverse effects and the duration of action of any effects (desirable or adverse). Onset of sedation is 20–30 min after i.m. administration; clinical doses cause sedation for up to 6 hours. The oral dose of ACP tablets required to produce sedation varies between individual animals and high doses can lead to very prolonged sedation.

Safety and handling: Normal precautions should be observed.

Contraindications: Hypotension due to shock, trauma or cardiovascular disease. Avoid in animals <3 months old and animals with liver disease. Avoid in gerbils as lowers the seizure threshold in susceptible strains. Not recommended in birds.

Adverse reactions: Rarely, healthy animals may develop profound hypotension following administration of phenothiazines. Supportive therapy to maintain body temperature and fluid balance is indicated until the animal is fully recovered. Can lead to seizures in gerbils.

Drug interactions: Other CNS depressant agents (e.g. barbiturates, propofol, alfaxalone, volatile anaesthetics) will cause additive CNS depression if used with ACP. Doses of other anaesthetic drugs should be reduced when ACP has been used for premedication. Quinidine given with phenothiazines may cause additional cardiac depression. Increased levels of both drugs may result if propranolol is administered with phenothiazines. As phenothiazines block alpha-adrenergic receptors, concomitant use with adrenaline may lead to unopposed beta activity, thereby causing vasodilation and tachycardia. Antidiarrhoeal mixtures (e.g. kaolin/pectin, bismuth salicylate) and antacids may cause reduced GI absorption of oral phenothiazines.

DOSES

When used for sedation is generally given as part of a combination. See Appendix for sedation protocols in all species.

Mammals: **Ferrets:** 0.2–0.5 mg/kg i.m., s.c., p.o.; **Rabbits:** 0.1–1.0 mg/kg i.m., s.c.; **Guinea pigs:** 0.5–5 mg/kg i.m., s.c., p.o.; **Rats:** 0.5–2.5 mg/kg i.m., s.c., p.o.; **Mice:** 0.5–5 mg/kg i.m., s.c., p.o.; **Hamsters:** 0.5–5 mg/kg i.m., s.c., p.o.; **Gerbils:** Not recommended; **Primates (small):** 0.5–1 mg/kg p.o., s.c., i.m.; **Marsupials:** 0.2 mg/kg i.m., s.c., p.o.; **Hedgehogs:** 0.1–1 mg/kg p.o., s.c., i.m. The higher doses should only be given orally.
Birds: Not recommended.
Reptiles: 0.1–0.5 mg/kg i.m. [a]
Amphibians, Fish: No information available.

References
[a] Alves-Junior JR, Bosso AC, Andrade MB *et al.* (2012) Association of acepromazine with propofol in giant Amazon turtles (*Podocnemis expansa*) reared in captivity. *Acta Cirurgica Brasileira* **27(8)**, 552–556

Acetaminophen see **Paracetamol**

Acetazolamide
(Diamox*, Diamox SR*) **POM**

Formulations: Injectable: 500 mg vial (powder for reconstitution). Oral: 250 mg tablets, capsules.

Action: Systemic carbonic anhydrase inhibitor.

Use: Treatment of gas bubble disease in seahorses but also requires the correction of contributing causes such as faulty air pumps and algal overgrowth. Has also been used to treat ocular gas bubbles (both intraocular and retrobulbar) in fish caused by supersaturation of the water or suspected disorders of the pseudobranch or choroidal rete.

Safety and handling: Normal precautions should be observed.

Contraindications: No information available.

Adverse reactions: In fish, the drug may interfere with normal carbonic anhydrase activity in the vascular rete of other organs such as the swim bladder and result in disturbance of normal buoyancy.

Drug interactions: No information available.

DOSES
Fish: Seahorses: 6 mg/l by immersion, change daily for 4–8 days; 2–3 mg/kg i.m., intracoelomic for gas bubble disease; **Other species:** 6 mg/kg by peribulbar injection.
Mammals, Birds, Reptiles, Amphibians: No information available.

Acetic acid

Formulations: Available in a variety of concentrations including glacial acetic acid (100%) and vinegar formulations (5–20%).

Action: Not known.

Use: Treatment of ectoparasites (e.g. protozoans, monogeneans, hirudinea, crustaceans) in fish. Other treatments are considered safer to use. Management of intestinal dysbiosis in birds.

Safety and handling: Corrosive to skin and irritant to mucous membranes.

Contraindications: No information available.

Adverse reactions: May be toxic to small tropical fish.

Drug interactions: No information available.

DOSES
Birds: 15 ml apple cider vinegar/l drinking water.
Fish: 2 ml/l by immersion in glacial acetic acid for 30–60 seconds.
Mammals, Reptiles, Amphibians: No information available

Acetylcysteine
(Ilube*, Parvolex*) **POM**

Formulations: Injectable: 200 mg/ml solution. **Topical:** 5% ophthalmic solution in combination with 0.35% hypromellose ophthalmic drops in 10 ml bottle.

Action: Decreases the viscosity of bronchial secretions, maintains glutathione levels in the liver and has some anticollagenase activity.

Use: As a mucolytic in respiratory disease. Reduces the extent of liver injury in cases of paracetamol poisoning but no reports on this use in exotic species. In rabbits direct application into the ear has been reported as beneficial in cases of secretory otitis media, reducing inflammation and preventing long-term fibrotic changes. In birds, used as a mucolytic agent via nebulization for respiratory disease and to improve penetration of nebulized drugs through mucus exudates. In reptiles, it may be applied to retained spectacles to aid removal.

Safety and handling: Normal precautions should be observed.

Contraindications: No information available.

Adverse reactions: Acetylcysteine has caused hypersensitivity and bronchospasm when used in the pulmonary tree. When given orally for paracetamol poisoning it may cause GI effects (nausea, vomiting) and, rarely, urticaria.

Drug interactions: In cases of paracetamol poisoning the concurrent administration of activated charcoal is controversial as it may also reduce acetylcysteine absorption.

DOSES

Mammals: Ferrets, Rabbits, Rodents, Primates: Mucolytic: 20 mg/ml solution (dilute with saline) nebulized for 30–60 min as required (e.g. q6–12h); Otic lavage: 1–2 ml of a 20% solution.

Birds: Mucolytic: 22 mg/ml sterile water for nebulization. May be combined with other drugs (e.g. amikacin at 6 mg/ml, gentamicin at 10 mg/ml or kanamycin at 3–15 mg/ml).

Reptiles: Mucolytic: 20 mg/ml solution (dilute with saline) nebulized for 15–30 min as required.

Amphibians, Fish: No information available.

Acetylsalicyclic acid see Aspirin

Aciclovir
(Aciclovir*, Zovirax*) **POM**

Formulations: Ophthalmic: 3% ointment in 4.5 g tubes. Oral: 200 mg, 800 mg tablets; 200 mg/5 ml, 400 mg/5 ml suspension. Injectable: 250 mg, 500 mg vials for reconstitution. Skin: 5% ointment in 10 g, 25 g tubes.

Action: Inhibits viral replication (viral DNA polymerase); depends on viral thymidine kinase for phosphorylation.

Use: Management of ocular herpesvirus lesions in mammals although unable to eradicate latent viral infection. Used to treat systemic herpesvirus infections in various avian species (e.g. Pacheco's disease in psittacine birds) and also for prophylaxis of psittacine herpesvirus in outbreaks. In reptiles, it is used to treat chelonian herpesvirus infections.

Safety and handling: Normal precautions should be observed.

Contraindications: No information available.

Adverse reactions: Ocular irritation may occur and the frequency of application should be reduced if this develops. Treatment should not be continued for >3 weeks. May cause vomiting in birds.

Drug interactions: No information available.

DOSES

Mammals: Rabbits: topically, 1–5 times daily [a].

Birds: Raptors: 330 mg/kg p.o. q12h for 7–14 days; **Psittacids:** 20–40 mg/kg i.m. q12h or 80 mg/kg p.o. q8h for 7 days [b] or 400 mg/kg in food in aviaries.

Reptiles: Testudo species: 80 mg/kg p.o. q8–24h; topically to oral lesions q8–24h [c]; *Terrapene* species: 40 mg/kg p.o. q24h [d].

Amphibians, Fish: No information available.

References

[a] Trousdale MD, Dunkel EC, Nesburn AB (1980) Effect of acyclovir on acute and latent herpes simplex virus infections in the rabbit. *Investigative Ophthalmology & Visual Science* **19(11)**, 1336–1341

[b] Norton TM, Gaskin J, Kollias GV *et al.* (1991) Efficacy of acyclovir against herpesvirus infection in Quaker parakeets. *American Journal of Veterinary Research* **52(12)**, 2007–2009

[c] Gaio C, Rossi T, Villa R *et al.* (2007) Pharmacokinetics of acyclovir after a single oral administration in marginated tortoises (*Testudo marginata*). *Journal of Herpetological Medicine and Surgery* **17**, 8–11

[d] Allender MC, Mitchell MA, Yarborough J and Cox S (2013) Pharmacokinetics of a single oral dose of acyclovir and valacyclovir in North American box turtles (*Terrapene* species). *Journal of Veterinary Pharmacology and Therapeutics* **36(2)**, 205–208

ACP see **Acepromazine**

Acriflavine (Acriflavinium chloride)
(Acriflavin, Acriflavine) **ESPA**

Formulations: Immersion: dry powder. **Liquid**: proprietary liquid formulations, occasionally mixed with proflavine.

Action: No information available.

Use: Treatment of external fungal, bacterial and parasitic diseases in fish. Some bacterial resistance exists and acriflavine is considered to be less effective than other medications. It is strongly recommended that a proprietary formulation is used initially to avoid problems related to purity and enable accurate dosing.

Safety and handling: Powdered formulation is irritant and potentially mutagenic.

Contraindications: No information available.

Adverse reactions: May cause reproductive failure in some species (e.g. guppies). Will kill aquatic plants.

Drug interactions: No information available.

DOSES
Fish: 5 mg/l by immersion for 3–5 days, 10 mg/l by immersion for 2 h or 500 mg/l for 30 min; use proprietary formulations at the manufacturer's recommended dose rate.
Mammals, Birds, Reptiles, Amphibians: No information available.

Acfiflavinium chloride see **Acriflavine**
ACTH see **Tetracosactide**
Activated charcoal see **Charcoal**

Adrenaline (Epinephrine)
(Adrenaline*, Epinephrine*) **POM**

Formulations: Injectable: Range of concentrations for injection: 0.1–10 mg/ml, equivalent to 1:10,000 to 1:100.

Action: Adrenaline exerts its effects via alpha-1 and -2, and beta-1 and -2 adrenoreceptors.

Use: Cardiac resuscitation, status asthmaticus and to offset the effects of histamine release in severe anaphylactoid reactions. The effects of adrenaline vary according to dose. Infusions of low doses mainly result in beta-adrenergic effects (increases in cardiac output, myocardial oxygen consumption, and a reduced threshold for arrhythmias with peripheral vasodilation and a fall in diastolic blood pressure). At high doses alpha-1 effects predominate, causing a rise in systemic vascular resistance, diverting blood to the central organs; however, this may improve cardiac output and blood flow. Adrenaline is not a substitute for fluid replacement therapy. Respiratory effects include bronchodilation and an increase in pulmonary vascular resistance. Renal blood flow is moderately decreased. The duration of action of adrenaline is short (2–5 min). Beware of using in animals with diabetes mellitus (monitor blood glucose concentration), hypertension or hyperthyroidism. Use with caution in hypovolaemic animals. Overdosage can be fatal so check dose, particularly in small patients. Intracardiac injection is not recommended. Used for the treatment of cardiac arrest in fish. Use in anaesthetized reptiles is debatable as it has been suggested to increase hypoxia by diverting blood away from the lungs.

Safety and handling: Do not confuse adrenaline vials of different concentrations. Adrenaline is sensitive to light and air: do not use if it is pink, brown or contains a precipitate. It is unstable in 5% dextrose.

Contraindications: The use of human adrenaline pen injections is not recommended for the treatment of suspected anaphylaxis. The doses in such pens are usually too small to be effective in most normal animals and by the time the animal has collapsed would be unlikely to have any effect on outcome. If such pen injections are administered by owners, then, in common with medical practice, patients must be carefully monitored for at least 6 hours.

Adverse reactions: Increases myocardial oxygen demand and produces arrhythmias including ventricular fibrillation. These may be ameliorated by administering oxygen and slowing the heart rate with beta-2 antagonists. Other adverse effects include tachycardia, arrhythmias, dry mouth and cold extremities. Repeated injections can cause necrosis at the injection site.

Drug interactions: Toxicity may occur if used with other sympathomimetic amines because of additive effects. The effects of adrenaline may be potentiated by antihistamines and thyroxine.

Propranolol may block the beta effects of adrenaline, thus facilitating an increase in blood pressure. Alpha blocking agents or diuretics may negate or diminish the pressor effects. When adrenaline is used with drugs that sensitize the myocardium (e.g. high doses of digoxin) monitor for signs of arrhythmias. Hypertension may result if adrenaline is used with oxytocic agents.

DOSES
Mammals: Ferrets: 20 µg (micrograms)/kg s.c., i.m., i.v., intratracheal; Rabbits: cardiac resuscitation: 100 µg/kg i.v., repeated and/or higher doses (up to 200 µg/kg) may be required at intervals of 2–5 min; Guinea pigs: 3 µg/kg i.v.; **Other rodents:** 10 µg/kg i.v. as required.
Birds: 0.1–1.0 mg/kg i.m., i.v., intraosseous, intracardiac, intratracheal.
Reptiles: Resuscitation: 0.5 mg/kg i.v., intraosseous; 1 mg/kg intratracheal diluted in 1 ml saline/100 g body weight; To speed recovery from anaesthesia: 0.1 mg/kg i.m. [a]
Fish: 0.2–0.5 mg/kg i.m., i.v., intraperitoneal, intracardiac.
Amphibians: No information available.

References
[a] Goe A, Shmalberg J, Gatson B *et al.* (2016) Epinephrine or GV-26 electrical stimulation reduces inhalant anesthetic recovery time in common snapping turtles (*Chelydra serpentina*). *Journal of Zoo and Wildlife Medicine* **47(2)**, 501–507

Aglepristone
(Alizin) **POM-V**

Formulations: Injectable: 30 mg/ml solution.

Action: Progesterone receptor blockage leads to reduced progesterone support for pregnancy.

Use: Termination of pregnancy in mammals. No specific information is available for exotic mammal species. In bitches confirmed as pregnant, a partial abortion may occur in up to 5% and a similar situation may occur in other mammals; owners should be warned. A clinical examination (uterine palpation) is always recommended after treatment in order to confirm termination. After induced abortion an early return to oestrus is frequently observed (the oestrus-to-oestrus interval may be significantly shortened). Can also be used for the treatment of pyometra in some mammals, although recurrence is fairly common.

Safety and handling: Use with care. Accidental injection may be a hazard to women who are pregnant or intending to become pregnant.

Contraindications: Consider avoiding in animals with diagnosed or suspected hypoadrenocorticism or diabetes mellitus.

Adverse reactions: Transient pain at the injection site; any local inflammation produced resolves uneventfully. In animals treated in the later stages of gestation, abortion may be accompanied by the physiological signs of parturition, i.e. fetal expulsion, anorexia, mammary congestion.

Drug interactions: Aglepristone binds to glucocorticoid receptors and may therefore interfere with the actions of glucocorticoids; however, the clinical significance of this is unclear.

DOSES

Mammals: Rabbits: pregnancy termination: 10 mg/kg on days 6 and 7 post implantation; **Guinea pigs:** pyometra/metritis: 10 mg/kg on days 1, 2 and 8; **Rats:** (10 mg/kg s.c. 24 hours apart) on Days 11 and 12 after mating (i.e., at midpregnancy) [a].
Birds, Reptiles, Amphibians, Fish: No information available.

References
[a] Gogny A and Fiéni F (2016) Aglepristone: A review on its clinical use in animals. *Theriogenology* **85(4)**, 555–566

Alfaxalone
(Alfaxan) **POM-V**

Formulations: Injectable: 10 mg/ml solution; the alfaxalone is solubilized in a cyclodextrin. Single or multidose bottles are available. Multidose bottles contain ethanol, chloroscresol and benzethonium chloride as preservative.

Action: Anaesthesia induced by the CNS depressant effect of the alfaxalone.

Use: Induction agent used before inhalational anaesthesia, or as a sole anaesthetic agent for examination or surgical procedures. As with all i.v. anaesthetic drugs, premedication will reduce the dose required for induction and maintenance of anaesthesia. Pre-oxygenation is recommended before i.v. induction as transient post-induction apnoea can occur. The drug should be given slowly and to effect in order to prevent inadvertent overdose. Analgesia is insufficient for surgery: other analgesic drugs such as opioids should be incorporated into the anaesthetic protocol. Alfaxalone is shorter acting and causes less excitement during recovery than the alfaxalone/alfadalone combination previously available. Alfaxalone can be given i.m. or s.c. to provide sedation. The drug should be administered in the cranial half in reptiles to avoid shunting to the liver and first-pass metabolism. Do not use in combination with other i.v. anaesthetic agents. Used for the induction and maintenance of anaesthesia in fish; the alfaxalone/alphadalone combination previously available has been used parenterally in large fish.

Safety and handling: The single-dose vial does not contain an antimicrobial preservative; thus it is recommended that the remainder of an opened bottle is discarded after single use within 24 hours.

Contraindications: No information available.

Adverse reactions: In mammals a slight increase in heart rate can occur immediately after i.v. injection as a compensatory response to maintain blood pressure in the face of mild hypotension. This effect can be minimized by slow i.v. injection. Transient post-induction apnoea can also occur. As with all anaesthetic drugs, respiratory depression can occur with overdoses.

Drug interactions: No information available.

DOSES

See Appendix for sedation protocols in all species.

Mammals:
- Unpremedicated: **Ferrets:** 9–12 mg/kg i.v., i.m.; **Guinea pigs:** 40 mg/kg i.m., i.p.; **Rats:** 2–5 mg/kg i.p., i.v.; **Other rodents:** 20 mg/kg i.m. or 120 mg/kg i.p.; **Small primates (e.g. Marmosets):** 12 mg/kg i.m. [a]
- Premedicated: **Rabbits:** licensed for use following premedication with opioid/alpha-2: 1–3 mg/kg i.v. or 3–6 mg/kg i.m. [b,c]; **Rats:** 2–3 mg/kg i.m. following premedication with opioid and midazolam.

Birds: For large birds and those with a dive response: 2–4 mg/kg i.v. to effect.

Reptiles: 5–9 mg/kg i.v., intraosseous for induction (light sedation) up to 30 mg/kg i.m. for surgical anaesthesia. Effects are dependent on species and temperature; **Chelonians:** 5 mg/kg i.v. [d] or 10 mg/kg i.m. (light sedation) up to 20 mg/kg i.m. for surgical anaesthesia; **Macquarie river turtles:** 9 mg/kg i.v.; **Lizards, Snakes:** <9 mg/kg i.v. [e]; **Green iguanas:** 10 mg/kg i.m. or 5 mg/kg i.v. (for sufficient sedation to allow intubation); **Veiled chameleons:** 5 mg/kg i.v. (for sufficient sedation to allow intubation); **Bearded dragons, Chinese water dragons, Leopard geckos:** 5 mg/kg i.v.; **Galliwasps:** 15 mg/kg i.m.; **Ball pythons:** 10–30 mg/kg i.m.; **Garter snakes:** 30 mg/kg intracoelomic.

Amphibians: Only provides light sedation when administed i.m. or by immersion bath. **Bullfrogs:** 10–17.5 mg/kg i.m.; **Australian green tree frogs:** 30 mg/kg i.m.; **Green and golden bell frogs, Booroolong frogs:** 20 mg/kg i.m. [f]; **Oriental fire-bellied toads:** 200 mg/l immersion bath.

Fish: 5–10 mg/l by immersion for induction of anaesthesia; 1–2.5 mg/l by immersion for maintenance of anaesthesia [g].

References

[a] Bakker J, Uilenreef JJ, Pelt ER *et al.* (2013) Comparison of three different sedative-anaesthetic protocols (ketamine, ketamine-medetomidine and alphaxalone) in common marmosets (*Callithrix jacchus*). *BMC Veterinary Research* **9(1)**, 113

[b] Grint NJ, Smith HE and Senior JM (2008) Clinical evaluation of alfaxalone in cyclodextrin for the induction of anaesthesia in rabbits. *Veterinary Record* **163(13)**, 395–396

[c] Huynh M, Poumeyrol S, Pignon C, Le Teuff G and Zilberstein L (2014) Intramuscular administration of alfaxalone for sedation in rabbits. *Veterinary Record* **176**, 255

[d] Knotek Z (2014) Alfaxalone as an induction agent for anaesthesia in terrapins and tortoises. *Veterinary Record* **175(13)**, 327

[e] Scheelings TF, Baker RT, Hammersley G *et al.* (2011) A preliminary investigation into the chemical restraint with alfaxalone of selected Australian squamate species. *Journal of Herpetological Medicine and Surgery* **21**, 63–67

f   Sladakovic I, Johnson RS and Vogelnest L (2014) Evaluation of intramuscular alfaxalone in three Australian frog species (*Litoria caerulea, Litoria aurea, Litoria booroolongensis*). *Journal of Herpetological Medicine and Surgery* **24(1)**, 36–42

g   Minter LJ, Bailey KM, Harms CA, Lewbart GA and Posner LP (2014) The efficacy of alfaxalone for immersion anesthesia in koi carp (*Cyprinus carpio*). *Veterinary Anaesthesia and Analgesia* **41(4)**, 398–405

Alfentanil
(Rapifen*) **POM CD SCHEDULE 2**

Formulations: Injectable: 0.5 mg/ml solution, available in 2 ml or 10 ml vials; 5 mg/ml solution.

Action: Pure mu agonist of the phenylpiperidine series.

Use: Very potent opioid analgesic (10–20 times more potent than morphine) used to provide intraoperative analgesia during anaesthesia. Use of such potent opioids during anaesthesia contributes to a balanced anaesthesia technique but they must be administered accurately. It has a rapid onset (15–30 seconds) and short duration of action. It is best given using continuous rate infusions. The drug is not suited to provision of analgesia in the postoperative period.

Safety and handling: Normal precautions should be observed.

Contraindications: No information available.

Adverse reactions: A reduction in heart rate is likely whenever alfentanil is given; atropine can be administered to counter bradycardia if necessary. Respiratory depression leading to cessation of spontaneous respiration is likely following administration. Do not use unless facilities for positive pressure ventilation are available (either manual or automatic). Rapid i.v. injection can cause a severe bradycardia, even asystole. In rabbits, seizures have been noted with the use of alfentanil as part of a midazolam, medetomidine and alfentanil combination.

Drug interactions: Alfentanil reduces the dose requirements of concurrently administered anaesthetics, including inhaled anaesthetics, by at least 50%. In humans it is currently recommended to avoid giving alfentanil to patients receiving monoamine oxidase inhibitors due to the risk of serotonin toxicity.

DOSES
Mammals: Rabbits: 0.03–0.07 mg/kg i.v.
Birds, Reptiles, Amphibians, Fish: No information available.

Allopurinol
(Zyloric*) **POM**

Formulations: Oral: 100 mg, 300 mg tablets.

Action: Xanthine oxidase inhibition decreases formation of uric acid by blocking the conversion of hypoxanthine to xanthine, and of xanthine to uric acid.

Use: Treatment of hyperuricaemia and articular gout in birds and reptiles. It should be remembered that, unlike mammals, uric acid is a natural end-product of protein metabolism in birds and reptiles. Therefore use of allopurinol is symptomatic only and the primary cause should be addressed. Ensure patients are adequately hydrated. Clinical response is variable in birds (e.g. studies in red-tailed hawks showed no significant effect on plasma uric acid levels). The dosage should be reduced as plasma uric acid levels decrease.

Safety and handling: Normal precautions should be observed.

Contraindications: No information available.

Adverse reactions: In red-tailed hawks, doses of 50 mg/kg and 100 mg/kg have been reported as toxic and causing renal failure.

Drug interactions: In humans, allopurinol may enhance the effects of azathioprine and theophylline.

DOSES
Birds: 10–30 mg/kg p.o. q12h (all species) [a,b]; **Pigeons:** 830 mg/l drinking water; **Psittacids:** 300 mg/l drinking water.
Reptiles: 10–20 mg/kg p.o. q24h (most species); **Chelonians:** 50 mg/kg p.o. q24h for 30 days then q72h [c]; **Green iguanas:** 25 mg/kg p.o. q24h [d].
Mammals, Amphibians, Fish: No information available.

References
[a] Lumeij JT, Sprang EPM and Redig PT (1998) Further studies on allopurinol-induced hyperuricaemia and visceral gout in Red-tailed hawks (*Buteo jamaicensis*). *Avian Pathology* **24(4)**, 390–393
[b] Poffers J, Lumeij JT, Timmermans-Sprang EP and Redig PT (2002) Further studies on the use of allopurinol to reduce plasma uric acid concentrations in the Red-tailed hawk (*Buteo jamaicensis*) hyperuricaemic model. *Avian Pathology* **31(6)**, 567–572
[c] Kolle P (2001) Efficacy of allopurinol in European tortoises with hyperuricaemia. *Proceedings of the Association of Reptilian and Amphibian Veterinarians*, p. 186
[d] Hernandez-Divers SJ, Martinez-Jimenez D, Bush S *et al.* (2008) Effects of allopurinol on plasma uric acid levels in normouricaemic and hyperuricaemic green iguanas (*Iguana iguana*). *Veterinary Record* **162(4)**, 112–115

Alphaxalone see Alfaxalone

Aluminium antacids
(Aluminium hydroxide)
(Alucap*. With alginate: Acidex*, Gastrocote*, Gaviscon Advance*, Peptac*. With magnesium salt: Asilone*, Maalox*, Mucogel*) **P, GSL**

Formulations: Oral: Aluminium hydroxide is available as a dried gel. Other products are composite preparations containing a variety of other compounds including magnesium oxide, hydroxide or trisilicate, potassium bicarbonate, sodium carbonate and bicarbonate, alginates and dimeticone. Aluminium hydroxide content varies.

Action: Neutralizes gastric hydrochloric acid. May also bind bile acids and pepsin and stimulate local prostaglandin (PGE-1) production. Also binds inorganic phosphate (PO_4^{3-}) in the GI tract, making it unavailable for absorption.

Use: Management of gastritis and gastric ulceration. In renal failure, to lower serum phosphate levels in animals with hyperphosphataemia. Frequent administration is necessary to prevent rebound acid secretion. Phosphate-binding agents are usually only used if low-phosphate diets are unsuccessful. Monitor serum phosphate levels at 10–14 day intervals and adjust dosage accordingly if trying to normalize serum concentrations. Thoroughly mix the drug with food to disperse it throughout the GI tract and to increase its palatability.

Safety and handling: Long-term use (many years) of oral aluminium products in humans has been associated with aluminium toxicity and possible neurotoxicity. This is unlikely to be a problem in veterinary medicine.

Contraindications: No information available.

Adverse reactions: Constipation may occur. This is an effect of the aluminium compound and is counteracted by inclusion of a magnesium salt. Reduced food intake and bodyweight may result at the higher doses used in rats.

Drug interactions: Do not administer digoxin, tetracycline or fluoroquinolone products orally within 2 hours of aluminium salts as their absorption may be impaired.

DOSES
Mammals: Rabbits: 30–60 mg/kg p.o. q8–12h; Guinea pigs: 20–40 mg/animal p.o. prn for hyperphosphataemia due to renal failure; Rats: 2.4–9.6 g/kg/day for chronic renal failure [a].
Birds: 30–90 mg/kg p.o. q12h.
Reptiles: 100 mg/kg p.o. q24h.
Amphibians, Fish: No information available.

References
[a] Sanai T, Okuda S, Onoyama K et al. (1991) Effect of different doses of aluminium hydroxide on renal deterioration and nutritional state in experimental chronic renal failure. *Mineral and Electrolyte Metabolism* **17(3)**, 160–165

Aluminium hydroxide see **Aluminium antacids**

Amantadine
(Lysovir*, Symmetrel*) **POM**

Formulations: Oral: 100 mg capsule; 10 mg/ml syrup.

Action: Provides analgesia through NMDA antagonist action which may potentiate the effects of other analgesics. Anti-viral activity proposed for avian influenza and bornavirus infections.

Use: Adjunctive analgesic in animals that are unresponsive to opioids, or that require chronic pain relief in a home environment (e.g. osteoarthritis or cancer pain). Proventricular dilatation disease (PDD) in parrots.

Safety and handling: Normal precautions should be observed.

Contraindications: No information available.

Adverse reactions: In humans, minor GI and CNS effects have been reported, although these have not been reported in animals.

Drug interactions: No information available.

DOSES
Mammals: Ferrets: 3–5 mg/kg. May have a role in the treatment of neuropathic pain in rabbits and rodents at canine doses (3–5 mg/kg p.o. q24h).
Birds: 25 mg/kg p.o. q12h. Doses of 1 mg/kg reported as ineffective in PDD.
Reptiles, Amphibians, Fish: No information available.

Amethocaine see **Tetracaine**

Amikacin
(Amikacin*, Amikin*) **POM**

Formulations: Injectable: 50 mg/ml, 250 mg/ml solutions.

Action: Aminoglycosides inhibit bacterial protein synthesis. They are bactericidal and their mechanism of killing is concentration-dependent, leading to a marked post-antibiotic effect, allowing prolonged dosing intervals (which may reduce toxicity).

Use: Active against many Gram-negative bacteria, *Staphylococcus aureus* and *Nocardia* spp., including some that may be resistant to gentamicin. Streptococci and anaerobes are usually resistant. Its use is only indicated after sensitivity testing has been performed and the organism shown to be resistant to other aminoglycosides such as gentamicin. Activity at low oxygen sites may be limited. Movement across biological membranes may also be limited, hence systemic levels require parenteral administration, and access to sites such as the CNS and ocular fluids is very limited. Monitoring serum amikacin levels should be considered to ensure therapeutic levels and minimize toxicity, particularly in neonates, geriatric patients and those with reduced renal function. Monitoring renal function is also advisable during treatment of any animal. Intravenous doses should be given slowly, generally over 30–60 min. Concurrent fluid therapy is advised.

Safety and handling: Normal precautions should be observed.

Contraindications: If possible avoid use in animals with reduced renal function. Avoid oral administration in small herbivores (e.g. rabbits).

Adverse reactions: Nephrotoxic and ototoxic. Oral doses can cause fatal enterotoxaemia in small herbivores. Use with caution in birds, as it is toxic.

Drug interactions: Synergism may occur *in vivo* when aminoglycosides are combined with beta-lactam antimicrobials. Avoid the concurrent use of other nephrotoxic, ototoxic or neurotoxic agents (e.g. amphotericin B, furosemide). Aminoglycosides may be inactivated *in vitro* by beta-lactam antibiotics (e.g. penicillins, cephalosporins) or heparin; do not give these drugs in the same syringe. Can potentiate neuromuscular blockade so avoid use in combination with neuromuscular blocking agents.

DOSES
See Appendix for guidelines on responsible antibacterial use.
Mammals: Ferrets: 8–16 mg/kg i.v., i.m., s.c. q8–24h; Rabbits: 2–10 mg/kg i.v., i.m., s.c. q8–12h; Rodents: 5–15 mg/kg i.v., i.m., s.c. q8–12h. Concurrent fluid therapy advised, especially if hydration status poor or uncertain. Nebulization: 10 mg in 10 ml of water for injection over 15–30 minutes q6–12h.
Birds: 10–20 mg/kg i.m., s.c., i.v. q8–12h or 6 mg/ml via nebulization (may be given in combination with acetylcysteine) [a,b].
Reptiles: Gopher tortoises: 5 mg/kg i.m. q48h [c]; Gopher snakes: 5 mg/kg i.m. once, then 2.5 mg/kg i.m. q72h at 25°C [d]; concurrent fluid therapy is advised due to potential nephrotoxicity; Ball pythons: 3.48 mg/kg i.m. once [e]. Can also be administered at 5 mg/ml via nebulization for 15–30 minutes q12h.
Amphibians: 5–10mg/kg s.c., i.m. q24–48h [f].
Fish: 5 mg/kg i.m., intracoelomic q72h for 3 treatments.

References
[a] Gronwall R, Brown MP and Clubb S (1989) Pharmacokinetics of amikacin in African grey parrots. *American Journal of Veterinary Research* **50(2)**, 250–252
[b] Ramsay EC and Vulliet R (1993) Pharmacokinetic properties of gentamicin and amikacin in the cockatiel. *Avian Diseases* **37(2)**, 628–634
[c] Caligiuri R, Kollias GV, Jacobson E et al. (1990) The effects of ambient temperature on amikacin pharmacokinetics in gopher tortoises. *Journal of Veterinary Pharmacology and Therapeutics* **13**, 287–291

^d Mader DR, Conzelman GM Jr and Baggot JD (1985) Effects of ambient temperature on the half-life and dosage regimen of amikacin in the gopher snake. *Journal of the American Veterinary Medical Association* **187(11)**, 1134–1136

^e Johnson JH, Jensen JM, Brumbaugh GW and Booth DM (1997) Amikacin pharmacokinetics and the effects of ambient temperature on the dosing regimen in ball pythons (*Python regius*). *Journal of Zoo Wildlife and Medicine* **28(1)**, 80–88

^f Letcher J and Papich M (1994) Pharmacokinetics of intramuscular administration of three antibiotics in bullfrogs (*Rana catesbeiana*). *Proceedings of the Association of Reptilian and Amphibian Veterinarians/American Association of Zoo Veterinarians Conference*, pp. 79–93

Amino acid solutions
(Duphalyte, Aminoplasmal*, Aminoven*, Clinimix*, Glamin*, Hyperamine*, Intrafusin*, Kabiven*, Kabiven Peripheral*, Nutriflex*) **POM, POM-V**

Formulations: Injectable: synthetic crystalline l-amino acid solutions for i.v. use only. Numerous human products are available, varying in concentrations of amino acids. Most products also contain electrolytes. Some products contain varying concentrations of glucose.

Action: Support protein anabolism, arrest protein and muscle wasting, and maintain intermediary metabolism.

Use: Amino acid solutions supply essential and non-essential amino acids for protein production. They are used parenterally in patients requiring nutritional support but unable to receive enteral support. The authorized veterinary preparation (Duphalyte) contains insufficient amino acids to meet basal requirements for protein production and is intended as an aid for i.v. fluid support. All products are hyperosmolar. The use of concentrated amino acid solutions for parenteral nutrition support should not be undertaken without specific training and requires central venous access and intensive care monitoring. Parenteral nutrition may also be able to meet the patient's requirements for fluids, essential electrolytes (sodium, potassium, magnesium) and phosphate. Additionally, if treatment is prolonged, vitamins and trace elements may need to be given. Intravenous lines for parenteral nutrition should be dedicated for that use alone and not used for other medications. As many of the available amino acids solutions contain potassium, the maximal acceptable rates of infusion will depend on the potassium content of the amino acid preparation.

Safety and handling: Normal precautions should be observed.

Contraindications: Dehydration, hepatic encephalopathy, severe azotaemia, shock, congestive heart failure and electrolyte imbalances.

Adverse reactions: The main complications of parenteral nutrition are metabolic, including hyperglycaemia, hyperlipidaemia, hypercapnia, acid–base disturbances and electrolyte disturbances. Other complications include catheter-associated thrombophlebitis, bacterial colonization of the catheter and resulting bacteraemia and septicaemia. Potentially life-threatening electrolyte imbalances including hypophosphataemia may also be seen (also referred to as refeeding syndrome). As with other hyperosmolar solutions, severe tissue damage could occur if extravasated, though this has not been reported.

Drug interactions: Consult specific product data sheet(s).

DOSES
Mammals: Rabbits, Rodents: Anecdotally, these products have been used either alone or diluted with lactated Ringer's solution at a 1:5 ratio and given at a total volume of approximately 100 ml/kg/day.
Birds: Up to 10 ml/kg/day.
Reptiles, Amphibians, Fish: No information available.

Aminophylline
(Aminophylline*) **POM**

Formulations: Injectable: 25 mg/ml solution. **Oral:** 100 mg tablet. For modified-release preparations **see Theophylline** (100 mg of aminophylline is equivalent to 79 mg of theophylline).

Action: Aminophylline is a stable mixture of theophylline (q.v.) and ethylenediamine. Causes inhibition of phosphodiesterase, alteration of intracellular calcium, release of catecholamine, and antagonism of adenosine and prostaglandin, leading to bronchodilation and other effects.

Use: Spasmolytic agent and has a mild diuretic action. It is used in the treatment of small airway disease. Beneficial effects include bronchodilation, enhanced mucociliary clearance, stimulation of the respiratory centre, increased sensitivity to P_aCO_2, increased diaphragmatic contractility, stabilization of mast cells and a mild inotropic effect. Aminophylline has a low therapeutic index and should be dosed on a lean body weight basis. Administer with caution in patients with severe cardiac disease, gastric ulcers, hyperthyroidism, renal or hepatic disease, severe hypoxia or severe hypertension. Therapeutic plasma aminophylline values are 5–20 µg/ml.

Safety and handling: Do not mix aminophylline in a syringe with other drugs.

Contraindications: Patients with known history of arrhythmias or seizures.

Adverse reactions: Vomiting, diarrhoea, polydipsia, polyuria, reduced appetite, tachycardia, arrhythmias, nausea, twitching, restlessness, agitation, excitement and convulsions. Most adverse effects are related to the serum level and may be symptomatic of toxic serum concentrations. The severity of these effects may be decreased by the use of modified-release preparations. They are more likely to be seen with more frequent administration. Aminophylline causes intense local pain when given i.m. and is very rarely used or recommended via this route.

Drug interactions: Agents that may increase the serum levels of aminophylline include cimetidine, diltiazem, erythromycin, fluoroquinolones and allopurinol. Phenobarbital may decrease the serum concentration of aminophylline. Aminophylline may decrease the effects of pancuronium. Aminophylline and beta-adrenergic blockers (e.g. propranolol) may antagonize each other's effects. Aminophylline administration with halothane may cause an increased incidence of cardiac dysrhythmias, and with ketamine an increased incidence of seizures.

DOSES
Mammals: Ferrets: 4.4–6.6 mg/kg p.o., i.m. q12h; **Rabbits:** 2.0 mg/kg i.v. q12h (slowly for emergency bronchodilation); **Guinea pigs:** 50 mg/kg p.o. q12h.
Birds: 4–5 mg/kg i.m., i.v. q6–12h; **Raptors:** 8–10 mg/kg p.o., i.m., i.v. q6–8h.
Reptiles: 2–4 mg/kg i.m. once.
Amphibians, Fish: No information available.

Amitraz
(Aludex, Promeris Duo) **POM-V**

Formulations: Topical: 5% w/v concentrated liquid; spot-on 150 mg/ml amitraz combined with metaflumizone in pipettes of various sizes.

Action: Increases neuronal activity through its action on octopamine receptors of mites.

Use: To treat generalized mite infestation, including demodicosis and sarcoptic acariasis. Used for generalized demodicosis in ferrets and hamsters and for acariasis in rodents. Dip to be left on coat. Clipping long hair coats will improve penetration. Ensure accurate dilution and application, especially for smaller rodents. Concurrent bacterial skin infections should be treated appropriately.

Safety and handling: Do not store diluted product.

Contraindications: No information available.

Adverse reactions: Sedation and bradycardia; can be reversed with an alpha-2 antagonist, e.g. atipamezole. Can cause irritation of the skin.

Drug interactions: No information available.

DOSES
Mammals: Ferrets, Guinea pigs: 0.3% solution (1 ml Aludex concentrated liquid in 17 ml water) applied topically to skin q14d for

3–6 treatments; **Hamsters, Rats, Mice:** 1.4 ml/l topically applied with a cotton bud q7d; **Gerbils:** 0.007% solution (1.4 ml Aludex concentrated liquid in 1000 ml water) applied with a cotton bud q14d for 3–6 treatments.
Birds, Reptiles, Amphibians, Fish: No information available.

Amitriptyline
(Amitriptyline*) **POM**

Formulations: Oral: 10 mg, 25 mg, 50 mg tablets; 5 mg/ml, 10 mg/ml solutions.

Action: Blocks noradrenaline and serotonin re-uptake in the brain, resulting in antidepressive activity.

Use: Management of chronic anxiety problems, including 'compulsive disorders', separation anxiety and psychogenic alopecia. Used for a minimum of 30 days for feather plucking in birds. Amitriptyline is bitter and can be distasteful. Some caution and careful monitoring is warranted in patients with cardiac or renal disease.

Safety and handling: Normal precautions should be observed.

Contraindications: Hypersensitivity to tricyclic antidepressants, glaucoma, history of seizures or urinary retention, severe liver disease.

Adverse reactions: Sedation, dry mouth, vomiting, excitability, arrhythmias, hypotension, syncope, increased appetite, weight gain and, less commonly, seizures and bone marrow disorders have been reported in humans. The bitter taste may cause ptyalism. Extrapyramidal side effects have been seen in a macaw.

Drug interactions: Should not be used with monoamine oxidase inhibitors or drugs metabolized by cytochrome P450 2D6, e.g. chlorphenamine, cimetidine. If changing medication from one of these compounds, a minimal washout period of 2 weeks is recommended (the washout period may be longer if the drug has been used for a prolonged period of time).

DOSES
Mammals: Rats: 5–20 mg/kg p.o. q24h.
Birds: 1–9 mg/kg p.o. q12h. Studies suggest higher dose rates generally needed. However, dosing should be started low and titrated upwards given the occurrence of severe extrapyramidal signs seen at 5mg/kg [a,b].
Reptiles, Amphibians, Fish: No information available.

References
[a] Barboza T and Beaufrere H (2017) Extrapyramidal side effects in a blue and gold macaw (Ara ararauna) treated with amitriptyline. *Journal of Veterinary Behavior* **22**, 19–23

[b] Visser M, Ragsdale MM and Boothe DM (2015) Pharmacokinetics of amitriptyline HCl and its metabolites in healthy African grey parrots (*Psittacus erithacus*) and Cockatoos (*Cacatua* species). *Journal of Avian Medicine and Surgery* **29(4)**, 275–281

Amoxicillin (Amoxycillin)
(Amoxinsol, Amoxycare, Amoxypen, Bimoxyl, Clamoxyl, Duphamox, **Vetremox Fish**) **POM-V**

Formulations: Injectable: 150 mg/ml suspension. **Oral:** 40 mg, 200 mg, 250 mg tablets; suspension which when reconstituted provides 50 mg/ml. **Topical:** 100% w/w powder for top dressing (Vetremox).

Action: Binds to penicillin-binding proteins involved in bacterial cell wall synthesis, thereby decreasing cell wall strength and rigidity, affecting cell division, growth and septum formation. These antimicrobials act in a time-dependent bactericidal fashion.

Use: Active against certain Gram-positive and Gram-negative aerobic organisms and many obligate anaerobes but not against those that produce penicillinases (beta-lactamases), e.g. *Escherichia coli*, *Staphylococcus aureus*. The more difficult Gram-negative organisms (*Pseudomonas*, *Klebsiella*) are usually resistant. Amoxicillin is excreted well in bile and urine. Oral amoxicillin may be given with or without food. Since amoxicillin works in a time-dependent fashion, it is important to maintain levels above the MIC for a high percentage of the time. In practical terms this means that the dosing interval is critical and missing doses can seriously compromise efficacy. In ferrets it is used in combination with bismuth subsalicylate, ranitidine or omeprazole and metronidazole ('triple therapy') for treatment of *Helicobacter mustelae* infection. Used to treat bacterial diseases in fish.

Safety and handling: Refrigerate oral suspension after reconstitution; discard if solution becomes dark or after 7 days.

Contraindications: Avoid oral antibiotics in critically ill patients, as absorption from the GI tract may be unreliable. Avoid use in animals with reported sensitivity to penicillins. Do not administer penicillins by any route to guinea pigs, chinchillas, hamsters, gerbils or degus. Do not administer oral penicillins to rabbits.

Adverse reactions: Nausea, diarrhoea and skin rashes are the commonest adverse effects. Oral doses can cause fatal enterotoxaemia in small herbivores (e.g. rabbits), hamsters and gerbils.

Drug interactions: Avoid concurrent use with bacteriostatic antibiotics (e.g. tetracycline, erythromycin, chloramphenicol). Do not mix in the same syringe as aminoglycosides. A synergistic effect is seen when beta-lactam and aminoglycoside antimicrobials are used concurrently.

DOSES
See Appendix for guidelines on responsible antibacterial use.
Mammals: **Ferrets:** 10–30 mg/kg s.c., p.o. q12h; **Rabbits:** 7 mg/kg s.c. q24h; **Rats, Mice:** 100–150 mg/kg i.m., s.c. q12h; **Primates:** 11 mg/kg p.o. q12h or 11 mg/kg s.c., i.m. q24h; **Sugar gliders:** 30 mg/kg p.o., s.c. q12–24h for 14 days; **Hedgehogs:** 15 mg/kg p.o., s.c., i.m. q8–12h. **Guinea pigs, Chinchillas, Hamsters, Gerbils, Degus;** do not use.

Birds: 150–175 mg/kg i.m., s.c. q8–12h (q24h for long-acting preparations); **Raptors, Parrots:** 175 mg/kg p.o. q12h; **Pigeons:** 1–1.5 g/l drinking water (Vetremox pigeon) q24h for 3–5 days or 100–200 mg/kg p.o. q6–8h; **Waterfowl:** 1 g/l drinking water (Amoxinsol soluble powder) alternate days for 3–5 days or 300–500 mg/kg p.o. (in soft food) for 3–5 days; **Passerines:** 1.5 g/l drinking water for 3–5 days.

Reptiles: 5–10 mg/kg i.m., p.o. q12–24h (most species); **Chelonians:** 5–50 mg/kg i.m., p.o. q12h.

Fish: 40–80 mg/kg in feed q24h for 10 days or 12.5 mg/kg i.m. once (long-acting preparation).

Amphibians: No information available.

Amoxicillin/Clavulanate see Co-amoxiclav
Amoxycillin see Amoxicillin

Amphotericin B
(Abelcet*, AmBisome*, Amphocil*, Fungizone*) **POM**

Formulations: Injectable: 50 mg/vial powder for reconstitution.

Action: Binds to sterols in fungal cell membrane creating pores and allowing leakage of contents.

Use: Management of systemic fungal infections and leishmaniosis. Given the risk of severe toxicity it is advisable to reserve use for severe/potentially fatal fungal infections only. Abelcet, AmBisome and Amphocil are lipid formulations that are less toxic. Physically incompatible with electrolyte solutions. Lipid formulations are far less toxic than conventional formulations for i.v. use because the drug is targeted to macrophages, but these preparations are far more expensive. Solutions are usually given i.v. but if regular venous catheterization is problematic then an s.c. alternative has been used for cryptococcosis and could potentially be used for other systemic mycoses. Renal values and electrolytes should be monitored pre- and post- each treatment; urinalysis and liver function tests weekly. If considering use in patients with pre-existing renal insufficiency (where other treatment options have failed and benefits outweigh risks), consider lipid formulations, concurrent saline administration and dose reduction. Has been used topically in reptiles to treat pulmonary candidiasis. In amphibians, amphotericin B has been used as a water treatment for the management of chytridiomycosis in adult animals.

Safety and handling: Keep in the dark, although loss of drug activity is negligible for at least 8 hours in room light. After initial reconstitution (but not further dilution), the drug is stable for 1 week if refrigerated and stored in the dark. Do not dilute in saline. Pre-treatment heating of the reconstituted concentrated solution to 70°C for 20 min produces superaggregates which are less nephrotoxic. To produce a lipid-formulated product if not commercially available mix 40 ml sterile saline, 10 ml of lipid infusion (q.v.) and 50 mg of the reconstituted concentrated solution.

Contraindications: Do not use in renal or hepatic failure.

Adverse reactions: Include hypokalaemia, leading to cardiac arrhythmias, phlebitis, hepatic failure, renal failure, vomiting, diarrhoea, pyrexia, muscle and joint pain, anorexia and anaphylactoid reactions. Nephrotoxicity is a major concern; do not use other nephrotoxic drugs concurrently. Nephrotoxicity may be reduced by saline infusion (20 ml/kg over 60 minutes) prior to administration of amphotericin B. Fever and vomiting may be decreased by pre-treating with aspirin, diphenhydramine or an antiemetic. Amphotericin B is toxic to birds when administered systemically; administer fluids and monitor carefully if giving i.v. Care is needed if amphotericin B is nebulized as birds may ingest it when preening. Can cause bronchospasm in humans if nebulized. Amphotericin B is acutely toxic to *Alytes muletensis* tadpoles at 8 µg/ml.

Drug interactions: Amphotericin may increase the toxic effects of fluorouracil, doxorubicin and methotrexate. Flucytosine is synergistic with amphotericin B *in vitro* against *Candida*, *Cryptococcus* and *Aspergillus*.

DOSES

Mammals: Ferrets: 0.4–0.8 mg/kg i.v. q7d for treatment of blastomycosis; **Rabbits:** 1 mg/kg i.v. q24h (desoxycholate form) or 5 mg/kg i.v. q24h (liposomal form); **Guinea pigs:** 1.25–2.5 mg/kg s.c. q24h for cryptococcosis; **Mice:** 0.11 mg/kg s.c. q24h or 0.43 mg/kg p.o. q24h.

Birds: Systemic fungal infections: 1–1.5 mg/kg i.v. q8–12h for 3–5 days (give with 10–15 ml/kg saline) or 1 mg/kg in 2 ml sterile water intratracheal q8–12h for 12 days then q48h for 5 weeks; **Parrots:** 100–300 mg/kg p.o. q12–24h for *Macrorhabdus* infection, although resistance has been reported [a]; **Passerines:** 100 mg/kg p.o. q8–12h or 1–5 g/l drinking water or 1 mg/ml in saline nebulized for 15 min q12h.

Reptiles: 0.5–1 mg/kg i.v., intracoelomic q24–72h for 2–4 weeks, concurrent fluid therapy is advised due to potential nephrotoxicity; Respiratory infections: Nebulize 5 mg in 150 ml saline for 30–60 min q12h; may also use topically on lesions q12h.

Amphibians: Internal mycoses: 1 mg/kg intracoelomic q24h; *Batrachochytrium dendrobatidis* sporangia and zoospores: 8–15 µg (micrograms)/ml in water for 48 h [b,c].

Fish: No information available.

References

[a] Baron HR, Leung KC, Stevenson BC, Gonzalez MS and Phalen DN (2018) Evidence of amphotericin B resistance in *Macrorhabdus ornithogaster* in Australian cage-birds. *Medical Mycology* **57(4)**, 421–428

[b] Holden WM, Ebert AR, Canning PF and Rollins-Smith LA (2014) Evaluation of amphotericin B and chloramphenicol as alternative drugs for treatment of chytridiomycosis and their impacts on innate skin defences. *Applied Environmental Microbiology* **80(13)**, 4034–4041

[c] Martel A, Van Rooij P, Vercauteren G *et al.* (2011) Developing a safe antifungal treatment protocol to eliminate *Batrachochytrium dendrobatidis* from amphibians. *Medical Mycology* **49(2)**, 143–149

A

B
C
D
E
F
G
H
I
J
K
L
M
N
O
P
Q
R
S
T
U
V
W
X
Y
Z

Ampicillin
(Amfipen, Ampicaps, Ampicare, Duphacillin)
POM-V

Formulations: Injectable: Ampicillin sodium 250 mg, 500 mg powders for reconstitution (human licensed product only); 150 mg/ml suspension, 100 mg/ml long-acting preparation. **Oral:** 500 mg tablets; 250 mg capsule.

Action: Binds to penicillin-binding proteins involved in bacterial cell wall synthesis, thereby decreasing cell wall strength and rigidity, affecting cell division, growth and septum formation. It acts in a time-dependent bactericidal fashion.

Use: Active against many Gram-positive and Gram-negative aerobic organisms and obligate anaerobes, but not against those that produce penicillinases (beta-lactamases), e.g. *Escherichia coli*, *Staphylococcus aureus*. The difficult Gram-negative organisms such as *Pseudomonas aeruginosa* and *Klebsiella* are usually resistant. Ampicillin is excreted well in bile and urine. Maintaining levels above the MIC is critical for efficacy and thereby prolonged dosage intervals or missed doses can compromise therapeutic response. Dose and dosing interval is determined by infection site, severity and organism. Oral bioavailability is reduced in the presence of food. Used to treat bacterial disease in fish

Safety and handling: After reconstitution the sodium salt will retain adequate potency for up to 8 hours if refrigerated, but use within 2 hours if kept at room temperature.

Contraindications: Avoid the use of oral antibiotic agents in critically ill patients, as absorption from the GI tract may be unreliable. Avoid use in animals with reported sensitivity to penicillins. Do not administer penicillins by any route to guinea pigs, chinchillas, hamsters, gerbils or degus. Do not administer oral penicillins to rabbits.

Adverse reactions: Nausea, diarrhoea and skin rashes are the commonest adverse effects. Oral doses can cause fatal enterotoxaemia in small herbivores (e.g. rabbits), hamsters and gerbils.

Drug interactions: Avoid the concurrent use of ampicillin with bacteriostatic antibiotics (e.g. tetracycline, erythromycin, chloramphenicol). Do not mix in the same syringe as aminoglycosides. A synergistic effect is seen when beta-lactam and aminoglycoside antimicrobials are used concurrently.

DOSES
See Appendix for guidelines on responsible antibacterial use.
Mammals: Ferrets: 5–30 mg/kg i.m., s.c. q12h; **Rats, Mice:** 25 mg/kg i.m., s.c. q12h or 50–200 mg/kg p.o. q12h; **Primates:** 20 mg/kg p.o., i.m., i.v. q8h; **Rabbits, Guinea pigs, Chinchillas, Hamsters, Gerbils, Degus:** do not use.

Birds: 50–100 mg/kg i.v., i.m. q8–12h, 150–200 mg/kg p.o. q8–12h, 1–2 g/l drinking water, 2–3 g/kg in soft feed[a].
Reptiles: 10–20 mg/kg s.c., i.m. q12–24h (most species); **Hermann's tortoises:** 50 mg/kg i.m. q12h.
Fish: 50–80 mg/kg in feed q24h for 10 days.
Amphibians: No information available.

References
[a] Ensley PK and Janssen DL (1981) A preliminary study comparing the pharmacokinetics of ampicillin given orally and intramuscularly to psittacines: Amazon parrots (*Amazona* spp.) and Blue-naped parrots (*Tanygnathus lucionensis*). *Journal of Zoo Animal Medicine* **12(2)**, 42–47

Amprolium
(Coxoid) **AVM-GSL**

Formulations: Oral: 3.84% solution for dilution in water.

Action: Thiamine analogue that disrupts protozoal metabolism.

Use: Coccidiosis in homing/racing pigeons and small mammals. Limit duration of therapy to 2 weeks.

Safety and handling: Normal precautions should be observed.

Contraindications: No information available.

Adverse reactions: Prolonged high doses can cause thiamine deficiency.

Drug interactions: No information available.

DOSES
Mammals: **Ferrets:** 19 mg/kg p.o. q72h; **Rabbits:** 20 mg/kg p.o. q24h for 2–4 weeks; **Chinchillas:** 10–15 mg/kg p.o. total daily dose divided q8–24h; **Gerbils, Hamsters, Rats, Mice:** 10–20 mg/kg p.o. total daily dose divided q8–24h.
Birds: **Pigeons:** 28 ml of the concentrated solution in 4.5 l of drinking water for 7 days; in severe outbreaks continue with half-strength solution (14 ml per 4.5 l) for a further 7 days; medicated water should be discarded after 24 hours; **Passerines:** 50–100 mg/l drinking water for 5 days or longer.
Reptiles, Amphibians, Fish: No information available.

Aniline green see **Malachite green**

Apomorphine
(Apovomin, Emedog) **POM-V**

Formulations: Injectable: 1 mg/ml solution (Emedog), 3 mg/ml solution (Apovomin).

Action: Stimulates emesis through D2 dopamine receptors in the chemoreceptor trigger zone.

Use: Induction of self-limiting emesis within a few minutes of administration in animals where vomiting is desirable, e.g. following the ingestion of toxic, non-caustic foreign material. Emesis generally occurs rapidly and within a maximum of 10 min. Further doses depress the vomiting centre and may not result in any further vomiting.

Safety and handling: Normal precautions should be observed.

Contraindications: Induction of emesis is contraindicated if strong acid or alkali has been ingested, due to the risk of further damage to the oesophagus. Induction of vomiting is contraindicated if the animal is unconscious, fitting, or has a reduced cough reflex, or if the poison has been ingested for >2 hours, or if the ingesta contains paraffin, petroleum products or other oily or volatile organic products, due to the risk of inhalation. Contraindicated in rabbits as they are unable to vomit. Contraindicated in rodents as their stomach walls lack the strength to tolerate forced emesis.

Adverse reactions: Apomorphine may induce excessive vomiting, respiratory depression and sedation.

Drug interactions: In the absence of compatibility studies, apomorphine must not be mixed with other products. Antiemetic drugs, particularly antidopaminergics (e.g. phenothiazines) may reduce the emetic effects of apomorphine. Additive CNS or respiratory depression may occur when apomorphine is used with opiates or other CNS or respiratory depressants.

DOSES
Mammals: Ferrets: 70 µg (micrograms)/kg s.c.
Birds, Reptiles, Amphibians, Fish: No information available.

Ara-C see **Cytarabine**
Ascorbic acid see **Vitamin C**
Asparaginase, L-Asparaginase see **Crisantaspase**

Aspirin (Acetylsalicyclic acid)
(Aspirin BP* and component of many others) P

Formulations: Oral: 75 mg, 300 mg tablets.

Action: Produces irreversible inhibition of cyclo-oxygenase (COX) by acetylation, thereby preventing the production of both prostaglandins and thromboxanes from membrane phospholipids.

Use: Prevention of arterial thromboembolism. Also can be used to control mild to moderate pain, although NSAIDs that are more selective for the COX-2 enzyme have a better safety profile; not an NSAID of choice for analgesia in small mammals. Administration of aspirin to animals with renal disease must be carefully evaluated. It is advisable to stop aspirin before surgery (at least 2 weeks) to allow recovery of normal platelet function and prevent excessive bleeding.

Safety and handling: Normal precautions should be observed.

Contraindications: Do not give aspirin to dehydrated, hypovolaemic or hypotensive patients or those with GI disease. Do not give to pregnant animals or animals <6 weeks old.

Adverse reactions: GI ulceration and irritation are common side effects of all NSAIDs. It is advisable to stop therapy if diarrhoea or nausea persists beyond 1–2 days. Stop therapy immediately if GI bleeding is suspected and begin symptomatic treatment. There is a small risk that NSAIDs may precipitate cardiac failure in humans and this risk in animals is unknown. All NSAIDs carry a risk of renal papillary necrosis due to reduced renal perfusion caused by a reduction in the production of renal prostaglandins. This risk is greatest when NSAIDs are given to animals that are hypotensive or animals with pre-existing renal disease.

Drug interactions: Do not administer concurrently or within 24 hours of other NSAIDs and glucocorticoids. Do not administer with other potentially nephrotoxic agents, e.g. aminoglycosides.

DOSES

Mammals: **Ferrets:** 10–20 mg/kg p.o. q24h; **Rabbits:** 100 mg/kg p.o. q12–24h; **Rodents:** 50–150 mg/kg p.o. q4–8h; **Primates:** 5–10 mg/kg p.o. q4–6h.
Birds: **Parrots:** 5 mg/kg p.o. q8h.
Reptiles, Amphibians, Fish: No information available.

Atenolol
(Atenolol*, Tenormin*) POM

Formulations: Oral: 25 mg, 50 mg, 100 mg tablets; 5 mg/ml syrup. Injectable: 0.5 mg/ml.

Action: Cardioselective beta-adrenergic blocker. It is relatively specific for beta-1 adrenergic receptors but can antagonize beta-2 receptors at high doses. Blocks the chronotropic and inotropic effects of beta-1 adrenergic stimulation on the heart, thereby reducing myocardial oxygen demand. Bronchoconstrictor, vasodilatory and hypoglycaemic effects are less marked due to its cardioselective nature.

Use: Cardiac tachyarrhythmias, hyperthyroidism, hypertrophic cardiomyopathy, obstructive cardiac disease (severe aortic or pulmonic stenosis) and systemic hypertension. Less effective when used alone for ventricular arrhythmias unless the arrhythmia is mediated by sympathetic tone. It is recommended to withdraw therapy gradually in patients who have been receiving the drug chronically. Alternatively, sotalol has been used in birds.

Safety and handling: Normal precautions should be observed.

Contraindications: Patients with bradyarrhythmias, acute or decompensated congestive heart failure. Relatively contraindicated in animals with medically controlled congestive heart failure as is poorly tolerated.

Adverse reactions: Most frequently seen in geriatric patients with chronic heart disease or in patients with acute or decompensated heart failure. Include bradycardia, AV block, myocardial depression, heart failure, syncope, hypotension, hypoglycaemia, bronchospasm and diarrhoea. Depression and lethargy may occur as a result of atenolol's high lipid solubility and its penetration into the CNS.

Drug interactions: Do not administer concurrently with alpha-adrenergic agonists (e.g. phenylpropanolamine). The hypotensive effect of atenolol is enhanced by many agents that depress myocardial activity including anaesthetic agents, phenothiazines, antihypertensive drugs, diuretics and diazepam. There is an increased risk of bradycardia, severe hypotension, heart failure and AV block if atenolol is used concurrently with calcium-channel blockers. Concurrent digoxin administration potentiates bradycardia. The metabolism of atenolol is accelerated by thyroid hormones; thus the dose of atenolol may need to be decreased when initiating carbimazole therapy. Atenolol enhances the effects of muscle relaxants (e.g. suxamethonium, tubocurarine). Hepatic enzyme induction by phenobarbital may increase the rate of metabolism of atenolol. The bronchodilatory effects of theophylline may be blocked by atenolol. Atenolol may enhance the hypoglycaemic effect of insulin.

DOSES

Mammals: Ferrets: 3.125–6.25 mg/animal p.o. q24h; **Rabbits:** 0.5–2 mg/kg p.o. q24h; **Rats:** 0.2–2 mg/kg q24h p.o.; **Mice:** 2–10 mg/kg i.v., i.p. q24h.

Birds: Atenolol 5–10 mg/kg p.o. q12–24h[1] or alternatively sotalol may be used at 1 mg/kg p.o. q12h[2].

References

[1] Beaufrere H, Schilliger L and Pauriat R (2016) Cardiovascular System. In: *Current Therapy in Exotic Pet Practice*, ed. MA Mitchell and TN Tully. Elsevier, St Louis
[2] Oster SC, Jung S and Moon R (2019) Resolution of supraventricular arrhythmia using sotalol in an adult golden eagle (*Aquila chrysaetos*) with presumed atherosclerosis. *Journal of Exotic Pet Medicine* **29**, 136–141

Atipamezole
(Alzane, Antisedan, Atipam, Revertor, Sedastop)
POM-V

Formulations: Injectable: 5 mg/ml solution.

Action: Selective alpha-2 adrenoreceptor antagonist.

Use: Reverses the sedative effects of medetomidine or dexmedetomidine; will also reverse other alpha-2 agonists to provide a quick recovery from anaesthesia and sedation. It also reverses other effects such as the analgesic, cardiovascular and respiratory effects of alpha-2 agonists. Atipamezole does not alter the metabolism of medetomidine or dexmedetomidine but occupies the alpha-2 receptor, preventing binding of the drug. The duration of action of atipamezole and medetomidine or dexmedetomidine are similar, so re-sedation is uncommon. Routine administration of atipamezole i.v. is not recommended because the rapid recovery from sedation is usually associated with excitation, though i.v. administration may be indicated in an emergency (e.g. excessive sedation from medetomidine or dexmedetomidine, or cardiovascular complications).

Safety and handling: Normal precautions should be observed.

Contraindications: No information available.

Adverse reactions: Transient over-alertness and tachycardia may be observed after overdosage. This is best handled by minimizing external stimuli and allowing the animal to recover quietly.

Drug interactions: No information available.

DOSES
Mammals: Ferrets, Rodents, Primates, Hedgehogs: Five times the previous medetomidine dose s.c., i.m.[a] or ten times the previous dexmedetomidine dose (i.e equal volume of solution to medetomidine or dexmedetomidine); **Rabbits, Marsupials:** Two and a half times the previous medetomidine dose or five times the previous dexmedetomidine dose (i.e. half the volume of medetomidine or dexmedetomidine). When medetomidine or dexmedetomidine has been administered at least an hour before, dose of atipamezole can be reduced by half and repeated if recovery is slow[b,c,d]; Amitraz toxicity: 25 μg (micrograms)/kg i.m. but if there is no benefit within half an hour this can be repeated or incrementally increased every 30 minutes up to 200 μg/kg.
Birds: 2.5–5 times the previous medetomidine or dexmedetomidine dose i.m., i.v.[e]
Reptiles
5 times the previous medetomidine or dexmedetomidine dose i.m., i.v.[f]
Fish: 0.2 mg/kg i.m.
Amphibians: No information available.

References

[a] Jang HS, Choi HS, Lee SH, Jang KH and Lee MG (2009) Evaluation of the anaesthetic effects of medetomidine and ketamine in rats and their reversal with atipamezole. *Veterinary Anaesthesia and Analgesia* **36(4)**, 319–327

[b] Baumgartner C, Bollerhey M, Ebner J et al. (2010) Effects of medetomidine-midazolam-fentanyl i.v. bolus injections and its reversal by specific antagonists on cardiovascular function in rabbits. *Canadian Journal of Veterinary Research* **74(4)**, 286–298

[c] Orr HE, Roughan JV and Flecknell PA (2005) Assessment of ketamine and medetomidine anaesthesia in the domestic rabbit. *Veterinary Anaesthesia and Analgesia* **32(5)**, 271–279

[d] Williams AM and Wyatt JD (2007) Comparison of subcutaneous and intramuscular ketamine-medetomidine with and without reversal by atipamezole in Dutch belted rabbits (*Oryctolagus cuniculus*). *Journal of the American Association of Laboratory Animal Science* **46(6)**, 16–20

[e] Sandmeier P (2000) Evaluation of medetomidine for short-term immobilization of domestic pigeons (*Columba livia*) and Amazon parrots (*Amazona* spp.). *Journal of Avian Medicine and Surgery* **14(1)**, 8–14

[f] Sleeman JM and Gaynor J (2000) Sedative and cardiopulmonary effects of medetomidine and reversal with atipamezole in Desert tortoises (*Gopherus agassizi*). *Journal of Zoo and Wildlife Medicine* **31(1)**, 28–35

Atracurium
(Tracrium*) POM

Formulations: Injectable: 10 mg/ml solution.

Action: Inhibits the actions of acetylcholine at the neuromuscular junction by binding competitively to the nicotinic acetylcholine receptor on the post-junctional membrane.

Use: Neuromuscular blockade during anaesthesia. This may be to improve surgical access through muscle relaxation, to facilitate positive pressure ventilation or for intraocular surgery. May also be used for mydriasis to allow ocular examination and/or surgery in birds. Atracurium has an intermediate duration of action (15–35 min) and is non-cumulative due to non-enzymatic (Hofmann) elimination. It is therefore suitable for administration to animals with renal or hepatic disease. Monitoring (using a nerve stimulator) and reversal of the neuromuscular blockade is recommended to ensure complete recovery before the end of anaesthesia. Hypothermia, acidosis and hypokalaemia will prolong the duration of action of neuromuscular blockade. Use the low end of the dose range in patients with myasthenia gravis and ensure that neuromuscular function is monitored during the period of the blockade and recovery using standard techniques.

Safety and handling: Store in refrigerator.

Contraindications: Do not administer unless the animal is adequately anaesthetized and facilities to provide positive pressure ventilation are available.

Adverse reactions: Can precipitate the release of histamine after rapid i.v. administration, resulting in bronchospasm and hypotension. Diluting the drug in normal saline and giving the drug slowly i.v. minimizes these effects.

Drug interactions: Neuromuscular blockade is more prolonged when atracurium is given in combination with volatile anaesthetics, aminoglycosides, clindamycin or lincomycin.

DOSES

Birds: 0.25 mg/kg i.v.; 1 mg/kg i.v. [a,b]

Mammals, Reptiles, Amphibians, Fish: No information available.

References

[a] Nicholson A and Ilkiw JE (1992) Neuromuscular and cardiovascular effects of atracurium in isoflurane-anesthetized chickens. *American Journal of Veterinary Research* **53**, 2337–2342

[b] Pascoe P and Hawkins M (2017) The effect of systemic atracurium on pupillary area in chickens. *Veterinary Anaesthesia and Analgesia* **44(5)**, 1262.e10

Atropine

(Atrocare) **POM-V**

Formulations: Injectable: 0.6 mg/ml. **Ophthalmic:** 0.5%, 1% solution in single-use vials, 5 ml bottle; 1% ointment.

Action: Blocks the action of acetylcholine at muscarinic receptors at the terminal ends of the parasympathetic nervous system, reversing parasympathetic effects and producing mydriasis, tachycardia, bronchodilation and general inhibition of GI function.

Use: Prevent or correct bradycardia and bradyarrhythmias, to dilate pupils, in the management of organophosphate and carbamate toxicities, and in conjunction with anticholinesterase drugs during antagonism of neuromuscular block. Routine administration prior to anaesthesia as part of premedication is no longer recommended; it is better to monitor heart rate and give atropine to manage a low heart rate if necessary. Some rabbits and rodents have endogenous plasma atropinesterase so efficacy may be reduced if used at standard doses. Ophthalmic use is ineffective in birds and reptiles because of the complex arrangement of musculature in the iris and ciliary body. Atropine has a slow onset of action (10 min i.m., 2–3 min i.v.), therefore it is important to wait for an adequate period of time for the desired effect before redosing. The ophthalmic solution tastes very bitter and can cause hypersalivation; therefore the ophthalmic ointment preparation is preferred. Used for the treatment of organophosphate poisoning in fish.

Safety and handling: The solution does not contain any antimicrobial preservative, therefore any remaining solution in the vial should be discarded after use. The solution should be protected from light.

Contraindications: Glaucoma, lens luxation, keratoconjunctivitis sicca.

Adverse reactions: Include sinus tachycardia (usually of short duration after i.v. administration), blurred vision from mydriasis, which may worsen recovery from anaesthesia, and drying of bronchial secretions. Atropine increases intraocular pressure and reduces tear production. Ventricular arrhythmias may be treated with lidocaine if severe. Other GI side effects such as ileus and vomiting are rare in small animals. May be associated with prolonged ileus in reptiles.

Drug interactions: Atropine is compatible (for at least 15 min) mixed with various medications but not with bromides, iodides, sodium bicarbonate, other alkalis or noradrenaline. The following may enhance the activity of atropine: antihistamines, quinidine, pethidine, benzodiazepines, phenothiazines, thiazide diuretics and sympathomimetics. Combining atropine and alpha-2 agonists is not recommended. Atropine may aggravate some signs seen with amitraz toxicity, leading to hypertension and gut stasis.

DOSES
Mammals: Ferrets: 0.02–0.04 mg/kg s.c., i.m., i.v.; **Rabbits:** 0.1–0.5 mg/kg i.m., i.v., endogenous atropinase levels may make repeat injections q10–15min necessary; **Chinchillas, Guinea pigs:** 0.1–0.2 mg/kg s.c., i.m.; **Rodents:** Organophosphate poisoning may require up to 10 mg/kg i.v., i.m. q20min; Bradyarrhythmias: 0.01–0.03 mg/kg i.v.; low doses may exacerbate bradycardia; repetition of the dose will usually promote an increase in heart rate; 0.03–0.04 mg/kg i.m. can be given to prevent development of bradycardia during administration of potent opioids such as fentanyl; **Primates:** 0.02–0.05 mg/kg s.c., i.m., i.v.; **Sugar gliders:** 0.01–0.02 mg/kg s.c., i.m.; **Hedgehogs:** 0.01–0.05 mg/kg s.c., i.m.; **Others:** 0.04–0.1 mg/kg i.m., s.c.

Birds: Organophosphate poisoning: 0.04–0.5 mg/kg i.v., i.m. q4h; Supraventricular bradycardia: 0.01–0.02 mg/kg i.v. once.

Reptiles: 0.01–0.04 mg/kg i.m., i.v.; May be ineffective in green iguanas[a].

Amphibians, Fish: 0.1 mg/kg s.c., i.m., i.v., intracoelomic as required (organophosphate toxicity).

References
[a] Pace L and Mader DR (2002) Atropine and glycopyrrolate, route of administration and response in the green iguana (*Iguana iguana*). *Proceedings of the Association of Reptilian and Amphibian Veterinarians*, pp. 79

Azathioprine
(Azathioprine*, Imuran*) **POM**

Formulations: Oral: 25 mg, 50 mg tablets.

Action: Inhibits purine synthesis, which is necessary for cell proliferation especially of leucocytes and lymphocytes. It suppresses cell-mediated immunity, alters antibody production and inhibits cell growth.

Use: Management of immune-mediated diseases. Often used in conjunction with corticosteroids. Routine haematology (including platelets) should be monitored closely: initially every 1–2 weeks; and every 1–2 months when on maintenance therapy. Use with caution in patients with hepatic disease. In animals with renal impairment, dosing interval should be extended. Clinical responses can take up to 6 weeks. Mycophenolic acid may be preferred if a more rapid response is required.

Safety and handling: Cytotoxic drug; see specialist texts for further advice on chemotherapeutic agents. Azathioprine tablets should be stored at room temperature in well closed containers and protected from light.

Contraindications: Do not use in patients with bone marrow suppression or those at high risk of infection.

Adverse reactions: Bone marrow suppression is the most serious adverse effect. This may be influenced by the activity of thiopurine s-methyltransferase, which is involved in the metabolism of the drug and which can vary between individuals due to genetic polymorphism. Avoid rapid withdrawal.

Drug interactions: Enhanced effects and increased azathioprine toxicity when used with allopurinol. Increased risk of azathioprine toxicity with aminosalicylates and corticosteroids.

DOSES
Mammals: Ferrets: 0.5 mg/kg p.o. q48h to 5 mg/kg p.o. q24h for eosinophilic gastroenteritis (limited evidence); 0.9 mg/kg p.o. q24–72h with prednisolone and dietary management for inflammatory bowel disease.
Birds, Reptiles, Amphibians, Fish: No information available.

Azithromycin
(Zithromax*) **POM**

Formulations: Oral: 250 mg capsule; 200 mg/5 ml suspension (reconstitute with water).

Action: Binds to the 50S bacterial ribosome (like erythromycin), inhibiting peptide bond formation and has bactericidal or bacteriostatic activity depending on the susceptibility of the organism. Azithromycin has a longer tissue half-life than erythromycin, shows better oral absorption and is better tolerated in humans.

Use: Alternative to penicillin in allergic individuals as it has a similar, although not identical, antibacterial spectrum. It is active against Gram-positive cocci (some *Staphylococcus* species are resistant), Gram-positive bacilli, some Gram-negative bacilli (*Haemophilus*, *Pasteurella*), mycobacteria, obligate anaerobes, *Chlamydia*, *Mycoplasma* and *Toxoplasma*. Some strains of *Actinomyces*, *Nocardia* and *Rickettsia* are also inhibited. Most strains of the Enterobacteriaceae (*Pseudomonas*, *Escherichia coli*, *Klebsiella*) are resistant. Useful in the management of respiratory tract, mild to moderate skin and soft tissue, and non-tubercular mycobacterial infections. Used to treat chlamydiosis in birds. Has been used in primates (macaques) as an anti-malarial. Doses are empirical and subject to change as experience with the drug is gained. More work is needed to optimize the clinically effective dose rate. Azithromycin activity is enhanced in an alkaline pH; administer on an empty stomach where possible.

Safety and handling: Normal precautions should be observed.

Contraindications: Avoid in renal and hepatic failure in all species.

Adverse reactions: In humans similar adverse effects to those of erythromycin are seen, i.e. vomiting, cholestatic hepatitis, stomatitis and glossitis, but the effects are generally less marked than with erythromycin.

Drug interactions: Azithromycin may increase the serum levels of methylprednisolone, theophylline and terfenadine. The absorption of digoxin may be enhanced.

DOSES
See Appendix for guidelines on responsible antibacterial use.

Mammals: Ferrets: 5 mg/kg p.o. q24h for 5 days as part of a protocol for treatment of *Helicobacter*; **Rabbits:** 4–5 mg/kg i.m. q48h for 7 days is effective against syphilis; 15–30 mg/kg p.o. q24h for respiratory infections; 50 mg/kg p.o. q24h azithromycin with 40 mg/kg p.o. q12h rifampin for staphylococcal osteomyelitis[a]; **Rats, Mice:** 50 mg/kg p.o. q12h for 14 days; **Prairie dogs:** 15–30 mg/kg p.o. q24h for 15 days; **Primates:** 25 mg/kg s.c. q24h[b,c].

Birds: Chlamydiosis: 40 mg/kg p.o. q24–48h for up to 45 days[d]; *Mycoplasma*: 50–80 mg/kg p.o. q24h for 3 days, then 4 days off; repeat for up to 3 weeks; **Blue-and-gold macaws:** 10 mg/kg p.o. q48h for susceptible infections[e].

Reptiles: 10 mg/kg p.o. q3d for skin infections; q5d for respiratory tract infections; q7d for liver and kidney infections[f].

Amphibians, Fish: No information available.

References

[a] Shirtliff ME, Mader JT and Calhoun J (1999) Oral rifampin plus azithromycin or clarithromycin to treat osteomyelitis in rabbits. *Clinical Orthopaedics and Related Research* **359**, 229–236

[b] Puri SK and Singh N (2000) Azithromycin: antimalarial profile against blood- and sporozoite-induced infections in mice and monkeys. *Experimental Parasitology* **94(1)**, 8–14

[c] Girard AE, Girard D, English AR et al. (1987) Pharmacokinetic and *in vivo* studies with azithromycin (CP-62,993), a new macrolide with an extended half-life and excellent tissue distribution. *Antimicrobial Agents and Chemotherapy* **31(12)**, 1948–1954

[d] Sanchez-Migallon Guzman D, Diaz-Figueroa O, Tully T Jr et al. (2010) Evaluating 21-day doxycycline and azithromycin treatments for experimental *Chlamydophila psittaci* infection in cockatiels (*Nymphicus hollandicus*). *Journal of Avian Medicine and Surgery* **24(1)**, 35–45

[e] Carpenter JW, Olsen JH, Randle-Port M, Koch DE, Isaza R and Hunter RP (2005) Pharmacokinetics of azithromycin in the blue-and-gold macaw (*Ara ararauna*) after intravenous and oral administration. *Journal of Zoo and Wildlife Medicine* **36(4)**, 606–609

[f] Coke RL, Hunter RP, Isaza R et al. (2003) Pharmacokinetics and tissue concentrations of azithromycin in ball pythons (*Python regius*). *American Journal of Veterinary Research* **64(2)**, 225–228

Aztreonam
(Azactam*, Squibb*) **POM**

Formulations: Injectable: 1 g, 2 g powder for solution.

Action: Bactericidal by interfering with cell wall synthesis.

Use: Treatment of Gram-negative bacterial infections in fish.

Safety and handling: Normal precautions should be observed.

Contraindications: No information available.

Adverse reactions: No information available.

Drug interactions: No information available.

DOSES
Fish: 100 mg/kg i.m., intracoelomic q48h for 7 treatments.
Mammals, Birds, Reptiles, Amphibians: No information available.

Benazepril

(Benefortin, Cardalis, Fortekor, Nelio, Prilben, Vetpril) **POM-V**

Formulations: Oral: 2.5 mg, 5 mg, 20 mg tablets. Available in a compound preparation with spironolactone (Cardalis tablets) in the following formulations: 2.5 mg benazepril/20 mg spironolactone, 5 mg benazepril/40 mg spironolactone, 10 mg benazepril/80 mg spironolactone.

Action: Angiotensin converting enzyme (ACE) inhibitor. It inhibits conversion of angiotensin I to angiotensin II and inhibits the breakdown of bradykinin. Overall effect is a reduction in preload and afterload via venodilation and arteriodilation, decreased salt and water retention via reduced aldosterone production and inhibition of the angiotensin-aldosterone-mediated cardiac and vascular remodelling. Efferent arteriolar dilation in the kidney can reduce intraglomerular pressure and therefore glomerular filtration. This may decrease proteinuria.

Use: Treatment of congestive heart failure in most species and chronic renal insufficiency (anecdotal only). Often used in conjunction with diuretics when heart failure is present as most effective when used in these cases. Can be used in combination with other drugs to treat heart failure (e.g. pimobendan, spironolactone, digoxin). May reduce blood pressure in hypertension. Benazepril undergoes significant hepatic metabolism and may not need dose adjustment in renal failure. ACE inhibitors are more likely to cause or exacerbate prerenal azotaemia in hypotensive animals and those with poor renal perfusion (e.g. acute, oliguric renal failure). Use cautiously if hypotension, hyponatraemia or outflow tract obstruction are present. Regular monitoring of blood pressure, serum creatinine, urea and electrolytes is strongly recommended with ACE inhibitor treatment. Hypotension, azotaemia and hyperkalaemia are all indications to stop or reduce ACE inhibitor treatment in rabbits. The use of ACE inhibitors in animals with cardiac disease stems mainly from extrapolation from theoretical benefits and studies showing a benefit in other species with heart failure and different cardiac diseases (mainly dogs and humans).

Safety and handling: Normal precautions should be observed.

Contraindications: Do not use in cases of cardiac output failure.

Adverse reactions: Potential adverse effects include hypotension, hyperkalaemia and azotaemia. Monitor blood pressure, serum creatinine and electrolytes when used in cases of heart failure. Dosage should be reduced if there are signs of hypotension (weakness, disorientation). Anorexia, vomiting and diarrhoea are rare. It is not recommended for breeding, pregnant or lactating animals, as safety has not been established. In rabbits, treatment with ACE inhibitors can be associated with an increase in azotaemia.

Drug interactions: Concomitant usage with potassium-sparing diuretics (e.g. spironolactone) or potassium supplements could result in hyperkalaemia. However, in practice, spironolactone and ACE inhibitors appear safe to use concurrently. There may be an increased risk of nephrotoxicity and decreased clinical efficacy when used with NSAIDs. There is a risk of hypotension with concomitant administration of diuretics, vasodilators (e.g. anaesthetic agents, antihypertensive agents) or negative inotropes (e.g. beta-blockers).

DOSES
Mammals: Ferrets: 0.25–0.5 mg/kg p.o. q24h; **Rabbits, Guinea pigs:** Starting dose 0.05 mg/kg p.o. q24h. Dose may be increased to a maximum of 0.1 mg/kg; **Rats:** ACE inhibitors have been used to mitigate protein losing nephropathy in rats at 0.5–1.0 mg/kg p.o. q24h [a].
Birds: 0.5 mg/kg p.o. q24h.
Reptiles, Amphibians, Fish: No information available

References
[a] Mudagal M, Patel J, Nagalakshmi NC and Asif Ansari M (2011) Renoprotective effects of combining ACE inhibitors and statins in experimental diabetic rats. *DARU Journal of Pharmaceutical Sciences* **19(5)**, 322–325

Benzalkonium chloride (Quaternary ammonium compound)
(Ark-Klens, **F10 Antiseptic Solution**) **ESPA**

Formulations: Various formulations including 12.5% liquid (Ark-Klens), benzalkonium chloride 5.4 g and polyhexanide 0.4 g liquid (F10 Antiseptic Solution Concentrate), benzalkonium chloride 0.4 g, polyhexanide 0.03 g and cypermethrin 0.25 g spray (F10® Germicidal Wound Spray with Insecticide). Also available in pre-diluted ready-to-use solution (1:250), barrier ointment and shampoo formulations.

Action: Biocidal action thought to cause damage to cell membranes and leakage of cell contents.

Use: Disinfection of equipment. May be used for nebulizing, nasal or sinus flushing and wound flushing at appropriate dilutions. Treatment of external bacterial infections of the skin and gills in fish. Quaternary ammonium compounds are more toxic at high temperatures and in water with low hardness, therefore dose rates should be reduced by 50%. Benzalkonium chloride has a low therapeutic index.

Safety and handling: Irritant to skin and eyes.

Contraindications: No information available.

Adverse reactions: No information available.

Drug interactions: No information available.

DOSES

Mammals, Birds, Reptiles, Amphibians: Nebulization, nasal, sinus, wound flushing; use 1:250 ml F10 Antiseptic solution[a].

Fish: 10 mg/l by immersion for 5–10 min; 0.5 mg/l by prolonged immersion.

References

[a] Drake GJ, Koeppel K and Barrows M (2010) Disinfectant (F10SC) nebulisation in the treatment of 'red leg syndrome' in amphibians. *Veterinary Record* **166**, 593–594

Benzocaine

Formulations: 100% powder for dissolution in acetone or ethanol.

Action: Benzocaine is lipid soluble and is rapidly absorbed across the gills and skin, resulting in anaesthesia by impeding peripheral nerve signal transmission to the CNS.

Use: Sedation, immobilization, anaesthesia and euthanasia of fish. Ideally, the drug should be used in water from the tank or pond of origin to minimize problems due to changes in water chemistry. The dry powder is poorly soluble in water and must be made into a stock solution with acetone or ethanol (e.g. 100 g/l) for more accurate dosing. Before use, the pH of the anaesthetic solution should be buffered with sodium bicarbonate to the same pH as the water of origin. The anaesthetic solution should be used on the day of preparation and be well aerated during use. Food should be withheld from fish for 12–24 h prior to anaesthesia to reduce the risk of regurgitation. The stage of anaesthesia reached is determined by the concentration used and the duration of exposure, since absorption continues throughout the period of immersion. Potency decreases with higher temperatures. Different species vary in their response and may require different concentrations. It is recommended to use the lower dose rates to test the selected drug concentration and exposure time with a small group before medicating large numbers. Fish may retain some movement during anaesthesia, making it less desirable to use during surgery. Anaesthetized fish should be returned to clean water from their normal environment to allow recovery. For euthanasia, use 5–10 times the normal anaesthetic dose and keep the fish in the solution for at least 60 minutes after respiration ceases.

Safety and handling: The powder should be stored dry and stock solutions should be stored in the dark.

Contraindications: No information available.

Adverse reactions: No information available.

Drug interactions: No information available.

DOSES

Fish: Induction of anaesthesia: 25–200 mg/l by immersion; Maintenance of anaesthesia: 15–40 mg/l by immersion[1].

Mammals, Birds, Reptiles, Amphibians: No information available.

References
[1] Sneddon LU (2012) Clinical anesthesia and analgesia in fish. *Journal of Exotic Pet Medicine* **21**, 32–43

Benzyl penicillin see **Penicillin G**

Betamethasone
(Fuciderm, Norbet, Otomax, Betnesol*, Maxidex*)
POM-V, POM

Formulations: Injectable: 4 mg/ml solution for i.v. or i.m. use. Oral: 0.25 mg tablet. **Topical:** 0.1% cream with 0.5% fusidic acid. Ophthalmic/Otic: 0.1% solution; 0.88 mg/ml suspension with clotrimazole and gentamicin. Betamethasone is also present in varying concentrations in several topical preparations with or without antibacterials.

Action: Alters the transcription of DNA, leading to alterations in cellular metabolism which cause reduction in inflammatory responses. Has high glucocorticoid but low mineralocorticoid activity. Betamethasone also antagonizes insulin and ADH.

Use: Short-term relief of many inflammatory but non-infectious conditions. Long duration of activity and therefore not suitable for long-term daily or alternate-day use. On a dose basis, 0.12 mg betamethasone is equivalent to 1 mg prednisolone. Prolonged use of glucocorticoids suppresses the hypothalamic–pituitary axis, resulting in adrenal atrophy. Animals on chronic corticosteroid therapy should be given tapered decreasing doses when discontinuing the drug. The use of long-acting steroids in most cases of shock is of no benefit, and may be detrimental.

Safety and handling: Wear gloves when applying cream.

Contraindications: Do not use in pregnant animals. Systemic corticosteroids are generally contraindicated in patients with renal disease and diabetes mellitus. Topical corticosteroids are contraindicated in ulcerative keratitis.

Adverse reactions: Catabolic effects of glucocorticoids lead to weight loss and cutaneous atrophy. Iatrogenic hyperadrenocorticism may develop. Vomiting, diarrhoea and GI ulceration may develop. Glucocorticoids may increase glucose levels and decrease serum T3 and T4 values. Impaired wound healing and delayed recovery from infections may be seen. Corticosteroids should be used with care in birds as there is a high risk of immunosuppression and side effects, such as hepatopathy and a diabetes mellitus-like syndrome. In rabbits, even small single doses can potentially cause severe adverse reactions. Ferrets are particularly susceptible to GI ulceration, and concurrent gastric protectants may be advisable, especially in stressed animals.

Drug interactions: There is an increased risk of GI ulceration if used concurrently with NSAIDs. Glucocorticoids antagonize the effect of insulin. Phenobarbital may accelerate the metabolism of corticosteroids and antifungals (e.g. itraconazole) may decrease it. There is an increased risk of hypokalaemia when used concurrently with acetazolamide, amphotericin and potassium-depleting diuretics (furosemide, thiazides).

DOSES
Mammals: 0.1 mg/kg s.c. q24h; Otic: 4 drops of polypharmaceutical to affected ear q12h; Ocular: 1 drop of ophthalmic solution to affected eye q6–8h; Skin: Apply cream to affected area q8–12h.
Birds: Not recommended.
Reptiles, Amphibians, Fish: No information available.

Bethanecol
(Myotonine*) **POM**

Formulations: Oral: 10 mg tablets.

Action: A muscarinic agonist (cholinergic or parasympathomimetic) that increases urinary bladder detrusor muscle tone and contraction.

Use: Management of urinary retention with reduced detrusor tone. It does not initiate a detrusor reflex and is ineffective if the bladder is areflexic. Best given on an empty stomach to avoid GI distress.

Safety and handling: Normal precautions should be observed.

Contraindications: Do not use when urethral resistance is increased unless in combination with agents that reduce urethral outflow pressure (e.g. phenoxybenzamine).

Adverse reactions: Vomiting, diarrhoea, GI cramping, anorexia, salivation and bradycardia (with overdosage). Treat overdoses with atropine.

Drug interactions: No information available.

DOSES
Mammals: Rabbits: 2.5–5 mg/kg p.o. q12h. Titrate doses upwards to avoid adverse effects.
Birds, Reptiles, Amphibians, Fish: Not indicated.

Bismuth salts (Bismuth carbonate, subnitrate and subsalicylate: tri-potassium di-citrato bismuthate (bismuth chelate))
(De-Noltab*, Pepto-Bismol*) **AVM-GSL, P**

Formulations: Oral: De-Noltab: tablets containing the equivalent of 120 mg bismuth oxide. Pepto-Bismol: bismuth subsalicylate suspension.

Action: Bismuth is a gastric cytoprotectant with activity against spiral bacteria. Bismuth chelate is effective in healing gastric and duodenal ulcers in humans, due to its direct toxic effects on gastric *Helicobacter pylori* and by stimulating mucosal prostaglandin and bicarbonate secretion. It is often used in conjunction with an H2 receptor antagonist. Bismuth subsalicylate has a mild anti-inflammatory effect.

Use: Acute oral poisoning, gastric ulceration and flatulent diarrhoea. Doses are empirical.

Safety and handling: Normal precautions should be observed.

Contraindications: Do not use where specific oral antidotes are being administered in cases of poisoning. Do not use if the patient is unconscious, fitting, or has a reduced cough reflex, or in cases of intestinal obstruction, or where enterotomy or enterectomy is to be performed.

Adverse reactions: Avoid long-term use (except chelates) as absorbed bismuth is neurotoxic. Bismuth chelate is contraindicated in renal impairment. Nausea and vomiting reported in humans.

Drug interactions: Absorption of tetracyclines is reduced by bismuth and specific antidotes may also be affected.

DOSES
Mammals: Ferrets: Pepto-Bismol: 17.6 mg/kg or 0.25–1.0 ml/kg p.o. q4–8h; Rabbits: Pepto-Bismol: 0.3–0.6 ml/kg p.o. q4–6h.
Birds, Reptiles, Amphibians, Fish: No information available.

Bright green see **Malachite green**
British anti-lewisite see **Dimercaprol**

Bromhexine
(Bisolvon) **POM-V**

Formulations: Injectable: 3 mg/ml solution. Oral: 10 mg/g powder.

Action: A bronchial secretolytic that disrupts the structure of acid mucopolysaccharide fibres in mucoid sputum and produces a less viscous mucus, which is easier to expectorate.

Use: To aid the management of respiratory diseases.

Safety and handling: Normal precautions should be observed.

Contraindications: No information available.

Adverse reactions: No information available.

Drug interactions: No information available.

DOSES
Mammals: 0.3 mg/animal p.o. q24h or via nebulizer as 0.15 mg/ml for 20–30 minutes, 1–3 times daily.
Birds: 1.5 mg/kg i.m., p.o. q12–24h [a].
Reptiles: 0.1–0.2 mg/kg p.o. q24h.
Amphibians, Fish: No information available.

References
[a] Sumano H, Gracia I, Capistrán A *et al.* (1995) Use of ambroxol and bromhexine as mucolytics for enhanced diffusion of furaltadone into tracheobronchial secretions in broilers. *British Poultry Science* **36(3)**, 503–507

Bronopol
(Pyceze) **POM-V**

Formulations: Immersion: 500 mg/l liquid.

Action: Inhibition of dehydrogenase activity, causing membrane damage.

Use: Treat and control external fungal infection in fish and fish eggs.

Safety and handling: Irritating to eyes, lungs and skin.

Contraindications: No information available.

Adverse reactions: No information available.

Drug interactions: No information available.

DOSES
Fish: 20 mg/l by immersion for 30 min q24h for 14 treatments; Eggs: 50 mg/l by immersion for 30 min [a].
Mammals, Birds, Reptiles, Amphibians: No information available.

References
[a] Branson E (2002) Efficacy of bronopol against infection of rainbow trout (*Oncorhynchus mykiss*) with the fungus *Saprolegnia* species. *Veterinary Record* **151(18)**, 539–541

Budesonide
(Budenofalk*, Budenofalk Rectal Foam*, Entocort*, Pulmicort*) **POM**

Formulations: Oral: 3 mg gastroresistant capsule, 3 mg capsule containing gastroresistant slow-release granules. **Rectal:** 2 mg (total dose) rectal foam, 0.02 mg/ml enema.

Action: Anti-inflammatory and immunosuppressive steroid.

Use: A novel steroid that is metabolized on its first pass through the liver in humans and therefore might be expected to have reduced systemic side effects. It has been suggested that it may be effective as a monotherapy in ferrets with inflammatory bowel disease when compared with other steroids (such as prednisolone). Systemic side effects were still seen in some patients. The dosing of this drug is unclear as it comes in a capsule of 0.3 mg and the dose is extrapolated from humans (no real pharmacokinetic data/hepatic metabolism data available in small animals). The uncoated powder for inhalant use in people (for which no information is available in small animals) should not be used for oral administration because of hydrolysis by gastric acid.

Safety and handling: Normal precautions should be observed.

Contraindications: Intestinal perforation; severe hepatic impairment.

Adverse reactions: In theory, the rapid metabolism should give minimal systemic adverse effects. However, signs of iatrogenic hyperadrenocorticism (hair loss, muscle wastage, elevation in liver enzymes, hepatomegaly, lethargy, polyphagia and polyuria/polydipsia) may develop. In theory, sudden transfer from other steroid therapy might result in signs related to reductions in steroid levels. Corticosteroids can potentially cause severe immunosuppression in rabbits; use with care.

Drug interactions: Additive effect if given with other corticosteroids. The metabolism of corticosteroids may be decreased by antifungals. Avoid using with antacids, erythromycin, cimetidine, itraconazole and other drugs that inhibit the liver enzymes that metabolize budesonide.

DOSES
Mammals: Ferrets: Doses of up to 1 mg/ferret p.o. q24h have been suggested for the management of IBD.
Birds, Reptiles, Amphibians, Fish: No information available.

Bupivacaine

(Marcain*, Sensorcaine*) **POM**

Formulations: Injectable: 2.5, 5.0, 7.5 mg/ml solutions, 2.5, 5.0 mg/ml solution with 1:200,000 adrenaline.

Action: Reversible blockade of the sodium channel in nerve fibres produces local anaesthesia.

Use: Provision of analgesia by perineural nerve blocks, regional and epidural techniques. Onset of action is significantly slower than lidocaine (20–30 min for epidural analgesia) but duration of action is relatively prolonged (6–8 h). Lower doses should be used when systemic absorption is likely to be high (e.g. intrapleural analgesia). Small volumes of bupivacaine can be diluted with normal saline to enable wider distribution of the drug for perineural blockade. Doses of bupivacaine up to 2 mg/kg q8h are unlikely to be associated with systemic side effects if injected perineurally, epidurally or intrapleurally. Combining bupivacaine with lidocaine can prolong the duration of the sensory block whilst limiting the duration of the motor block compared with administration of bupivacaine alone.

Safety and handling: Normal precautions should be observed.

Contraindications: Do not give i.v. or use for i.v. regional anaesthesia. Use of bupivacaine with adrenaline is not recommended when local vasoconstriction is undesirable (e.g. end arterial sites) or when a significant degree of systemic absorption is likely.

Adverse reactions: Inadvertent intravascular injection may precipitate severe cardiac arrhythmias that are refractory to treatment.

Drug interactions: All local anaesthetics share similar side effects, therefore the dose of bupivacaine should be reduced when used in combination with other local anaesthetics.

DOSES
Mammals:
- Perineural: volume of injection depends on the site of placement and size of the animal. As a guide: 0.1 ml/kg for femoral, radial and sciatic nerve block; 0.15 ml/kg for combined ulnar, musculocutaneous, median and ulnar nerve blocks; 0.3 ml/kg for brachial plexus nerve block; 0.25–1 ml total volume for blockade of the infraorbital, mental, maxillary and mandibular nerves. Choose an appropriate concentration of bupivacaine to achieve a 1–2 mg/kg dose within these volume guidelines.
- Epidural: 1.6 mg/kg (analgesia to level of L4), 2.3 mg/kg (analgesia to level of T11–T13); 1 mg/kg bupivacaine combined with preservative-free morphine 0.1 mg/kg. Limit the total volume of solution injected into the epidural space to 0.33 ml/kg in order to limit the cranial distribution of drugs in the epidural space and prevent adverse pressure effects.
- Interpleural: 1 mg/kg diluted with normal saline to a total volume of 1–5 ml depending on the size of the animal. The

solution can be instilled via a thoracotomy tube. Dilution reduces pain on injection due to the acidity of bupivacaine.
- **Ferrets:** 1–2 mg/kg local infusion; **Rabbits:** 1 mg/kg local infusion, do not exceed 2 mg/kg; **Guinea pigs:** 1–2 mg/kg for specific nerve blocks (may require dilution with saline for local infusion); **Rats:** 1–2 mg/kg local infusion or intradermally once.

Birds: <2 mg/kg local infusion [a,b]; may mix with dimethylsulfoxide (DMSO) for topical application preoperatively in bumblefoot.

Reptiles: 1–2 mg/kg local infusion or used in combination with lidocaine for intrathecal anaesthesia in chelonians [c].

Amphibians, Fish: No information available.

References

[a] Glatz PC, Murphy LB and Reston AP (1992) Analgesic therapy of beak-trimmed chickens. *Australian Veterinary Journal* **69(1)**, 18

[b] Machin KL and Livingston A (2001) Plasma bupivacaine levels in mallard duck (*Anas platyrhynchos*) following a single subcutaneous dose. *Proceedings of the Annual Conference of the AAZV/AAWV/ARAV/NAZWV*, pp. 159–163

[c] Mans C (2014) Clinical technique: Intrathecal drug administration in turtles and tortoises. *Journal of Exotic Pet Medicine* **23(1)**, 67–70

Buprenorphine

(Buprecare, Buprenodale, Vetergesic) **POM-V CD SCHEDULE 3**

Formulations: Injectable: 0.3 mg/ml solution; available in 1 ml vials that do not contain a preservative, or in 10 ml multidose bottle that contains chlorocresol as a preservative.

Action: Analgesia through high affinity, low intrinsic activity and slow dissociation with the mu receptor.

Use: Relief of mild to moderate perioperative pain. As a partial agonist it antagonizes the effects of full opioid agonists (e.g. methadone, fentanyl), although the clinical relevance of interactions between full mu agonists and buprenorphine has recently been questioned. However, in practice it is not recommended to administer buprenorphine when the subsequent administration of full mu agonists is likely. If analgesia is inadequate after buprenorphine, a full mu agonist may be administered without delay. Buprenorphine may be mixed with acepromazine or dexmedetomidine to provide sedation for minor procedures or pre-anaesthetic medication. Response to all opioids is variable between individuals; therefore assessment of pain after administration is imperative. Onset of action of buprenorphine may be slower than methadone (>15 min). Duration of effect is approximately 6 hours in rabbits and rodents. Buprenorphine is metabolized in the liver; some prolongation of effect may be seen with impaired liver function. The multidose preparation is unpalatable given sublingually due to the preservative. Be careful of species differences in effect in birds. Appears active for 2–5 hours in birds. Used for the relief of pain in fish, although it is considered to have poor analgesic properties in rainbow trout. In reptiles, studies show no evidence of analgesic efficacy.

Safety and handling: Normal precautions should be observed.

Contraindications: Combination with full mu agonists is not recommended for analgesia; therefore, do not use for premedication when administration of potent opioids during surgery is anticipated.

Adverse reactions: As a partial mu agonist, side effects are rare after clinical doses. Pain on i.m. injection of the multidose preparation has been anecdotally reported. The taste of the multidose preparation is aversive for some species.

Drug interactions: In common with other opioids, buprenorphine will reduce the doses of other drugs required for induction and maintenance of anaesthesia.

DOSES
When used for sedation is generally given as part of a combination. See Appendix for sedation protocols in all species.

Mammals: Analgesia: **Ferrets:** 0.01–0.05 mg/kg s.c., i.m., i.v. q6–8h[a]; **Rabbits:** 0.03–0.06 mg/kg s.c., i.m., i.v. q6–12h (doses <0.03 mg/kg have very limited analgesic effects but still have some sedative effects)[b]; **Most rodents:** 0.01–0.05 mg/kg i.m., s.c. q6–12h; **Guinea pigs, Chinchillas:** 0.05–0.2 mg/kg s.c., i.v. q4–8h[c,d]. The high end of the dose range may be needed for full analgesic effect, but use with caution as individual response is variable and sedation may be seen at higher doses; **Mice:** 0.05–0.1 mg/kg i.m., s.c. q6–12h; **Primates:** 0.01–0.03 mg/kg i.m, i.v q6–12h. Anecdotally, oral transmucosal delivery appears effective in rabbits, guinea pigs and chinchillas.

Birds: Analgesia: 0.01–0.05 mg/kg i.v., i.m. q8–12h. **Grey Parrots:** 0.25 mg/kg i.m. q8–12h; **Chickens:** 0.25–0.5 mg/kg i.m. q8–12h; **Cockatiels:** dose rates of 1.8 mg/kg or less had no effect on foot withdrawal following a thermal stimulus; **American kestrels:** a dose of 1.8 mg/kg s.c. using a sustained-relaease formulation provided apparent analgesic effects for up to 24 hours[e].

Reptiles: Analgesia: Doses of 0.01–0.1 mg/kg i.m. q24–48h have been suggested but analgesic efficacy is not established. Administration into the front limbs is recommended over the hind limbs for optimal systemic drug concentrations.

Amphibians: **Leopard frogs:** 38 mg/kg s.c.; **Newts:** 50 mg/kg intracoelomic q24h[f].

Fish: Analgesia: 0.01–0.1 mg/kg i.m.

References
[a] Katzenbach JE, Wittenburg LA, Allweiler SI, Gustafson DL and Johnston MS (2018) Pharmacokinetics of single-dose buprenorphine, butorphanol, and hydromorphone in the domestic ferret (*Mustela putorius furo*). *Journal of Exotic Pet Medicine* **27(2)**, 95–102
[b] Shafford HL and Schadt JC (2008) Effect of buprenorphine on the cardiovascular and respiratory response to visceral pain in conscious rabbits. *Veterinary Anaesthesia and Analgesia* **35(4)**, 333–340
[c] Sadar MJ, Knych HK, Drazenovich TL and Paul-Murphy JR (2018) Pharmacokinetics of buprenorphine after intravenous and oral transmucosal administration in guinea pigs (*Cavia porcellus*). *American Journal of Veterinary Research* **79(3)**, 260–266

d Fox L and Mans C (2018) Analgesic efficacy and safety of buprenorphine in chinchillas (*Chinchilla lanigera*). *Journal of the American Association for Laboratory Animal Science* **57(3)**, 286–290

e Guzman DSM, Ceulemans SM, Beaufrère H, Olsen GH and Paul-Murphy JR (2018) Evaluation of the Thermal Antinociceptive Effects of a Sustained-Release Buprenorphine Formulation After Intramuscular Administration to American kestrels (*Falco sparverius*). *Journal of Avian Medicine and Surgery* **32(1)**, 1–7

f Koeller CA (2009) Comparison of buprenorphine and butorphanol analgesia in the eastern red-spotted newt (*Notophthalmus viridescens*). *Journal of the American Association of Laboratory Animal Science* **48(2)**, 171–175

Buserelin
(Receptal) POM-V

Formulations: Injectable: 4 µg/ml solution. Authorized for use in rabbits, trout and certain large animal species.

Action: Synthetic GnRH (gonadotrophin releasing hormone) analogue that stimulates LH and FSH production, thus causing oestrus to develop and progress.

Use: To supplement natural LH in cases of ovulation failure or delay. Will also induce lactation postpartum in mammals. In males, it may stimulate testosterone secretion and is indicated in the management of genital hypoplasia and reduced libido. In ferrets it may be used in the management of signs of oestrus. In rabbits it is used to induce ovulation postpartum for insemination and to improve conception rates. In guinea pigs it can be used to resolve ovarian cysts if hormone-responsive. Used in birds for chronic egg laying (must be combined with husbandry changes). Used in trout to facilitate stripping in both male and female fish in spawning condition, and reduce mortality due to egg binding.

Safety and handling: Pregnant women should not administer the product.

Contraindications: No information available.

Adverse reactions: Anaphylactic reactions may occasionally occur.

Drug interactions: No information available.

DOSES
Mammals: Ferrets: 1.5 µg (micrograms)/animal i.m. q24h for 2 days; Rabbits: 0.8 µg/animal s.c. at time of insemination or mating; Guinea pigs: 25 µg/guinea pig, repeat in 2 weeks.
Birds: 0.5–1.0 µg (micrograms)/kg i.m. q48h, up to 3 times [a].
Fish: 3–4 µg (micrograms)/kg i.m. once, strip fish 2–3 days later [b].
Reptiles, Amphibians: No information available.

References
a Lovas EM, Johnston SD and Filippich LJ (2010) Using a GnRH agonist to obtain an index of testosterone secretory capacity in the cockatiel (*Nymphicus hollandicus*) and sulphur-crested cockatoo (*Cacatua galerita*). *Australian Veterinary Journal* **88**, 52–56

b Arabacı M, Diler İ and Sarı M (2004) Induction and synchronisation of ovulation in rainbow trout, Oncorhynchus mykiss, by administration of emulsified buserelin (GnRHa) and its effects on egg quality. *Aquaculture* **237(1–4)**, 475–484

Butorphanol
(Alvegesic, Dolorex, Torbugesic, Torbutrol, Torphasol) **POM-V**

Formulations: Injectable: 10 mg/ml solution. **Oral:** 5 mg, 10 mg tablets.

Action: Analgesia resulting from affinity for the kappa opioid receptor. Also has mu receptor antagonist properties and an antitussive action resulting from central depression of the cough mechanism.

Use: Management of mild perioperative pain. Provision of sedation through combination with acepromazine or alpha-2 agonists. Potent antitussive agent indicated for the relief of acute or chronic non-productive cough associated with tracheobronchitis, tracheitis, tonsillitis or laryngitis resulting from inflammatory conditions of the upper respiratory tract. Butorphanol has a very rapid onset and relatively short duration of action; in different models analgesia has been shown to last between 45 minutes and 4 hours. Butorphanol is metabolized in the liver and some prolongation of effect may be seen with impaired liver function. Butorphanol is unlikely to be adequate for the management of severe pain. Higher doses of full mu agonists may be needed to provide additional analgesia after butorphanol but it is not necessary to wait 4h after butorphanol administration to give other opioids. Response to all opioids appears to be very variable between individuals; therefore assessment of pain after administration is imperative. Be careful of species differences in effect in birds. There is limited evidence of analgesic efficacy in reptiles but does have sedative effects. Butorphanol has shown beneficial effects in koi following abdominal surgery but had no clear benefit in chain dogfish or zebrafish.

Safety and handling: Protect from light.

Contraindications: Animals with diseases of the lower respiratory tract associated with copious mucous production. Premedication when administration of potent opioids during surgery is anticipated. Decreased ventilation rate and buoyancy problems have been noted in koi.

Adverse reactions: As a kappa agonist/mu antagonist, side effects such as respiratory depression, bradycardia and vomiting are rare after clinical doses. Cough suppression following torbugesic tablets may be associated with mild sedation.

Drug interactions: In common with other opioids, butorphanol will reduce the doses of other drugs required for induction and maintenance of anaesthesia. Combination with full mu agonists is not recommended for analgesia, addition of butorphanol will reduce analgesia produced from the full mu agonist.

DOSES

When used for sedation is generally given as part of a combination. See Appendix for sedation protocols in all species.

Mammals: Analgesia: **Ferrets:** 0.1–0.5 mg/kg s.c. q4–6h; **Rabbits:** 0.1–0.5 mg/kg s.c. q4h; **Guinea pigs:** 0.2–2 mg/kg s.c. q4h; **Chinchillas:** 0.5–2 mg/kg s.c. q4h; **Gerbils, Hamsters, Rats, Mice:** 1–5 mg/kg s.c. q4h; **Primates:** 0.01–0.02 mg/kg i.v., s.c., p.o. q4–6h; **Sugar gliders:** 0.5 mg/kg i.m. q8h.

Birds: Analgesia: 0.3–4 mg/kg i.m., i.v. q2–12h[a,b]; Sedation: 3 mg/kg via the intranasal route combined with butorphanol. Use lower end doses for raptors. May prolong anaesthetic recovery.

Reptiles: Doses of 0.5–2 mg/kg i.m. q24h have been suggested for sedation but are not proven to provide analgesia. **Bearded dragons, Green iguanas:** 1.5 mg/kg i.m. q24h[c].

Amphibians: **Leopard frogs:** 0.2–0.4 mg/kg i.m.; **Newts:** 0.5 mg/l of water[d,e].

Fish: Analgesia: 0.25–5 mg i.m.; **Koi:** 10 mg/kg i.m.[f]

References

[a] Guzman DS, Flammer K, Paul-Murphy JR, Barker SA and Tully TN Jr (2011) Pharmacokinetics of butorphanol after intravenous, intramuscular and oral administration in Hispaniolan Amazon parrots (*Amazona ventralis*). *Journal of Avian Medicine and Surgery* **25(3)**, 185–191

[b] Paul-Murphy JR, Brunson DB and Miletic V (1999) Analgesic effects of butorphanol and buprenorphine in conscious African grey parrots (*Psittacus erithacus erithacus* and *Psittacus erithacus timneh*). *American Journal of Veterinary Research* **60(10)**, 1218–1221

[c] Greenacre CB, Takle G, Schmacher JP et al. (2006) Comparative anti-nociception of morphine, butorphanol and buprenorphine versus saline in the green iguana (*Iguana iguana*) using electrostimulation. *Journal of Herpetological Medicine and Surgery* **16**, 88–92

[d] Koeller CA (2009) Comparison of buprenorphine and butorphanol analgesia in the eastern red-spotted newt (*Notophthalmus viridescens*). *Journal of the American Association of Laboratory Animal Science* **48(2)**, 171–175

[e] Terril-Robb L, Suckow M and Grigdesby C (1996) Evaluation of the analgesic effects of butorphanol tartarate, xylazine hydrochloride and flunixin meglumine in leopard frogs (*Rana pipiens*). *Contemporary Topics in Laboratory Animal Science* **35**, 54–56

[f] Baker TR, Baker BB, Johnson SM and Sladky KK (2013) Comparative analgesic efficacy of morphine sulfate and butorphanol tartrate in koi (*Cyprinus carpio*) undergoing unilateral gonadectomy. *Journal of the American Veterinary Medical Association* **243(6)**, 882–890

Butylscopolamine (Hyoscine)
(Buscopan) **POM-V, P**

Formulations: Injectable: 4 mg/ml butylscopolamine + 500 mg/ml metamizole in 100 ml multidose bottle (Buscopan Compositum); 20 mg/ml butylscopolamine only, in 2 ml ampoules. **Oral:** 10 mg tablet containing butylscopolamine only.

Action: Inhibits M1 muscarinic acetylcholine receptors in the GI and urinary tracts causing smooth muscle relaxation but does not cross blood–brain barrier.

Use: Control of gastrointestinal pain in rabbits. Control of pain associated with urinary obstruction in rabbits. Must only be used in combination with investigations into the cause of abdominal pain or definitive relief of urinary obstruction.

Safety and handling: Avoid self-injection: metamizole can cause reversible but potentially serious agranulocytosis and skin allergies. Protect solution from light.

Contraindications: Intestinal obstruction. Contraindicated for the treatment of gastrointestinal ileus in rabbits.

Adverse reactions: Dry mouth, blurred vision, hesitant micturition and constipation at doses acting as gut neuromuscular relaxants. The i.m. route may cause a local reaction.

Drug interactions: Metamizole should not be given to animals that have been treated with a phenothiazine, as hypothermia may result. Effects may be potentiated by concurrent use of other anticholinergic or analgesic drugs.

DOSES
Mammals: Rabbits: 0.1 ml/kg i.v., i.m. q12h (Buscopan Compositum) as analgesic/antispasmolytic.
Birds, Reptiles, Amphibians, Fish: No information available.

Cabergoline
(Galastop) **POM-V**

Formulations: Oral: 50 µg/ml solution.

Action: Potent selective inhibition of prolactin.

Use: Has been used for pituitary adenomas in rats. May have beneficial effect in birds with chronic egg laying and other hormonal disorders related to high prolactin levels when combined with management changes. In birds it is also conjectured that its action could be mediated via its effect as a dopamine agonist. Carbergoline does not seem reliably effective in inducing abortion in the rat, mouse or rabbit. Generally ineffective if given for short periods in rabbits due to lack of clearly defined oestrus.

Safety and handling: Normal precautions should be observed.

Contraindications: Should not be used in combination with hypotensive drugs or in animals in a hypotensive state.

Adverse reactions: Not reported in exotic species. However, in dogs and cats vomiting or anorexia may occur after the first one or two doses in a small proportion of cases; there is no need to discontinue treatment unless vomiting is severe or it persists beyond the second dose. In some animals a degree of drowsiness may be seen in the first 2 days of dosing. May induce transient hypotension. Shown not to impair fertility in the male rat, non-teratogenic in mice and rabbits, and does not affect the latter phase of gestation or parturition in the female rat [a].

Drug interactions: Metoclopramide antagonizes the effects on prolactin.

DOSES
Mammals: Rats: 10–50 µg (micrograms)/kg p.o. q12–24h or 600 µg/kg p.o. q72h for pituitary adenoma and associated mammary pathology [b,c].
Birds: 10–50 µg (micrograms)/kg p.o. q24h [1].
Reptiles, Amphibians, Fish: No information available.

References
[a] Beltrame D, Longo M and Mazué G (1996) Reproductive toxicity of cabergoline in mice, rats and rabbits. *Reproductive Toxicology* **10(6)**, 471–483
[b] Eguchi K, Kawamoto K, Uozumi T *et al.* (1995) Effect of Cabergoline, a Dopamine Agonist, on Estrogen-Induced Rat Pituitary Tumors: *In Vitro* Culture Studies. *Endocrine Journal* **42(3)**, 413–420
[c] Mayer J, Sato A, Kiupel M, DeCubellis J and Donnelly T (2011) Extralabel use of cabergoline in the treatment of a pituitary adenoma in a rat. *Journal of the American Veterinary Medical Association* **239(5)**, 656–660
[1] Chitty J, Raftery A and Lawrie A (2006) Use of cabergoline in companion psittacine birds. *Proceedings of the Association of Avian Veterinarians*, pp. 65–57

CaEDTA see **Edetate calcium disodium**

Calcium salts (Calcium borogluconate, Calcium carbonate, Calcium chloride, Calcium gluconate, Calcium lactate)

(**Zolcal D**, Many cattle preparations, e.g. Calcibor. Minor component of **Aqupharm** No. 9 and **No. 11**. Several generic formulations) **POM-V, ESPA**

Formulations: There are many formulations available; a selection is given here.

* **Injectable:** 200 mg/ml calcium borogluconate solution equivalent to 15 mg/ml calcium formed from 168 mg/ml of calcium gluconate and 34 mg/ml boric acid (Calcibor 20); 100 mg/ml (10%) calcium chloride solution containing 27.3 mg/ml elemental calcium (= 1.36 mEq calcium/ml = 680 µmol/ml); 100 mg/ml calcium gluconate solution 10 ml ampoules containing 9 mg elemental calcium/ml (= mEq calcium/ml).
* **Oral solution:** 35 mg/ml calcium gluconate, 25 IU/ml cholecalciferol, 2 mg/ml magnesium (Zolcal-D).
* **Note on other formulations:** 11.2 mg calcium gluconate, 13.3 mg calcium borogluconate, 7.7 mg calcium lactate, 3.6 mg calcium chloride; each contains 1 mg elemental calcium = 0.5 mEq calcium.

Action: Calcium is an essential element involved in maintenance of numerous homeostatic roles and key reactions including activation of key enzymes, cell membrane potentials and nerve and musculoskeletal function.

Use: Management of hypocalcaemia and hyperkalaemic cardiotoxicity associated with urinary obstruction. Calcium gluconate and borogluconate are preferred for this. Serum calcium levels and renal function tests should be assessed before starting therapy. ECG monitoring during i.v. infusions is advised. Avoid using mixed electrolyte solutions intended for cattle use if possible. Treatment of hyperkalaemic cardiotoxicity with calcium rapidly corrects arrhythmias but effects are short-lived (5–10 min to effect) and i.v. glucose 0.5–1 g/kg $\pm$ insulin may be needed to decrease serum potassium. Parenteral calcium should be used very cautiously in dehydrated birds and reptiles and in patients receiving digitalis glycosides or those with cardiac or renal disease. Used before oxytocin in medical treatment of birds and reptiles with egg retention/dystocia. Calcium salts are given to many captive birds and reptiles as a routine dietary supplement for prevention of nutritional secondary hyperparathyroidism.

Safety and handling: Normal precautions should be observed.

Contraindications: Ventricular fibrillation or hypercalcaemia. Calcium should be avoided in pregnancy unless there is a deficient state. Hyperkalaemia associated with hypoadrenocorticism is often associated with hypercalcaemia and therefore additional calcium is not recommended in those cases.

Adverse reactions: Hypercalcaemia can occur, especially in renal impairment or cardiac disease. Tissue irritation is common and can occur with injectable preparation regardless of route. Rapid injection may cause hypotension, cardiac arrhythmias and cardiac arrest. Perivascular administration is treated by stopping the infusion, infiltrating the tissue with normal saline and topical application of corticosteroids. Be careful using i.v. in dehydrated reptiles and birds as has been suggested to precipitate gout.

Drug interactions: Patients on digitalis glycosides are more prone to develop arrhythmias if given i.v. calcium. All calcium salts may antagonize verapamil and other calcium-channel blockers. Calcium borogluconate is compatible with most i.v. fluids except those containing other divalent cations or phosphorus. Calcium borogluconate is reportedly compatible with lidocaine, adrenaline and hydrocortisone. Calcium chloride is incompatible with amphotericin B, cefalotin sodium and chlorphenamine. Calcium gluconate is incompatible with many drugs, including lipid emulsions, propofol, amphotericin B, cefamandole, naftate, cefalotin sodium, dobutamine, methylprednisolone sodium succinate and metoclopramide. Consult manufacturers' data sheets for incompatibilities with other solutions.

DOSES
Mammals: Guinea pigs, Chinchillas: 100 mg/kg calcium gluconate i.m., i.p. once, repeat as necessary; **Primates:** 200 mg/kg calcium gluconate s.c., i.m., i.v. once, repeat if necessary; 10–20 mg/kg calcium chloride i.v. slow infusion; **Sugar gliders:** 100 mg/kg calcium gluconate s.c. q12h x 3–5 days (dilute in saline to 10 mg/ml) for nutritional secondary hyperparathyroidism; 150 mg/kg p.o. q24h calcium glubionate; **Hedgehogs:** Hypocalcaemia: 50 mg/kg calcium gluconate i.m.

Birds: Egg retention, hypocalcaemia: 150–200 mg/kg calcium borogluconate i.m., s.c., slow i.v. once; Hypocalcaemia: 5–10 mg/kg calcium gluconate i.m. q12h.

Reptiles: Dystocia, hypocalcaemia: 100 mg/kg calcium borogluconate i.v., i.m., s.c. or 50–100 mg/kg calcium gluconate i.m., s.c. once, repeat as necessary.

Amphibians: 1 mg/kg calcium glubionate p.o. q24h; Hypocalcaemic tetany: 100–200 mg/kg calcium gluconate s.c. once; Nutritional secondary hyperparathyroidism: 2.3% bath of calcium gluconate (with 2–3 IU/ml vitamin D3).

Fish: No information available.

Carbimazole
(Vidalta) **POM-V**

Formulations: Oral: 10 mg, 15 mg tablets in a sustained-release formulation.

Action: Carbimazole is metabolized to the active drug methimazole, which interferes with the synthesis of thyroid hormones.

Use: Control of thyroid hormone levels in guinea pigs.

Safety and handling: Normal precautions should be observed.

Contraindications: No information available.

Adverse reactions: Vomiting (in relevant species) and inappetence/anorexia may be seen but are often transient. Jaundice, cytopenias, immune-mediated diseases and dermatological changes (pruritus, alopecia and self-induced trauma) are reported but rarely seen. Treatment of hyperthyroidism can decrease glomerular filtration rate, thereby raising serum urea and creatinine values, and can occasionally unmask occult renal failure. Animals that have an adverse reaction to methimazole are likely also to have an adverse reaction to carbimazole.

Drug interactions: Carbimazole should be discontinued before iodine-131 treatment. Do not use with low iodine prescription diets.

DOSES
Mammals: Guinea pigs: 1–2 mg/kg p.o. q24h[1].
Birds, Reptiles, Amphibians, Fish: No information available.

References
[1] Künzel F, Hierlmeier B, Christian M and Reifinger M (2013) Hyperthyroidism in four guinea pigs: clinical manifestations, diagnosis and treatment. *Journal of Small Animal Practice* **54(12)**, 667–671

Carbomer 980
(Lubrithal) **P, general sale**

Formulations: Ophthalmic: 0.2% (10 g tube, single-use vial), 0.25% (10 g tube) gel. This formulation is marketed specifically for small animals. Other formulations are widely available for general sale.

Action: Mucinomimetic, replacing both aqueous and mucin components of the tear film.

Use: Tear replacement and beneficial for management of quantitative (keratoconjunctivitis sicca (KCS) or dry eye) and qualitative tear film disorders. It has longer corneal contact time than the aqueous tear substitutes.

Safety and handling: Normal precautions should be observed.

Contraindications: No information available.

Adverse reactions: It is tolerated well and ocular irritation is unusual.

Drug interactions: No information available.

DOSES
Mammals: 1 drop per eye q4–6h. Use during anaesthesia: apply every 15 minutes or so to avoid ocular drying, especially if ketamine combinations are used or forced warm air warming is employed.
Birds, Reptiles, Amphibians, Fish: No information available.

Carboplatin
(Carboplatin*, Paraplatin*) **POM**

Formulations: Injectable: 10 mg/ml solution.

Action: Binds to DNA to form intra- and interstrand crosslinks and DNA-protein crosslinks, resulting in inhibition of DNA synthesis and function.

Use: May be of use in a number of neoplastic diseases including anal adenocarcinoma, squamous cell carcinoma, ovarian carcinoma, mediastinal carcinoma, pleural adenocarcinoma, nasal carcinoma and thyroid adenocarcinoma. The drug is highly irritant and must be administered via a preplaced i.v. catheter. Do not use needles or i.v. sets containing aluminium as precipitation of the drug may occur. This drug is generally now preferred over cisplatin due to reduced GI and renal toxicity. Use with caution in patients with abnormal renal function, active infections, hearing impairment or pre-existing hepatic disease. Has been used in renal adenocarcinoma in Budgerigars and squamous cell carcinoma (mixed with bird's own plasma for intralesional use) and bile duct carcinoma in Amazon parrots. The health risks to owners of (particularly indoor) birds from such treatments need to be considered carefully before recommending chemotherapy in birds.

Safety and handling: Potent cytotoxic drug that should only be prepared and administered by trained personnel. See specialist texts for further advice on chemotherapeutic agents.

Contraindications: No information available.

Adverse reactions: Include myelosuppression, nephrotoxicity, ototoxicity, nausea, vomiting, electrolyte abnormalities, neurotoxicity and anaphylactic reactions. However, produces fewer adverse reactions than cisplatin.

Drug interactions: Concomitant use of aminoglycosides or other nephrotoxic agents may increase risk of nephrotoxicity. May adversely affect the safety and efficacy of vaccinations.

DOSES

Birds: 5 mg/kg i.v., intraosseous over 3 minutes; 5 mg/kg intralesional use (mixed with plasma to make a concentration of 10 mg/ml) for squamous cell carcinoma [a,b].

Mammals, Reptiles, Amphibians, Fish: No information available.

References

[a] Filippich LJ, Charles BG, Sutton RH and Bucher AM (2004) Carboplatin pharmacokinetics following a single-dose infusion in sulphur-crested cockatoos (*Cacatua galerita*). *Australian Veterinary Journal* **82(6)**, 366–369

[b] Antonissen G, Devreese M, De Baere S *et al.* (2015) Comparative pharmacokinetics and allometric scaling of carboplatin in different avian species. *PLOS One* **10(7)**, e0134177

Carnidazole
(Spartrix) **AVM-GSL**

Formulations: Oral: 10 mg tablet.

Action: Coccidiocidal; mode of action not known.

Use: Pigeon canker (*Trichomonas columbae*); treat all birds in loft simultaneously. It should be used in conjunction with good loft hygiene, including disinfection of feed and water bowls.

Safety and handling: Direct contact with the product must be avoided. Wear impermeable gloves when handling.

Contraindications: Not to be used in birds intended for human consumption.

Adverse reactions: No information available.

Drug interactions: None known.

DOSES

Birds: Raptors: 25–30 mg/kg p.o., one dose normally sufficient but can be repeated next day if needed; **Psittacids:** 30–50 mg/kg p.o., repeat after 2 weeks; **Pigeons:** 12.5–25 mg/kg p.o. once; **Other birds:** 20–30 mg/kg p.o. once.

Mammals, Reptiles, Amphibians, Fish: No information available.

Carprofen
(Canidryl, Carprodyl, Dolagis, Rimadyl, Rimifin) **POM-V**

Formulations: Injectable: 50 mg/ml. Oral: 20 mg, 50 mg, 100 mg tablets (in plain and palatable formulations).

Action: Preferentially inhibits COX-2 enzyme, thereby limiting the production of prostaglandins involved in inflammation. Other non-COX-mediated mechanisms are suspected to contribute to the anti-inflammatory effect but these have not yet been identified.

Use: Control of postoperative pain and inflammation following surgery and reduction of chronic inflammation, e.g. degenerative joint disease, osteoarthritis. All NSAIDs should be administered cautiously in the perioperative period. Although carprofen preferentially inhibits COX-2, it may still adversely affect renal perfusion during periods of hypotension. If hypotension during anaesthesia is anticipated, delay carprofen administration until the animal is fully recovered from anaesthesia and is normotensive. Liver disease will prolong the metabolism of carprofen, leading to the potential for drug accumulation and overdose with repeated dosing. Prolonged long-term treatment should be under veterinary supervision. Use with caution in birds with dehydration, shock and renal dysfunction. Carprofen has induced some analgesic effects in rainbow trout.

Safety and handling: Formulations that use palatable tablets can be extremely palatable. Animals have been reported to eat tablets spontaneously, resulting in overdose. Ensure that tablets are stored out of animal reach. Store injectable solution in the refrigerator; once broached the product is stable for use at temperatures up to 25°C for 28 days.

Contraindications: Do not give to dehydrated, hypovolaemic or hypotensive patients or those with GI disease or blood clotting abnormalities. Administration of carprofen to animals with renal disease must be carefully evaluated and is not advisable in the perioperative period. Do not give to pregnant animals or animals <6 weeks old. Care may be needed when using in vultures[a].

Adverse reactions: GI signs may occur in all animals after NSAID administration. Stop therapy if this persists beyond 1–2 days. Some animals develop signs with one NSAID and not another. A 1–2 week wash-out period should be allowed before starting another NSAID after cessation of therapy. Stop therapy immediately if GI bleeding is suspected. There is a small risk that NSAIDs may precipitate cardiac failure in humans and this risk in animals is unknown. Fish may exhibit depressed activity at higher dose rates.

Drug interactions: Different NSAIDs should not be administered within 24 hours of each other or glucocorticoids as they are more ulcerogenic when used concurrently. The nephrotoxic tendencies of all NSAIDs are significantly increased when administered concurrently with other nephrotoxic agents, e.g. aminoglycosides.

DOSES

Mammals: Ferrets: 1–5 mg/kg total daily dose p.o.; **Rabbits:** 2–4 mg/kg s.c. q24h or 1.5 mg/kg p.o. q24h[b]; **Rodents:** 2–5 mg/kg total daily dose i.v., i.m., s.c., p.o. in single or two divided doses [c,d]; **Others:** 2–4 mg/kg i.v., i.m., s.c. q24h.

Birds: 1–5 mg/kg i.m., s.c., p.o. q12–24h (higher rate appears effective for 24 hours). (Note: 3 mg/kg i.m. q12h was not sufficient to provide analgesia in experimentally induced arthritis[e].)

Reptiles: 4 mg/kg s.c., i.m., p.o. once, then 2 mg/kg s.c., i.m., p.o. q24h; **Bearded dragons:** 2 mg/kg i.m. q24h.

Fish: 1–5 mg i.m. [1]

Amphibians: No information available.

References

[a] Cuthbert R, Parry-Jones J, Green RE and Pain DJ (2007) NSAIDs and scavenging birds: potential impacts beyond Asia's critically endangered vultures. *Biology Letters* **3(1)**, 91–94

[b] Hawkins MG, Taylor IT, Craigmill AL and Tell LA (2008) Enantioselective pharmacokinetics of racemic carprofen in New Zealand white rabbits. *Journal of Veterinary Pharmacology and Therapeutics* **31(5)**, 423–430

[c] Roughan JV and Flecknell PA (2004) Behaviour-based assessment of the duration of laparotomy-induced abdominal pain and the analgesic effects of carprofen and buprenorphine in rats. *Behavioural Pharmacology* **15**, 461–472

[d] Zegre Cannon C, Kissling GE, Goulding DR, King-Herbert AP and Blankenship-Paris T (2011) Analgesic effects of tramadol, carprofen or multimodal analgesia in rats undergoing ventral laparotomy. *Laboratory Animal* **40(3)**, 85–93

[e] Paul-Murphy JR, Sladky KK, Krugner-Higby LA *et al.* (2009) Analgesic effects of carprofen and liposome-encapsulated butorphanol tartrate in Hispaniolan parrots (*Amazona ventralis*) with experimentally induced arthritis. *American Journal of Veterinary Research* **70(10)**, 1201–1210

[1] Sneddon LU (2012) Clinical anaesthesia and analgesia in fish. *Journal of Exotic Pet Medicine* **21**, 32–43

Carvedilol
(Cardevidol*, Eucardic*) POM

Formulations: Oral: 3.125 mg, 6.25 mg, 12.5 mg, 25 mg tablets.

Action: Non-selective beta-adrenergic blocker with the afterload reduction properties of an alpha-1 adrenergic blocker. Additional antioxidant properties may decrease the oxidant stress associated with heart failure.

Use: Has been advocated for use as an adjunctive therapy in the management of chronic heart failure due to valvular disease or DCM and as an antihypertensive drug in patients that do not respond to first-line therapy. Veterinary experience is limited and benefit has not been established. Limited data on pharmacokinetics and pharmacodynamics in animals. Treatment should not be started until congestive heart failure has been stabilized for at least 2 weeks initially. Since it undergoes extensive hepatic metabolism, caution should be exercised in patients with hepatic insufficiency.

Safety and handling: Normal precautions should be observed.

Contraindications: Patients with bradyarrhythmias, acute or decompensated heart failure and bronchial disease. Do not administer concurrently with alpha-adrenergic agonists (e.g. adrenaline).

Adverse reactions: Potential side effects include lethargy, diarrhoea, bradycardia, AV block, myocardial depression, exacerbation of heart failure, syncope, hypotension and bronchospasm. A reduction in the glomerular filtration rate may exacerbate pre-existing renal impairment.

Drug interactions: The hypotensive effect of carvedilol is enhanced by many agents that depress myocardial activity including anaesthetic agents, phenothiazines, antihypertensive drugs, diuretics and diazepam. There is an increased risk of bradycardia, severe hypotension, heart failure and AV block if carvedilol is used concurrently with calcium-channel blockers. Hypotensive effect may be antagonized by NSAIDs. Concurrent digoxin administration potentiates bradycardia. Carvedilol may enhance the hypoglycaemic effect of insulin. Carvedilol increases plasma concentration of ciclosporin. Rifampin can decrease carvedilol plasma concentrations.

DOSES
Mammals: Rats: 2–30 mg/kg p.o. q24h [a]; **Hamsters:** 1–11 mg/kg p.o. q24h [b,c,d].
Birds: 1–9 mg/kg p.o. q12–24h.
Reptiles, Amphibians, Fish: No information available.

References
[a] Watanabe K, Ohta Y, Nakazawa M *et al.* (2000) Low dose carvedilol inhibits progression of heart failure in rats with dilated cardiomyopathy. *Pharmacology* **130(7)**, 1489–1495

[b] Cruz N, Arocho L, Rosario L and Crespo MJ (2007) Chronic administration of carvedilol improves cardiac function in 6-month-old Syrian cardiomyopathic hamsters. *Pharmacology* **80**, 144–150

[c] Nanjo S, Yamazaki J, Yoshikawa K, Ishii T and Togane Y (2006) Carvedilol prevents myocardial fibrosis in hamsters. *International Heart Journal* **47(4)**, 607–616

[d] Zendaoui A, Lachance D, Roussel E, Couet J and Arsenault M (2011) Usefulness of carvedilol in the treatment of chronic aortic valve regurgitation. *Circulation: Heart Failure* **4(2)**, 207–213

CCNU see **Lomustine**

Cefalexin (Cephalexin)
(Cefaseptin, Cephacare, Ceporex, Rilexine, Therios) **POM-V**

Formulations: Injectable: 180 mg/ml (18%) suspension.
Oral: 50 mg, 75 mg, 120 mg, 250 mg, 300 mg, 500 mg, 600 mg, 750 mg tablets; granules which, when reconstituted, provide a 100 mg/ml oral syrup.

Action: A 1st generation cephalosporin that binds to proteins involved in bacterial cell wall synthesis, thereby decreasing cell wall strength and rigidity, and affecting cell division. Resistant to some bacterial beta-lactamases, particularly those produced by *Staphylococcus* spp. As for other beta-lactam antibacterials, works in a time-dependent fashion.

Use: Active against several Gram-positive and Gram-negative organisms (e.g. *Staphylococcus*, *Pasteurella* and *Escherichia coli*). *Pseudomonas* and *Proteus* are often resistant. Maintaining levels above the MIC is critical for efficacy and prolonged dosage intervals or missed doses can compromise therapeutic response. Dose and dosing interval is determined by infection site, severity and organism. In severe or acute conditions, doses may be doubled or given at more frequent intervals.

Safety and handling: Reconstituted oral drops should be stored in the refrigerator and discarded after 10 days.

Contraindications: Patients hypersensitive to penicillins may also be sensitive to cephalosporins (cross-hypersensitivity in <10% of human patients); avoid use in animals with reported sensitivity to other beta-lactam antimicrobials. Avoid oral administration in small herbivores (e.g. rabbits).

Adverse reactions: Vomiting (where species are susceptible) and diarrhoea most common; administration with food may reduce these. Can cause fatal enterotoxaemia in small herbivores especially if given via the oral route which should be avoided. Injection may be painful.

Drug interactions: Bactericidal activity may be affected by concomitant use of bacteriostatic agents (e.g. erythromycin, oxytetracycline). May be an increased risk of nephrotoxicity if cephalosporins are used with amphotericin or loop diuretics (e.g. furosemide); monitor renal function. Do not mix in the same syringe as aminoglycosides.

DOSES
See Appendix for guidelines on responsible antibacterial use.
Mammals: Ferrets: 15–30 mg/kg p.o. q8–12h; **Rabbits:** 15–20 mg/kg s.c. q12–24h; **Guinea pigs:** 25 mg/kg i.m. q12–24h; **Primates:** 20–30 mg/kg p.o. q12h; **Sugar gliders:** 30 mg/kg s.c. q24h; **Hedgehogs:** 25 mg/kg p.o. q8h; **Others:** 15–30 mg/kg i.m. q8–12h.
Birds: 35–100 mg/kg p.o., i.m. q6–8h[a].
Reptiles: 20–40 mg/kg p.o. q12h.
Amphibians, Fish: No information available.

References
[a] Bush M, Locke D, Neal LA and Carpenter JW (1981) Pharmacokinetics of cephalothin and cephalexin in selected avian species. *American Journal of Veterinary Research* **42**, 1014–1017

Cefotaxime
(Cefotaxime*) **POM**

Formulations: Injectable: 500 mg, 1 g, 2 g powders for reconstitution.

Action: A 3rd generation cephalosporin that binds to proteins involved in bacterial cell wall synthesis, thereby decreasing cell wall strength and rigidity, and affecting cell division. Resistant to many bacterial beta-lactamases, particularly those produced by *Staphylococcus* spp. As other beta-lactam antibacterials, works in a time-dependent fashion.

Use: Good activity against many Gram-negative organisms, especially Enterobacteriaceae (not *Pseudomonas*) but lower activity against many Gram-positive organisms than 1st and 2nd generation cephalosporins. It is important to maintain tissue concentrations above the MIC. Use should be reserved for: patients with acute sepsis or serious infections; where cultures are pending or culture and sensitivity testing shows sensitivity; or where licensed preparations are not appropriate, and the animal is not a good candidate for intensive aminoglycoside therapy (e.g. pre-existing renal dysfunction). Use with care in patients with renal disease and consider increasing dose interval. *Escherichia coli* resistance reported in feral birds [a].

Safety and handling: The reconstituted solution is stable for 10 days when refrigerated.

Contraindications: Patients hypersensitive to penicillins may also be sensitive to cephalosporins (cross-hypersensitivity in <10% of human patients); avoid use in animals with reported sensitivity to other beta-lactam antimicrobials. Avoid oral administration in small herbivores (e.g. rabbits).

Adverse reactions: May produce pain on injection. GI disturbance and superinfection with resistant microorganisms is a potential risk. Can cause fatal enterotoxaemia in small herbivores especially if given via the oral route, which should be avoided.

Drug interactions: Bactericidal activity may be affected by concomitant use of bacteriostatic agents (e.g. oxytetracycline, erythromycin). The cephalosporins are synergistic with the aminoglycosides, but should not be mixed in the same syringe. May be increased risk of nephrotoxicity if cephalosporins are used with amphotericin or loop diuretics (e.g. furosemide); monitor renal function.

DOSES
See Appendix for guidelines on responsible antibacterial use.
Mammals: Rabbits, Primates: 50 mg/kg i.m., i.v. q8h.
Birds: 50–100 mg/kg i.m. q6–8h.
Reptiles: 20–40 mg/kg i.m. q24h.
Amphibians, Fish: No information available.

References
[a] Zurfluh K, Nüesch-Inderbinen M, Stephan R and Hächler H (2013) Higher generation cephalosporin-resistant *Escherichia coli* in feral birds in Switzerland. *International Journal of Antimicrobial Agents* **41(30)**, 296–297

Cefovecin
(Convenia) **POM-V**

Formulations: Injectable: Lyophilized powder which when reconstituted contains 80 mg/ml cefovecin.

Action: A 3rd generation cephalosporin that binds to proteins involved in bacterial cell wall synthesis, thereby decreasing cell wall strength and rigidity, and affecting cell division. Resistant to some bacterial beta-lactamases. Assumed to work in a time-dependent fashion as other beta-lactam antibacterials.

Use: In line with rational antimicrobial use, cefovecin should not be considered if a 14 day course of antimicrobial would not ordinarily be required for the infection being treated. Specifically indicated for the prolonged treatment of skin and soft tissue infections and for infections of the urinary tract. Also used as part of the management of severe periodontal disease. Good efficacy against organisms commonly associated with these conditions (e.g. *Staphylococcus, Streptococcus, Escherichia coli, Pasteurella multocida, Proteus*). Activity against anaerobes such as *Prevotella, Fusobacterium, Bacteroides* and *Clostridium* also appears to be good. Not active against *Pseudomonas*. Due to unique pharmacokinetic profile, cefovecin has an extremely long half-life in some mammals but not in birds or reptiles. Cefovecin concentrations were detectable for 4 days in white bamboo sharks and 7 days in copper rockfish following a single subcutaneous injection.

Safety and handling: Store in the refrigerator even prior to reconstitution; use reconstituted drug within 28 days.

Contraindications: Patients hypersensitive to penicillins may also be sensitive to cephalosporins (cross-hypersensitivity in <10% of human patients); avoid use in animals with reported sensitivity to other beta-lactam antimicrobials. Do not use in rabbits, guinea pigs and other small herbivores. Avoid use during lactation and in pregnant animals, as safety has not been established.

Adverse reactions: Appears to be relatively safe but has not been assessed in renal disease. Reported adverse reactions include mild GI disturbance and transient swelling at the injection site. Can cause fatal enterotoxaemia in small herbivores especially if given via the oral route, which should be avoided.

Drug interactions: Highly bound to plasma proteins, therefore it would be prudent to exhibit caution when using in conjunction with other highly protein-bound drugs such as furosemide and NSAIDs.

DOSES
See Appendix for guidelines on responsible antibacterial use.
Mammals: Ferrets: 8 mg/kg s.c. q48–72h. **Hedgehogs:** 8 mg/kg s.c. q5–6d.
Birds, Reptiles: Initial data appear to show it is not practicable (half-life <2h in poultry, <4h in hens and green iguanas[a], <7h in red-eared sliders[b], ~20h in Hermann's tortoises[c]). Further data show that the half-life in parrots is similar to that in chickens.
Fish: White bamboo sharks: 8 mg/kg s.c. q4d[d]; **Copper rockfish:** 16 mg/kg s.c. q7d[e].
Amphibians: No information available.

References
[a] Thuesen R, Bertelsen MF, Brimer L and Skaanild MT (2009) Selected pharmacokinetic parameters for cefovecin in hens and green iguanas. *Journal of Veterinary Pharmacology and Therapeutics* **32(6)**, 631–617
[b] Sypniewski LA, Maxwell LK, Murray JK, Brandão JL and Papich MG (2017) Cefovecin Pharmacokinetics in the Red-Eared Slider. *Journal of Exotic Pet Medicine* **26(2)**, 108–113

^c Nardini G, Barbarossa A, Dall'Occo A *et al.* (2014) Pharmacokinetics of cefovecin sodium after subcutaneous administration to Hermann's tortoises (*Testudo hermanni*). *American Journal of Veterinary Research* **75(10)**, 918–923

^d Steeil JC, Schumacher J, George RH *et al.* (2014) Pharmacokinetics of cefovecin (Convenia®) in white bamboo sharks (*Chiloscyllium plagiosum*) and Atlantic horseshoe crabs (*Limulus polyphemus*). *Journal of Zoo and Wildlife Medicine* **45(2)**, 389–392

^e Seeley KE, Wolf KN, Bishop MA, Turnquist M and KuKanich B (2016) Pharmacokinetics of long-acting cefovecin in copper rockfish (*Sebastes caurinus*). *American Journal of Veterinary Research* **77(3)**, 260–264

Ceftazidime
(Fortum*, Kefadim*) **POM**

Formulations: Injectable: 500 mg, 1 g, 2 g, 3 g powders for reconstitution.

Action: A 3rd generation cephalosporin that binds to proteins involved in bacterial cell wall synthesis, thereby decreasing cell wall strength and rigidity, and affecting cell division. Resistant to some bacterial beta-lactamases. As other beta-lactam antibacterials, works in a time-dependent fashion.

Use: Higher activity against many Gram-negative organisms but lower activity against many Gram-positives when compared to 1st and 2nd generation cephalosporins. Very good activity against *Pseudomonas* in humans. Use should be limited to cases with a confirmed susceptibility and acute sepsis or serious infections where licensed preparations are found to be inappropriate. Limited information on clinical pharmacokinetics in animal species and doses given below are empirical. Important to maintain tissue concentrations above the MIC with regular doses. Used for the treatment of bacterial disease in fish.

Safety and handling: Normal precautions should be observed.

Contraindications: Patients hypersensitive to penicillins may also be sensitive to cephalosporins (cross-hypersensitivity in <10% of human patients); avoid use in animals with reported sensitivity to other beta-lactam antimicrobials. Avoid oral administration in small herbivores (e.g. rabbits).

Adverse reactions: GI disturbances associated with drug use in humans. Pain may be noted following injection. Can cause fatal enterotoxaemia in small herbivores especially if given via the oral route, which should be avoided.

Drug interactions: Bactericidal activity may be affected by concomitant use of bacteriostatic agents (e.g. oxytetracycline, erythromycin). May be an increased risk of nephrotoxicity if cephalosporins are used with amphotericin or loop diuretics (e.g. furosemide); monitor renal function. Do not mix in the same syringe as aminoglycosides. Ceftazidime is synergistic with the aminoglycoside antimicrobials *in vivo* (often used in humans for pseudomonal infection in neutropenic patients).

DOSES

See Appendix for guidelines on responsible antibacterial use.

Mammals: Rabbits: 100 mg/kg i.m. q12h; **Primates:** 50 mg/kg i.m., i.v. q8h.

Birds: 75–200 mg/kg i.v., i.m. q6–12h.

Reptiles: **Most species:** 20 mg/kg i.m., s.c., i.v. q72h[a]; More frequent dosing (q24–48h) has been suggested in chameleons. Less frequent dosing (q120h) has been suggested in Eastern box turtles, yellow-bellied sliders and river cooters[b].

Amphibians: 20 mg/kg s.c., i.m. q48–72h.

Fish: 20 mg/kg i.m. q72h for 3–5 treatments[c].

References

[a] Lawrence K, Muggleton PW and Needham J (1984) Preliminary study on the use of ceftazidime, a broad spectrum cephalosporin antibiotic, in snakes. *Research in Veterinary Science* **36(1)**, 16–20

[b] Cerreta AJ, Lewbart GA, Dise DR and Papich MG (2018) Population pharmacokinetics of ceftazidime after a single intramuscular injection in wild turtles. *Journal of veterinary pharmacology and therapeutics* **41(4)**, 495–501

[c] Govett PD, Buur J, Krein A, McDowell T and Weber ES (2009) Pharmacokinetics of ceftazidime in koi (*Cyprinus carpio*) after a single dose intramuscular or intracoelomic administration. *Proceedings of the International Association of Aquatic Animal Medicine 40th annual conference*, p.19

Ceftiofur

(Excenel) **POM-V**

Formulations: Injectable: 1 g, 4 g powder for reconstitution; 50 mg/ml suspension.

Action: A 3rd generation cephalosporin that binds to proteins involved in bacterial cell wall synthesis, thereby decreasing cell wall strength and rigidity and affecting cell division. Resistant to many bacterial beta-lactamases, particularly those produced by *Staphylococcus* spp. Uniquely among the cephalosporins, ceftiofur is metabolized to desfuroylceftiofur which is an active metabolite. Action is time-dependent.

Use: Higher activity against many Gram-negative organisms, especially Enterobacteriaceae (not *Pseudomonas*) but lower activity against many Gram-positives than 1st and 2nd generation cephalosporins. Use should be reserved for patients suffering from acute sepsis or serious infections where cultures are pending, other licensed preparations are not appropriate and the animal is not a good candidate for intensive aminoglycoside therapy (pre-existing renal dysfunction). Important to maintain tissue concentrations above the MIC. Use with care in patients with renal disease and consider increasing dose interval.

Safety and handling: Store powder in the refrigerator; once reconstituted store in the refrigerator and discard after 7 days or within 12 hours if stored at room temperature.

Contraindications: Patients hypersensitive to penicillins may also be sensitive to cephalosporins (cross-hypersensitivity in <10% of human patients); avoid use in animals with reported sensitivity to other beta-lactam antimicrobials. Avoid oral administration in small herbivores (e.g. rabbits).

Adverse reactions: May produce pain on injection. GI disturbance and superinfection with resistant microorganisms is a potential risk. May be an increased risk of nephrotoxicity if cephalosporins are used with amphotericin or loop diuretics (e.g. furosemide); monitor renal function. Can cause fatal enterotoxaemia in small herbivores especially if given via the oral route, which should be avoided.

Drug interactions: Bactericidal activity may be affected by concomitant use of bacteriostatic agents (e.g. oxytetracycline, erythromycin). The cephalosporins are synergistic with the aminoglycosides, but should not be mixed in the same syringe.

DOSES
See Appendix for guidelines on responsible antibacterial use.
Mammals: Primates: 2.2 mg/kg i.m. q24h; **Hedgehogs:** 20 mg/kg s.c. q12–24h.
Birds: Amazons: 10 mg/kg i.m. q8–12h; **Cockatiels:** 10 mg/kg i.m. q4h; in some cases, higher doses (up to 100 mg/kg) may be necessary [a,b]. In red-tailed hawks dose administration frequencies for infections with Gram-negative and Gram-positive organisms were estimated as every 36 and 45 hours for the 10 mg/kg dose and every 96 and 120 hours for the 20 mg/kg dose, respectively [c].
Reptiles: Chelonians: 4 mg/kg i.m. q24h; **Green iguanas:** 5 mg/kg i.m., s.c. q24h [d]; **Bearded dragons:** 30 mg/kg i.m, s.c. lasts 12 days [e]; **Ball pythons:** 15 mg/kg i.m. lasts >5 days [f].
Amphibians, Fish: No information available.

References
[a] Al-Kheraije KA (2013) Studies on the antibacterial activity of ceftiofur sodium *in vitro* and birds. *Open Journal of Veterinary Medicine* **3(1)**, 16–21

[b] Tell L, Harrenstien L, Wetzlich S *et al.* (1998) Pharmacokinetics of ceftiofur sodium in exotic and domestic avian species. *Journal of Veterinary Pharmacology and Therapeutics* **21(2)**, 85–91

[c] Sadar MJ, Hawkins MG, Byrne BA *et al.* (2015) Pharmacokinetics of a single intramuscular injection of ceftiofur crystalline-free acid in red-tailed hawks (*Buteo jamaicensis*). *American Journal of Veterinary Research* **76(12)**, 1077–1084

[d] Benson KG, Tell LA, Young LA, Wetzlich S and Craigmill AL (2003) Pharmacokinetics of ceftiofur sodium after intramuscular or subcutaneous administration in green iguanas (*Iguana iguana*). *American Journal of Veterinary Research* **64(10)**, 1278–1282

[e] Churgin SM, Musgrave KE, Cox SK and Sladky KK (2014) Pharmacokinetics of subcutaneous *versus* intramuscular administration of ceftiofur crystalline-free acid to bearded dragons (*Pogona vitticeps*). *American Journal of Veterinary Research* **75(5)**, 453–459

[f] Adkesson MJ, Fernandez-Varon E, Cox S and Martín-Jiménez T (2011) Pharmacokinetics of a long-acting ceftiofur formulation (ceftiofur crystalline free acid) in the ball python (*Python regius*). *Journal of Zoo and Wildlife Medicine* **42(3)**, 444–450

Cefuroxime
(Zinacef*, Zinnat*) **POM**

Formulations: Injectable: 250 mg, 750 mg, 1.5 g powders for reconstitution (sodium salt). **Oral (as cefuroxime axetil):** 125 mg, 250 mg tablets; 125 mg/5 ml suspension.

Action: A 2nd generation cephalosporin that binds to proteins involved in bacterial cell wall synthesis, thereby decreasing cell wall strength and rigidity, and affecting cell division. Resistant to some bacterial beta-lactamases. As other beta-lactam antibacterials, works in a time-dependent fashion. Cefuroxime axetil is hydrolysed in intestinal mucosa and liver to yield active drug giving oral bioavailability.

Use: Higher activity against many Gram-negative organisms when compared to 1st generation cephalosporins. Good activity against a wider spectrum of Enterobacteriaceae (not *Pseudomonas*). Many obligate anaerobes also susceptible. It is a time-dependent antimicrobial, so maintaining levels above the MIC is important for efficacy. Limited applications in veterinary species and limited pharmacokinetic data make appropriate dose selection problematic.

Safety and handling: Normal precautions should be observed.

Contraindications: Patients hypersensitive to penicillins may also be sensitive to cephalosporins (cross-hypersensitivity in <10% of human patients); avoid use in animals with reported sensitivity to other beta-lactam antimicrobials. Avoid oral administration in small herbivores (e.g. rabbits).

Adverse reactions: May cause pain on i.m. and s.c. injection. GI disturbance has been reported in humans, particularly associated with the oral axetil formulation. Can cause fatal enterotoxaemia in small herbivores especially if given via the oral route, which should be avoided.

Drug interactions: Bactericidal activity may be affected by concomitant use of bacteriostatic agents (e.g. oxytetracycline, erythromycin). May be an increased risk of nephrotoxicity if cephalosporins are used with amphotericin or loop diuretics (e.g. furosemide); monitor renal function. Synergistic with aminoglycosides, do not mix in the same syringe.

DOSES
See Appendix for guidelines on responsible antibacterial use.
Mammals: Rabbits: 18.75 mg/kg i.v. q8h[a].
Reptiles: 100 mg/kg i.m. q24h for 10 days at 30°C.
Birds, Amphibians, Fish: No information available.

References
[a] Pützler J, Arens D, Metsemakers W *et al.* (2017) Duration of antibiotic prophylaxis with intravenous cefuroxime affects infection rate with *Staphylococcus aureus* in an open fracture model in rabbits. *Orthopaedic Proceedings* **99-B(S22)**, 63

Celecoxib

(Celebrex*, Celecoxib*) **POM**

Formulations: Oral: 100 mg, 200 mg capsules.

Action: Preferentially inhibits COX-2 enzyme, thereby limiting the production of prostaglandins involved in inflammation.

Use: Used in the management of proventricular dilatation disease in parrots and for analgesia in the management of arthritis in rats.

Safety and handling: Normal precautions should be observed.

Contraindications: Do not give to dehydrated, hypovolaemic or hypotensive patients, or those with GI disease or clotting problems. Administration of celecoxib to animals with renal disease must be carefully evaluated and is not advisable in the perioperative period. Do not give to animals <6 weeks of age.

Adverse reactions: GI signs may occur in all animals after NSAID administration. Stop therapy if this persists beyond 1–2 days. Some animals develop signs with one NSAID and not another. A 1–2 week wash-out period should be allowed before starting another NSAID after cessation of therapy. Stop therapy immediately if GI bleeding is suspected. There is a small risk that NSAIDs may precipitate cardiac failure in humans and this risk in animals is unknown.

Drug interactions: No information available.

DOSES

Mammals: Rats: 10–20 mg/kg p.o.[a]
Birds: 10–20 mg/kg p.o. q24h[b,c].
Reptiles, Amphibians, Fish: No information available.

References
[a] Millecamps M, Jourdan D, Leger S et al. (2005) Circadian pattern of spontaneous behavior in monarthritic rats: a novel global approach to evaluation of chronic pain and treatment effectiveness. *Arthritis & Rheumatology* **52(11)**, 3470–3478
[b] Dahlhausen R, Aldred S and Colaizzi E (2002) Resolution of clinical proventricular dilatation disease by cyclooxygenase 2 inhibition. *Proceedings of the Annual Conference of the Association of Avian Veterinarians*, pp. 9–12
[c] Hawkins MG (2006) The use of analgesics in birds, reptiles and small exotic mammals. *Journal of Exotic Pet Medicine* **15(3)**, 177–191

Cephalexin see Cefalexin

Charcoal (Activated charcoal)

(Actidose-Aqua*, Charcodote*, Liqui-Char*) **AVM-GSL**

Formulations: Oral: 50 g activated charcoal powder or premixed slurry (200 mg/ml).

Action: Absorbs toxins, fluids and gases in the GI tract. Activated charcoal has increased porosity and enhanced absorptive capacity.

Use: In acute poisoning with organophosphates, carbamates, chlorinated hydrocarbons, strychnine, ethylene glycol, inorganic and organic arsenical and mercurial compounds, polycyclic organic compounds (most pesticides) and dermal toxicants that may be ingested following grooming. As a general rule administer at a dose of at least 10 times the volume of intoxicant ingested. Repeat dosing as required if emesis or massive toxin ingestion occurs. Repeated dosing necessary if highly lipid-soluble toxins, which are likely to undergo enterohepatic recirculation, have been ingested. Used in the treatment of oiled birds.

Safety and handling: Activated charcoal powder floats, covering everything in the area; prepare very carefully as it will stain permanently. Paste forms are available which are more controllable.

Contraindications: Activated charcoal should not be used prior to the use of emetics.

Adverse reactions: Charcoal colours stools black, which is medically insignificant but may be alarming to the owner.

Drug interactions: Activated charcoal reduces the absorption and therefore efficacy of orally administered drugs.

DOSES
Mammals: 0.5–5 g/kg p.o.
Birds: 3.75 g/kg p.o.
Reptiles: Chelonians: 2–8 g/kg by stomach tube.
Amphibians, Fish: No information available.

Chitosan
(Ipakitine) **GSL**

Formulations: Oral: powder containing 8% chitosan, 10% calcium carbonate and 82% lactose.

Action: Adsorbent for intestinal uraemic toxins, including phosphate.

Use: The combination has been suggested to reduce serum urea and phosphate in chronic renal disease in ferrets, based on its use in cats. Phosphate-binding agents are usually only used if low phosphate diets are unsuccessful. Monitor serum phosphate levels at 10–14 day intervals and adjust dosage accordingly if trying to normalize serum concentrations. As formulation contains lactose, use with care in diabetic and lactose-intolerant animals.

Safety and handling: Normal precautions should be observed.

Contraindications: Not advised in rabbits due to the risk of hypercalcuria.

Adverse reactions: Hypercalcaemia, possibly due to the calcium carbonate component.

Drug interactions: None noted.

DOSES

Mammals: Ferrets: 0.5 mg/kg on food q12h; **Rats:** 200 mg/kg chitosan p.o. q24h has been shown to have hepatic protective effects[a]; 165–825 mg/kg chitosan p.o. q24h has been shown to have renal protective effects[b].

Birds, Reptiles, Amphibians, Fish: No information available.

References

[a] Ozcelik E, Uslu S, Erkasap N and Karimi H (2014) Protective effect of chitosan treatment against acetaminophen-induced hepatotoxicity. *The Kaohsiung Journal of Medical Sciences* **30(6)**, 286–290

[b] Chou CK, Li YC, Chen SM, Shih YM and Lee JA (2015) Chitosan Prevents Gentamicin-Induced Nephrotoxicity via a Carbonyl Stress-Dependent Pathway. *BioMed Research International* **2015**, 675714

Chlorambucil
(Leukeran*) **POM**

Formulations: Oral: 2 mg tablet.

Action: Alkylating agent that inhibits DNA synthesis and function through cross-linking with cellular DNA. Cell cycle non-specific.

Use: Management of some malignancies, lymphoproliferative, myeloproliferative and immune-mediated diseases. Immunosuppressive effect is not well defined and therefore it should only be considered where more established therapies such as prednisolone and azathioprine have failed. Has been used for treatment of lymphosarcoma in cockatoos.

Safety and handling: Cytotoxic drug; see specialist texts for further advice on chemotherapeutic agents. Tablets should be stored in a closed, light-protected container under refrigeration (2–8°C).

Contraindications: Bone marrow suppression, factors predisposing to infection.

Adverse reactions: Anorexia, nausea, vomiting, leucopenia, thrombocytopenia, anaemia (rarely), neurotoxicity, alopecia (rarely) and slow regrowth of clipped hair coat.

Drug interactions: Drugs that stimulate hepatic cytochrome P450 system increase cytotoxic effects. Prednisolone has a synergistic effect in the management of lymphoid neoplasia.

DOSES

See Appendix for chemotherapy protocols in ferrets.

Mammals: Ferrets: Used as part of a multi-drug protocol for lymphoma.

Birds: Lymphosarcoma: 1–2 mg/kg p.o. twice weekly[a]; 2 mg/kg p.o. twice weekly for thymic lymphoma in a Java Sparrow[b].

Reptiles, Amphibians, Fish: No information available.

References

a Rivera S, McClearen JR and Reacill DR (2009) Treatment of non-epitheliotropic cutaneous B-cell lymphoma in an Umbrella cockatoo (*Cacatua alba*). *Journal of Avian Medicine and Surgery* **23(4)**, 294–302

b Yu PH and Chi CH (2015) Long-term management of thymic lymphoma in a Java sparrow (*Lonchura oryzivora*). *Journal of Avian Medicine and Surgery* **29(1)**, 51–55

Chloramine-T (Sodium N-chloro 4-methylbenzenesulfonamide, Sodium N-chloro-para-toluenesulfonylamide) (Chloramine T, Halamid) ESPA

Formulations: 100% white powder.

Action: The chemical slowly decomposes in water to the hypochlorite anion to produce weak hypochlorous acid, which decomposes further to active chlorine and oxygen to provide a disinfectant effect.

Use: For the treatment of external water-borne bacterial infections, particularly bacterial gill disease, and some protozoan and trematode ectoparasites in fish. It should not be mixed in metal containers or ones in which other chemicals have been previously mixed. Do not use in bright sunlight or in water <12°C. Turn off UV and carbon filter systems for 24 hours. More toxic in water with low hardness and low pH. Make up fresh solution immediately prior to use since product degrades in water. Do not dispose of product in drains or waterways.

Safety and handling: Corrosive. Wear gloves and eye protection.

Contraindications: No information available.

Adverse reactions: Hyperplastic thickening and oedema of respiratory epithelia at significantly higher dose rates causing increased respiratory rates.

Drug interactions: The chemical should not be used with other chemicals (other than salt), particularly reducing agents such as formalin.

DOSES

Fish: 1–2 mg/l by prolonged immersion; repeat daily for 4 days if necessary.

Mammals, Birds, Reptiles, Amphibians: No information available.

Chloramphenicol

(Chloramphenicol*, Chloromycetin Ophthalmic Ointment*, Chloromycetin Redidrops*, Kemicetine*) **POM**

Formulations: Injectable: 1 g powder for reconstitution. Ophthalmic: 1% ointment; 0.5% solution. Oral: 250 mg capsules.

Action: Bacteriostatic antimicrobial that acts by binding to the 50S ribosomal subunit of susceptible bacteria, preventing bacterial protein synthesis.

Use: Broad spectrum of activity against Gram-positive (e.g. *Streptococcus*, *Staphylococcus*), Gram-negative (e.g. *Brucella*, *Salmonella*, *Haemophilus*) and obligate anaerobic bacteria (e.g. *Clostridium*, *Bacteroides fragilis*). Other sensitive organisms include *Chlamydia*, *Mycoplasma* (unreliable in treatment of ocular mycoplasmosis) and *Rickettsia*. Used in amphibians for chytridiomycosis; safe for larvae, metamorphs and adults. Resistant organisms include *Nocardia* and *Mycobacterium*. Acquired resistance may occur in Enterobacteriaceae. High lipid solubility makes it suitable for the treatment of intraocular infections. It will also access the CNS. However, due to concerns of resistance development and human toxicity, use should be restricted to individual animals where there is a specific indication such as salmonellosis resistant to other antimicrobials or deep infections of the eye. Patients with hepatic or renal dysfunction may need adjustment to dose. Decrease dose or increase dosing interval in neonates. Use with caution or avoid in nursing animals, especially those with neonates, as crosses into milk.

Safety and handling: Humans exposed to chloramphenicol may have an increased risk of developing a fatal aplastic anaemia. Products should be handled with care; use impervious gloves and avoid skin contact.

Contraindications: In amphibians, chloramphenicol might dramatically alter the protective natural skin microbiome when used as an antifungal agent.

Adverse reactions: Dose-related reversible bone marrow suppression can develop in all species. Unlike humans, the development of irreversible aplastic anaemia in veterinary species does not appear to be a significant problem. Other adverse effects include nausea, vomiting, diarrhoea and anaphylaxis.

Drug interactions: Irreversible inhibitor of a large number of hepatic cytochrome P450-dependent enzymes and so increases plasma levels of pentobarbital, phenobarbital and oral hypoglycaemic agents. Recovery requires synthesis of new liver enzymes and can take up to 3 weeks. Rifampin accelerates the metabolism of chloramphenicol, thus decreasing serum levels. Chloramphenicol may inhibit activity of bactericidal antimicrobials such as the aminoglycosides and beta-lactams. May also be an inhibitory effect if used in combination with macrolide or lincosamide antimicrobials.

DOSES
See Appendix for guidelines on responsible antibacterial use.
Mammals: **Ferrets:** 25–50 mg/kg p.o., s.c., i.m., i.v. q12h; **Rabbits:** 50 mg/kg p.o., s.c. q12–24h; **Guinea pigs:** 0.83 mg/ml drinking water; **Mice:** 50 mg/kg i.m., p.o. q12h, 200 mg/kg p.o. q12h or 0.5 mg/ml drinking water; **Gerbils:** 1 mg/ml drinking water; **Other rodents:** 30–50 mg/kg i.v., i.m., s.c., p.o. q8–12h; **Primates:** 50–100 mg/kg s.c., i.m., i.v. q8h; **Sugar gliders:** 50 mg/kg p.o. q12h; **Hedgehogs:** 30–50 mg/kg p.o., s.c, i.m, i.v. q12h. Ophthalmic: 1 drop q4–8h; ointment q8–12h.
Birds: 50 mg/kg i.v., i.m. q8h or 75 mg/kg p.o. q8h; **Pigeons:** 25 mg/kg p.o. q12h.
Reptiles: **Most species:** 40–50 mg/kg i.m., s.c., p.o. q24h; **Rat snakes, King snakes, Indigo snakes:** 50 mg/kg i.m. q12h; **Boids:** 50 mg/kg i.m. q12–24h; **Water snakes** (*Nerodia* spp.): 50 mg/kg i.m. q12–72h[a].
Amphibians: 50 mg/kg s.c., i.m., intracoelomic q12–24h or 10–20 mg/l as a bath[b,c,d].
Fish: No information available.

References
[a] Clark CH, Rogers ED and Milton JL (1985) Plasma concentrations of chloramphenicol in snakes. *American Journal of Veterinary Research* **46(12)**, 2654–2657
[b] Bishop PJ, Speare R, Poulter R et al. (2009) Elimination of the amphibian chytrid fungus *Batrachochytrium dendrobatidis* by Archey's frog (*Leiopelma archeyi*). *Diseases of Aquatic Organisms* **84(1)**, 9–15
[c] Holden WM, Ebert AR, Canning PF and Rollins-Smith LA (2014) Evaluation of amphotericin B and chloramphenicol as alternative drugs for treatment of chytridiomycosis and their impacts on innate skin defences. *Applied Environmental Microbiology* **80(13)**, 4034–4041
[d] Young S, Speare R, Berger L and Skerratt LF (2012) Chloramphenicol with fluid and electrolyte therapy cures terminally ill green tree frogs (*Litoria caerulea*) with chytridiomycosis. *Journal of Zoo and Wildlife Medicine* **43(2)**, 330–337

Chlorhexidine
(Hibiscrub, Malaseb, Microbex, Savlon, Chlorohex*, CLX wipes*, Otodine*, TrizChlor*, Viatop*) **POM-V, AVM-GSL**

Formulations: Topical shampoo: 2% chlorhexidine + 2% miconazole (Malaseb); 31.2 mg/ml chlorhexidine (Microbex); **Cleansing solution:** 1.5% chlorhexidine + cetrimide (Savlon); **Surgical scrub solution:** 4% chlorhexidine + isopropyl alcohol (Hibiscrub); **Mouthwash:** 0.12% chlorhexidine (Chlorohex); **Topical gel:** 0.06% chlorhexidine, aqua, raffinose, propylene glycol, saponins, triethanolamine, acrylates, phenoxyethanol, benzoic acid esters, allantoin (Viatop); **Topical skin cleaner:** Chlorhexidine, Tris-EDTA, zinc gluconate, glycerine, climbazole, benzyl alcohol, propylene glycol (CLX wipes); **Ear cleaner:** 0.15% chlorhexidine + EDTA (TrizChlor); Chlorhexidine, Tris-EDTA, lactic acid (Otodine).

Action: Chemical antiseptic that disrupts bacterial cell membrane.

Use: Topical treatment of bacterial, dermatophyte and *Malassezia* skin infections in animals as a shampoo (Malaseb). Topical treatment of *Malassezia* infections (Microbex). Washing surgical instruments, routine antisepsis for surgical operations (Savlon, Hibiscrub) and dental hygiene (Chlorohex). Topical treatment of mild pruritus (Viatop). Concurrent systemic antibacterial therapy is generally advised when treating bacterial skin infections. Leave in contact with the skin for 5–10 minutes prior to washing off. Ear cleaners for cleansing and removal of cerumen. Chlorhexidine as a single agent is not consistently effective as an antifungal. Use diluted, but very sparingly to reduce gross contamination only in the preparation of surgical sites in fish.

Safety and handling: Normal precautions should be observed.

Contraindications: Do not instil into ears where the integrity of the tympanum is unknown. Do not use on eyes. Has been associated with skin damage in amphibians so use not recommended[a].

Adverse reactions: Ototoxic. May irritate mucous membranes.

Drug interactions: Not known.

DOSES

Mammals: Apply to affected area q8h at 0.5–2.0% concentrations. 0.05% solution in water can be used as a safe wound flush. When treating dermatophytosis continue treatment for 2 weeks after apparent clinical cure and negative fungal culture results. Otic: Dilute topical products to a 1.0% concentration and apply topically q8–12h.

Birds: Apply 2–3 times weekly. May be used less frequently once infection is controlled.

Reptiles: 0.05% solution in water has been suggested as a safe wound flush q24h.

Amphibians: Not recommended.

Fish: Use 0.025% solution very sparingly to remove gross contamination only[1].

References

[a] Philips BH, Crim MJ, Hankenson FC *et al.* (2015) Evaluation of presurgical skin preparation agents in African clawed frogs (*Xenopus laevis*). *Journal of the American Association for Laboratory Animal Science* **54(6)**, 788–798

[1] Harms CA and Lewbart GA (2000) Surgery in fish. *Veterinary Clinics: Exotic Animal Practice* **3(3)**, 759–774

Chloroquine (Chloroquine diphosphate, Chloroquine phosphate)
(Avloclor*) **POM**

Formulations: Oral: 250 mg tablets.

Action: Antiprotozoal; mode of action not known but may enter the cell of marine protozoan ectoparasites causing cell lysis due to disruption of normal cell membrane function.

Use: Treatment of haemoparasites, most commonly *Plasmodium* in a variety of zoo and wild animal species, although rarely indicated in exotic pets. Treatment of skin and gill disease due to infestation with marine protozoan ectoparasites (e.g. *Cryptocaryon irritans* (marine white spot), *Brooklynella*, *Uronema*) and dinoflagellates (e.g. *Amyloodinium ocellatum* (marine velvet)). When using in aquatic set-ups, do not use activated carbon, UV sterilization, ozone or protein skimmer during treatment. Change 25% of the water before each dose.

Safety and handling: Normal precautions should be observed.

Contraindications: Highly toxic to micro- and macroalgae and various invertebrates, particularly corals, clams and echinoderms. Do not use in reef tanks.

Adverse reactions: May cause reduced appetite.

Drug interactions: No information available.

DOSES
Birds: Raptors: 10–20 mg/kg p.o., then 5–10 mg/kg at 6, 24, 48h. May be combined with primaquine.
Reptiles: Tortoises: 125 mg/kg p.o. q48h for 3 doses.
Fish: For *Amyloodinium*: 10 mg/l by immersion, repeat after 21 days prn[1]; For protozoans: 10–15 mg/l by immersion then 10 mg/l q7–10d for 3 doses (more effective if salinity is reduced to 12–13 ppt)[2,3]. Add activated carbon to remove the drug if no relapse apparent after 21 days.
Mammals, Amphibians: No information available.

References
1. Noga EJ (2010) *Fish Disease – Diagnosis and Treatment, 2nd edn.* Wiley-Blackwell, Oxford
2. Goemans B and Ichinotsubo L (2008) Parasitic Infestations. In: *The Marine Fish – Health & Feeding Handbook*, ed. B Goemans and L Ichinotsubo, pp. 142–171. TFH Publications, New Jersey
3. Goemans B (2014) Expert Advice: Marine Ich. *Marine Habitat* **20**, 12

Chlorphenamine (Chlorpheniramine)
(Piriton*) **POM, GSL**

Formulations: Injectable: 10 mg/ml solution. Oral: 4 mg tablet, 0.4 mg/ml syrup.

Action: Binds to H1 histamine receptors to prevent histamine binding.

Use: Management of allergic disease and prevention and early treatment of anaphylaxis. Commonly used as premedication before transfusions and certain chemotherapeutic agents. Specific doses for animals have not been determined by pharmacokinetic studies. Use with caution in cases with urinary retention, angle-closure glaucoma and pyloroduodenal obstruction.

Safety and handling: Normal precautions should be observed.

Contraindications: No information available.

Adverse reactions: May cause mild sedation. May reduce seizure threshold.

Drug interactions: No information available.

DOSES
Mammals: Ferrets: 1–2 mg/kg p.o. q8–12h; **Rabbits:** 0.2–0.4 mg/kg p.o. q12h; **Rodents:** 0.6 mg/kg p.o. q24h; **Primates:** 0.5 mg/kg p.o. q24h.
Birds, Reptiles, Amphibians, Fish: No information available.

Cholestyramine see **Colestyramine**

Chorionic gonadotrophin (Human chorionic gonadotrophin, hCG)
(Chorulon) **POM-V**

Formulations: Injectable: 1500 IU powder for reconstitution.

Action: In females, induces follicular maturation, ovulation and development of the corpus luteum. In males, stimulates testosterone secretion.

Use: Used to supplement or replace LH in cases of ovulation failure or delay, to induce lactation post-partum, or in females who fail to hold to mating. Used in ferrets to treat persistent oestrus. In guinea pigs it can be used to resolve ovarian cysts if hormone-responsive. In male animals it may increase libido; may also assist the treatment of cryptorchidism before surgical castration, provided inguinal canal remains patent and therapy is started early. May have an effect in preventing egg laying in birds. Used in amphibians for mating or release of sperm in males, followed with GnRH in 8–24h, and induction of ovulation in females (can be used with progesterone or PMSG).

Safety and handling: Reconstituted vials do not contain any preservative and so should be discarded within 24 hours.

Contraindications: No information available.

Adverse reactions: Anaphylactic reactions may occasionally occur.

Drug interactions: No information available.

DOSES

Mammals: Ferrets: 100 IU/animal i.m. q14d for 2 doses; **Rabbits:** 20–25 IU/animal i.v. once to induce ovulation; **Guinea pigs:** 100 IU/kg i.m. weekly for 3 doses; **Primates:** 250 IU i.m. once.

Birds: 500–1000 IU/kg i.m. on days 1, 3 and 7 q3–6wk to inhibit egg laying [a].

Amphibians: 300–400 IU s.c., i.m. [b]

Reptiles, Fish: No information available.

References

[a] Lightfoot TL (2000) Clinical use and preliminary data of chorionic gonadotropin administration in psittacines. *Proceedings of the Annual Conference of the American Avian Veterinarians*, pp. 17–21

[b] Kouba AJ, del Barco-Trillo J, Vance CK, Milam C and Carr M (2012) A comparison of human chorionic gonadotropin and luteinizing hormone releasing hormone on the induction of spermiation and amplexus in the American toad (*Anaxyrus americanus*). *Reproductive Biology and Endocrinology* **10**, 59

Ciclosporin (Cyclosporin(e))
(Atopica, Optimmune, Neoral*, Sandimmun*)
POM-V, POM

Formulations: Ophthalmic: 0.2% ointment (Optimmune). **Oral:** 10 mg, 25 mg, 50 mg, 100 mg capsules; 100 mg/ml solution. Injectable: 50 mg/ml solution.

Action: T lymphocyte inhibition.

Use: Used for disseminated idiopathic myositis and pure red cell aplasia in ferrets, and sebaceous adenitis in rabbits. May be of use in the treatment of bornavirus in cockatiels. No evidence of systemic or ocular toxicity following ocular administration but systemic absorption has been reported. Recommended that bacterial and fungal infections are treated before use. Whilst the nephrotoxicity seen in human patients does not appear to be common in animals, care should be taken in treating animals with renal impairment, and creatinine levels should be monitored regularly. Use with caution in patients with pre-existing infections and monitor for opportunistic infections.

Safety and handling: Use gloves to prevent cutaneous absorption.

Contraindications: Do not use in progressive malignant disorders. Do not give live vaccines during treatment or within a 2-week interval before or after treatment. The manufacturer does not recommend use in diabetic animals.

Adverse reactions: Hypertrichosis is common. There may be immediate discomfort on topical application (blepharospasm). Transient vomiting and diarrhoea may follow systemic administration; these are usually mild and do not require cessation of treatment. Infrequently observed adverse effects include: anorexia; mild to moderate gingival hyperplasia; papillomatous lesions of the skin; red and swollen pinnae; muscle weakness; and muscle cramps. These effects resolve spontaneously after treatment is stopped. Systemic treatment may be associated with an increased risk of malignancy.

Drug interactions: The metabolism of ciclosporin is reduced, and thus serum levels increased, by various drugs that competitively inhibit or induce enzymes involved in its metabolism, particularly cytochrome P450, including diltiazem, doxycycline and imidazole antifungal drugs. In humans there is an increased risk of nephrotoxicity if ciclosporin is administered with aminoglycosides, NSAIDs, quinolones, or trimethoprim/sulphonamides; concomitant use of ciclosporin not recommended. Increased risk of hyperkalaemia if used with ACE inhibitors. As a substrate and inhibitor of the *MDR-1* P-glycoprotein transporter, co-administration of ciclosporin with P-glycoprotein substrates such as macrocyclic lactones (e.g. ivermectin and milbemycin) could decrease the efflux of such drugs from blood—brain barrier cells, potentially resulting in signs of CNS toxicity. Ciclosporin has been shown to affect glucose metabolism and decrease the effects of insulin and to do so as much as low doses of glucocorticoids; therefore, use with caution in diabetic patients.

DOSES
Mammals: **Ferrets:** 5 mg/kg p.o. q24h; **Rabbits:** 5 mg/kg p.o. q24h for idiopathic sebaceous adenitis; **Rats:** 10 mg/kg p.o. q24h.

Birds: **Cockatiels:** 0.2 mg/animal p.o. to stop development of avian bornavirus[a]. For anti-inflammatory activity, doses of 30—60 mg/kg p.o. q12—24h have been used in various parrot species, however, in a Harris' hawk these dose rates produced toxic signs — pharmacokinetic study showed that a dose rate of 5 mg/kg was required to maintain plasma levels without toxicity[b].

Reptiles, Amphibians, Fish: No information available.

References
[a] Hameed SS, Guo J, Tizard I, Shivaprasad HL and Payne S (2018) Studies on immunity and immunopathogenesis of parrot bornaviral disease in cockatiels. *Virology* **515**, 81—91

[b] Chitty J (2017) An Update on Pyoderma in Harris' Hawks. *Proceedings of the International Conference on Avian, Reptile and Exotic Mammals*. Venice, pp. 354—355

Cimetidine
(Zitac, Cimetidine*, Dyspamet*, Tagamet*)
POM-V, POM

Formulations: Injectable: 100 mg/ml solution in 2 ml ampoule. Oral: 100 mg, 200 mg, 400 mg, 800 mg tablets; 40 mg/ml syrup.

Action: Histamine (H2) receptor antagonist, blocking histamine-induced gastric acid secretion. Rapidly absorbed with high bioavailability; undergoes hepatic metabolism and renal excretion. Plasma half-life is about an hour.

Use: Management of idiopathic, uraemic or drug-related erosive gastritis, gastric and duodenal ulcers, oesophagitis, and hypersecretory conditions secondary to gastrinoma or mast cell neoplasia. Efficacy against NSAID-induced ulcers is controversial. Reduction of vomiting due to gastritis and gastric ulceration is typically achieved in about 2 weeks but animals should be treated for at least 2 weeks after the remission of clinical signs, so minimum of 28 days recommended. If considered successful, medication can then be stopped. Rebound gastric acid secretion may be seen on cessation of cimetidine, so therapy should be tapered. A 2-week medication-free period should be allowed to see if vomiting occurs again. If the animal starts vomiting again after a medication-free period, treatment can be re-initiated, without risk for intolerance. Depending on the response, treatment can be adapted to the individual animal until the response is considered to be adequate and then continued at this level. Concomitant treatment with sucralfate may be helpful, and dietary measures should always be maintained. If used i.v., should be administered over 30 min to prevent cardiac arrhythmias and hypotension. Dosage should be reduced for animals with renal impairment. Less effective at reducing gastric acidity than more modern H2 blockers and proton pump inhibitors. Cimetidine has minimal prokinetic effects.

Safety and handling: Normal precautions should be observed.

Contraindications: No information available.

Adverse reactions: Rare, although hepatotoxicity and nephrotoxicity have been reported in humans. Adverse reactions are generally minor even at high doses. In humans cimetidine has been associated with headache, gynaecomastia and decreased libido.

Drug interactions: Retards oxidative hepatic drug metabolism by binding to the microsomal cytochrome P450. May increase plasma levels of beta-blockers (e.g. propranolol), calcium-channel blockers (e.g. verapamil), diazepam, lidocaine, metronidazole, pethidine and theophylline. When used with other agents that cause leucopenia may exacerbate the problem. Sucralfate may decrease bioavailability; although there is little evidence to suggest this is of clinical importance it may be a wise precaution to administer sucralfate at least 2 hours before cimetidine. Stagger oral doses by 2 hours when used with other antacids, digoxin, itraconazole or maropitant.

DOSES
Mammals: Ferrets: 5–10 mg/kg i.m., s.c., p.o. q8h; **Rabbits:** 5–10 mg/kg p.o. q6–8h; **Rodents:** 5–10 mg/kg p.o., s.c., i.m., i.v. q6–12h; **Primates:** 10 mg/kg p.o., s.c., i.m. q8h; **Hedgehogs:** 10 mg/kg p.o. q8h.
Birds: 5 mg/kg i.m., p.o. q8–12h.
Reptiles: 4 mg/kg i.m., p.o. q8–12h.
Amphibians, Fish: No information available.

Ciprofloxacin
(Ciloxan*, Ciproxin*) **POM**

Formulations: Oral: 100 mg, 250 mg and 500 mg tablets; 50 mg/ml suspension. **Injectable:** 2 mg/ml for i.v. infusion. **Ophthalmic:** 0.3% solution in 5 ml bottle; 0.3% ointment in 3.5 g tube.

Action: Bactericidal through inhibition of bacterial DNA gyrase.

Use: Ideally fluoroquinolone use should be reserved for infections where culture and sensitivity testing predicts a clinical response and where first- and second-line antimicrobials would not be effective. Broad-spectrum activity against wide range of Gram-negative and some Gram-positive aerobes; some activity against *Mycoplasma* and *Chlamydia*. Active against many ocular pathogens, including *Staphylococcus* and *Pseudomonas aeruginosa*, although there is increasing resistance amongst staphylococci and streptococci. The eye drop formulation is also used in reptiles for the topical management of wounds or stomatitis.

Safety and handling: Normal precautions should be observed.

Contraindications: No information available.

Adverse reactions: May cause local irritation after application. In humans the following are reported: local burning and itching; lid margin crusting; hyperaemia; taste disturbances; corneal staining, keratitis, lid oedema, lacrimation, photophobia, corneal infiltrates; nausea; and visual disturbances.

Drug interactions: No information available.

DOSES
See Appendix for guidelines on responsible antibacterial use.

Mammals: Ferrets: 10–30 mg/kg p.o. q24h; Rabbits: 10–20 mg/kg p.o. q24h or 1 drop to affected eye q6h; loading dose can be used 1 drop to affected eye q15min for 4 doses; **Guinea pigs, Chinchillas:** 5–25 mg/kg p.o. q12h; **Hamsters:** 10–20 mg/kg p.o. q12h; **Other rodents:** 7–25 mg/kg p.o. q12h; **Primates:** 10–20 mg/kg p.o. q12h[a]; **Sugar gliders:** 10 mg/kg p.o. q12h; **Hedgehogs:** 5–20 mg/kg p.o. q12h.

Birds: 5–20 mg/kg i.v., i.m., p.o. q12h[b]; **Raptors:** 50 mg/kg p.o. q12h[c].

Reptiles: Topical: 1 drop to affected eyes or in wounds or topical application for stomatitis; Systemic: 5–10 mg/kg p.o., s.c., i.m. q24h.

Amphibians: 10 mg/kg p.o. q24–48h for 7 days; 500–750 mg/75 litres as a bath for 6–8h q24h.

Fish: 15 mg/kg i.v., i.m. q2–5days[d].

References
[a] Nelson M, Stagg AJ, Stevens DJ *et al.* (2011) Post-exposure therapy of inhalational anthrax in the common marmoset. *International Journal of Antimicrobial Agents* **38(1)**, 60–64

[b] Atta AH and Sharif L (1997) Pharmacokinetics of ciprofloxacin following intravenous and oral administration is broiler chickens. *Journal of Veterinary Pharmacology and Therapeutics* **20(4)**, 326–329

c   Isaza R, Budsberg SC, Sundlof SF and Baker B (1993) Disposition of ciprofloxacin in red-tailed hawks (*Buteo jamaicensis*) following a single oral dose. *Journal of Zoo and Wildlife Medicine* **24(4)**, 498–502

d   Nouws JFM, Grondel JL, Schutte AR and Laurensen J (1988) Pharmacokinetics of ciprofloxacin in carp, African catfish and rainbow trout. *Veterinary Quarterly* **10(3)**, 211–216

Cisapride
(Cisapride) **POM-V**

Formulations: Various formulations (including tablets and suspensions) available as a veterinary special depending on requirements.

Action: Gastrointestinal prokinetic agent related to metoclopramide but has no central antiemetic activity.

Use: Primarily used in GI stasis in rabbits and herbivorous rodents (e.g. guinea pigs, chinchillas). Its licence for humans was withdrawn due to potentially fatal cardiac arrhythmias and it is solely available to the veterinary profession on a named patient or named veterinary surgeon 'special basis'.

Safety and handling: Normal precautions should be observed.

Contraindications: In humans, simultaneous administration of cisapride and ranitidine may cause nausea. In rabbits it is difficult to judge whether this is a significant issue, but should be considered if the patient exhibits signs of inappetence or discomfort or suspected nausea, and the doses staggered by at least 2 hours.

Adverse reactions: Abdominal cramps and diarrhoea may develop, especially at higher doses or if used alongside other prokinetic agents. Fatal cardiac arrhythmias have not been reported in rabbits or rodents.

Drug interactions: Opioid analgesics and antimuscarinics (e.g. atropine) may antagonize the effects of cisapride. In humans, it is known that drugs inhibiting the cytochrome P450 3A4 enzymes which metabolize cisapride (clarithromycin, erythromycin, itraconazole) when taken alongside cisapride have led to fatal arrhythmias.

DOSES
Mammals: Rabbits, Guinea pigs, Chinchillas: 0.1–1.0 mg/kg (typically 0.5 mg/kg) p.o. q8–12h; **Primates:** 0.2 mg/kg p.o. q12h[a]; **Sugar gliders:** 0.25 mg/kg p.o., s.c. q8–24h.
Birds, Reptiles, Amphibians, Fish: No information available.

References
a   Yogo K, Onoma M, Ozaki K *et al.* (2008) Effects of oral mitemcinal (GM-611), erythromycin, EM-574 and cisapride on gastric emptying in conscious rhesus monkeys. *Digestive Diseases and Sciences* **53(4)**, 912–918

Clarithromycin
(Klaricid*) **POM**

Formulations: Oral: 250 mg, 500 mg tablets; 125 mg/5 ml suspension; 250 mg/5 ml suspension; 250 mg granules sachet (to be dissolved in water). **Injectable:** 500 mg vial for reconstitution.

Action: Derived from erythromycin and with greater activity. Bactericidal (time-dependent) or bacteriostatic properties, depending on concentration and susceptibility. Binds to the 50S ribosome, inhibiting peptide bond formation.

Use: Alternative to penicillin in penicillin-allergic humans as it has a similar, although not identical, antibacterial spectrum. Active against Gram-positive cocci (some *Staphylococcus* spp. resistant), Gram-positive bacilli, some Gram-negative bacilli (e.g.*Pasteurella*) and some spirochaetes (e.g. *Helicobacter*). Some strains of *Actinomyces*, *Nocardia*, *Chlamydia*, *Mycoplasma* and *Rickettsia* also inhibited. Most strains of Enterobacteriaceae (*Pseudomonas*, *Escherichia coli*, *Klebsiella*) are resistant. Highly lipid-soluble and useful against intracellular pathogens. Particularly useful in management of respiratory tract infections, mild to moderate skin and soft tissue infections, and non-tubercular mycobacterial infections. For the latter used in combination with enrofloxacin and rifampin. Activity is enhanced in an alkaline pH; administer on an empty stomach. There is limited information regarding use in animals. Use with caution in animals with hepatic dysfunction. Reduce dose in animals with renal impairment. In ferrets it has been used successfully to treat pneumonia due to *Mycobacterium abscessus* and it can be used in combination with omeprazole or ranitidine and bismuth plus amoxicillin or metronidazole for treatment of *Helicobacter mustelae*. In tortoises it has been used to resolve clinical signs in severe cases of mycoplasmosis.

Safety and handling: Normal precautions should be observed.

Contraindications: No information available.

Adverse reactions: In humans similar adverse effects to those of erythromycin are seen, i.e. vomiting, cholestatic hepatitis, stomatitis and glossitis.

Drug interactions: May increase serum levels of several drugs, including methylprednisolone, theophylline, omeprazole and itraconazole. The absorption of digoxin may be enhanced.

DOSES
See Appendix for guidelines on responsible antibacterial use.
Mammals: Ferrets: 50 mg/kg p.o. q12–24h; **Rabbits:** 80 mg/kg p.o. q12h with rifampin at 40 mg/kg p.o. q12h for *Staphylococcus* osteomyelitis; **Rats:** 3.5–10 mg/kg p.o. q8–12h; **Primates:** 10 mg/kg p.o. q12h[a], 20 mg/kg p.o. q24h[b]; **Hedgehogs:** 5.5 mg/kg p.o. q12h.
Birds: 85 mg/kg p.o. q24h.

Reptiles: Desert tortoises: 15 mg/kg p.o. q48−72h [c,d].
Amphibians, Fish: No information available.

References

[a] Dubois A, Berg DE, Fiala N *et al.* (1998) Cure of *Helicobacter pylori* infection by omepraxole-clarithromycin-based therapy in non-human primates. *Journal of Gastroenterology* **33**, 18−22

[b] Badyal DK, Garg SK (2000) Effects of clarithromycin on the pharmacokinetics of carbamazepine in rhesus monkeys. *Methods and Findings in Experimental and Clinical Pharmacology* **22**, 581−584

[c] Wimsatt JH, Johnson J, Mangone BA *et al* (1999) Clarithromycin pharmacokinetics in the desert tortoise (*Gopherus agassizii*). *Journal of Zoo and Wildlife Medicine* **30(1)**, 36−43

[d] Wimsatt J, Tothill A, Offermann CF, Sheehy JG and Peloquin CA (2008) Long-term and per rectum disposition of clarithromycin in the desert tortoise (*Gopherus agassizzi*). *Journal of the American Association of Laboratory Animal Science* **47(4)**, 41−45

Clazuril
(Harkers CoxiTabs) **AVM-GSL**

Formulations: Oral: 2.5 mg tablet.

Action: Coccidiocidal; mode of action unclear.

Use: Treatment and control of coccidiosis (*Eimeria labbeana, E. columbarum*) in homing and show pigeons. Birds should be treated following transportation to shows or races where they may have been exposed to coccidia.

Safety and handling: Normal precautions should be observed.

Contraindications: Do not use in birds intended for human consumption.

Adverse reactions: No information available.

Drug interactions: Do not administer with drugs that may cause vomiting.

DOSES

Birds: Raptors: 30 mg/kg once; **Pigeons:** 5−10 mg/kg once (treat all birds in loft simultaneously) [a,b]; **Psittacids:** 7 mg/kg p.o. q2d for 2 doses.
Mammals, Reptiles, Amphibians, Fish: No information available.

References

[a] Maes L, Coussement W, Desplenter L and Marsboom R (1988) Safety of a new anticoccidial agent, clazuril, during reproduction in carrier pigeons. *Tijdschr Diergeneeskd* **113(4)**, 195−204

[b] Vercruysse J (1990) Efficacy of toltrazuril and clazuril against experimental infections with *Eimeria labbeana* and *E. columbarum* in racing pigeons. *Avian Diseases* **34(1)**, 73−79

Clindamycin

(Antirobe, Clinacin, Clindacyl, Clindaseptin)
POM-V

Formulations: Oral: 25 mg, 75 mg, 150 mg, 300 mg capsules and tablets; 25 mg/ml solution.

Action: Lincosamide antibiotic that binds to the 50S ribosomal subunit, inhibiting peptide bond formation. May be bactericidal or bacteriostatic depending on susceptibility.

Use: Bone and joint infections associated with Gram-positive bacteria; pyoderma; toxoplasmosis and infections associated with the oral cavity. Active against Gram-positive cocci (including penicillin-resistant staphylococci), many obligate anaerobes, *Mycoplasma*s and *Toxoplasma gondii*. Attains high concentrations in bone and bile. Being a weak base, it becomes ion-trapped (and therefore concentrated) in fluids that are more acidic than plasma, such as prostatic fluid, milk and intracellular fluid. There is complete cross resistance between lincomycin and clindamycin, and partial cross resistance with erythromycin. Use with care in individuals with hepatic or renal impairment.

Safety and handling: Normal precautions should be observed.

Contraindications: Do not administer lincosamides to rabbits, other small herbivores or hamsters.

Adverse reactions: Colitis, vomiting and diarrhoea are reported. Lincosamides can cause fatal enterotoxaemia in small herbivores and hamsters.

Drug interactions: May enhance the effect of non-depolarizing muscle relaxants (e.g. tubocurarine) and may antagonize the effects of neostigmine and pyridostigmine. Do not administer with macrolide, chloramphenicol or other lincosamide antimicrobials as these combinations are antagonistic.

DOSES
See Appendix for guidelines on responsible antibacterial use.
Mammals: Ferrets: 5.5–11 mg/kg p.o. q12h (toxoplasmosis: 12.5–25 mg/kg p.o. q12h). Rats: 7.5–25 mg/kg p.o. q24h[a]; **Primates:** 10 mg/kg p.o. q12h; **Sugar gliders, Hedgehogs:** 5.5–10 mg/kg p.o. q12h.
Birds: 25 mg/kg p.o. q8h, 50 mg/kg p.o. q12h or 100 mg/kg p.o. q24h. **Pigeons:** 100 mg/kg p.o. q6h[b].
Reptiles: 2.5–5 mg/kg p.o. q24h.
Amphibians, Fish: No information available.

References
[a] Yang SH, Lee MG (2007) Dose-independent pharmacokinetics of clindamycin after intravenous and oral administration to rats: contribution of gastric first-pass effect to low bioavailability. *International Journal of Pharmaceutics* **332(1–2)**, 17–23
[b] Lenarduzzi T, Langston C and Ross MK (2011) Pharmacokinetics of clindamycin administered orally to pigeons. *Journal of Avian Medicine and Surgery* **25(4)**, 259–265

Clomipramine
(Clomicalm) **POM-V**

Formulations: Oral: 5 mg, 20 mg, 80 mg tablets.

Action: Both clomipramine and its primary metabolite desmethylclomipramine are active in blocking serotonin and noradrenaline re-uptake in the brain, with resultant anxiolytic, antidepressant and anticompulsive effects.

Use: Used in association with a behaviour modification plan for the management of anxiety-related disorders in animals, including 'compulsive behaviours', noise fears and urine spraying. Care required before use in animals with a history of constipation, epilepsy, glaucoma, urinary retention or arrhythmias. Used in birds for feather plucking, especially if due to separation anxiety; should be used in association with a behaviour modification plan. Can be used with benzodiazepines.

Safety and handling: Normal precautions should be observed.

Contraindications: Patients sensitive to tricyclic antidepressants. Do not give with, or within 2 weeks of, monoamine oxidase inhibitors (e.g. selegiline). Not recommended for use in male breeding animals, as testicular hypoplasia may occur.

Adverse reactions: May cause sporadic vomiting, changes in appetite or lethargy. Vomiting may be reduced by co-administration with a small quantity of food.

Drug interactions: May potentiate the effects of the antiarrhythmic drug quinidine, anticholinergic agents (e.g. atropine), other CNS active drugs (e.g. barbiturates, benzodiazepines, general anaesthetics, neuroleptics), sympathomimetics (e.g. adrenaline) and coumarin derivatives. Simultaneous administration with cimetidine may lead to increased plasma levels of clomipramine. Plasma levels of certain antiepileptic drugs, e.g. phenytoin and carbamazepine, may be increased by co-administration with clomipramine.

DOSES
Mammals: Rats: 16–32 mg/kg p.o. q12h.
Birds: 0.5–1 mg/kg p.o. q6–8h or 3 mg/kg p.o. q12h[a].
Reptiles, Amphibians, Fish: No information available.

References
[a] Seibert LM, Crowell-Davis SL, Wilson GH and Ritchie BW (2004) Placebo-controlled clomipramine trial for the treatment of feather picking disorder in cockatoos. *Journal of the American Animal Hospital Association* **40(4)**, 261–269

Clotrimazole
(Canesten*, Clotrimazole*, Lotriderm*) **POM**

Formulations: Topical: 1% cream; 1% solution. Many other products available; some contain corticosteroids.

Action: Topical imidazole with an inhibitory action on the growth of pathogenic dermatophytes, *Aspergillus* and yeasts by inhibiting cytochrome P450-dependent ergosterol synthesis.

Use: Superficial fungal infections. Naso-sinal infections including aspergillosis, particularly in birds.

Safety and handling: Normal precautions should be observed.

Contraindications: No information available.

Adverse reactions: No information available.

Drug interactions: No information available.

DOSES
Mammals: Rabbits: Otic: Instil 3–5 drops in ear q12h; Topical: Apply to affected area and massage in gently q12h; if no improvement in 4 weeks re-evaluate therapy or diagnosis; **Guinea pigs, Chinchillas, Rats, Hamsters, Other small mammals:** Topical application to defined lesions q12h for 3–6 weeks.
Birds: Endoscopic: 10 mg/kg applied directly to fungal lesions. Nasal flush: 10 mg/ml (flush volume 20 ml/kg). Intratracheal: 2–3 ml of a 1% solution nebulized for periods of 1 hour q24h or topically.
Reptiles: Apply topically to lesion q12h.
Amphibians, Fish: No information available.

Cloxacillin
(Opticlox, Orbenin) **POM-V**

Formulations: Ophthalmic: Cloxacillin benzathine ester 16.7% suspension.

Action: Beta-lactamase-resistant penicillin which is bactericidal and works in a time-dependent fashion. Binds to penicillin-binding proteins involved in cell wall synthesis, thereby decreasing bacterial cell wall strength and rigidity, and affecting cell division, growth and septum formation.

Use: Narrow spectrum antimicrobial. Less active than penicillin G or V against *Streptococcus*. Specifically indicated for ocular infections with beta-lactamase-producing *Staphylococcus*.

Safety and handling: Normal precautions should be observed.

Contraindications: Avoid use in animals which have displayed hypersensitivity reactions to other antimicrobials within the beta-lactam family (which includes cephalosporins). Use of penicillins should be avoided in rabbits, other small herbivores, hamsters and gerbils, especially if there is a possibility of ingestion.

Adverse reactions: Avoid use in small herbivores (e.g. rabbits), hamsters and gerbils as ingestion of penicillins can cause fatal enterotoxaemia.

Drug interactions: Avoid the concomitant use of bacteriostatic antibiotics (chloramphenicol, erythromycin, tetracycline).

DOSES
See Appendix for guidelines on responsible antibacterial use.
Mammals: While topical cloxacillin is effective against *Treponema* localized to the eyelids, its use can treat local symptoms but leave the rabbit in a carrier state, and is not advised.
Birds: Apply 1/10th of a tube (0.3 g) q24h.
Reptiles, Amphibians, Fish: No information available.

Co-amoxiclav (Amoxicillin/Clavulanate, Amoxycillin/Clavulanic acid)
(Clavabactin, Clavaseptin, Clavucil, Clavudale, Combisyn, Kesium, Nisamox, Noroclav, Synulox, Augmentin*) **POM-V, POM**

Formulations: Injectable: 175 mg/ml suspension (140 mg amoxicillin, 35 mg clavulanate); 600 mg powder (500 mg amoxicillin, 100 mg clavulanate); 1.2 g powder (1 g amoxicillin, 200 mg clavulanate) for reconstitution (Augmentin). Oral: 50 mg, 250 mg, 500 mg tablets each containing amoxicillin and clavulanate in a ratio of 4:1; Palatable drops which when reconstituted with water provide 40 mg amoxicillin and 10 mg clavulanic acid per ml.

Action: Amoxicillin binds to penicillin-binding proteins involved in bacterial cell wall synthesis, thereby decreasing cell wall strength and rigidity, affecting cell division, growth and septum formation. The addition of the beta-lactamase inhibitor clavulanate increases the antimicrobial spectrum against those organisms that produce beta-lactamase, such as *Staphylococcus* and *Escherichia coli*.

Use: Active against Gram-positive and Gram-negative aerobic organisms and many obligate anaerobes. Penicillinase-producing *Escherichia coli* and *Staphylococcus* are susceptible, but difficult Gram-negative organisms such as *Pseudomonas aeruginosa* and *Klebsiella* are often resistant. Dose and dosing interval will be determined by infection site, severity and organism. The predominant bacterial infections in reptiles are Gram-negative and many are resistant to penicillins.

Safety and handling: Tablets are wrapped in foil moisture-resistant packaging; do not remove until to be administered. Refrigerate oral suspension and i.v. solution after reconstitution.

Discard oral suspension and i.v. formulation if they become dark or after 10 days. A small amount of discoloration of the i.v. solution is acceptable.

Contraindications: Avoid oral antibiotic agents in critically ill patients, as absorption from the GI tract may be unreliable; such patients may require i.v. formulation. Avoid use in animals which have displayed hypersensitivity reactions to other antimicrobials within the beta-lactam family (which includes cephalosporins). Use of penicillins should be avoided in rabbits, other small herbivores, hamsters and gerbils, especially via the oral route.

Adverse reactions: Nausea, diarrhoea and skin rashes are the commonest adverse effects. Oral doses of penicillins can cause fatal enterotoxaemia in small herbivores, hamsters and potentially gerbils.

Drug interactions: Avoid the concurrent use of amoxicillin with bacteriostatic antibiotics (e.g. tetracycline, erythromycin). Do not mix in the same syringe as aminoglycosides. Do not use with allopurinol in birds. Synergism may occur between the beta-lactam and aminoglycoside antimicrobials *in vivo*.

DOSES
See Appendix for guidelines on responsible antibacterial use.
Mammals: Ferrets: 12.5–20 mg/kg i.m., s.c. q12h; **Rats, Mice:** 100 mg/kg p.o., s.c. q12h; **Primates:** 15 mg/kg p.o. q12h; **Sugar gliders, Hedgehogs:** 12.5 mg/kg p.o., s.c. q12h.
Birds: 125–150 mg/kg p.o., i.v. q12h; 125–150 mg/kg i.m. q24h [a].
Reptiles, Amphibians, Fish: No information available.

References
[a] Orosz SE, Jones MO, Cox SK, Zagaya NK and Frazier DL (2000) Pharmacokinetics of amoxicillin plus clavulanic acid in blue-fronted Amazon parrots (*Amazona aestival aestival*). *Journal of Avian Medicine and Surgery* **14(2)**, 107–112

Colchicine
(Colchicine*) **POM**

Formulations: Oral: 0.5 mg tablet.

Action: Colchicine inhibits collagen synthesis, may enhance collagenase activity and blocks the synthesis and secretion of serum amyloid A.

Use: Management of fibrotic hepatic and pulmonary diseases, oesophageal stricture and renal amyloidosis. In birds, used for gout and hepatic cirrhosis/fibrosis. Due to the relatively high incidence of adverse reactions, this drug should be used with caution.

Safety and handling: Protect from light.

Contraindications: Pregnancy.

Adverse reactions: Commoner adverse effects include vomiting, abdominal pain and diarrhoea. Rarely, renal damage, bone marrow suppression, myopathy and peripheral neuropathy may develop. Colchicine may increase serum ALP, decrease platelet counts and cause false-positive results when testing urine for RBCs and haemoglobin. Overdoses can be fatal.

Drug interactions: Possible increased risk of nephrotoxicity and myotoxicity when colchicine given with ciclosporin. NSAIDs, especially phenylbutazone, may increase the risks of thrombocytopenia, leucopenia or bone marrow depression when used concurrently with colchicine. Many anticancer chemotherapeutics may cause additive myelosuppressive effects when used with colchicine.

DOSES
Birds: 0.04 mg/kg p.o. q12h [1,2].
Mammals, Reptiles, Amphibians, Fish: No information available.

References
[1] Hoefer H (1991) Hepatic fibrosis and colchicine therapy. *Journal of the Association of Avian Veterinarians* **5**, 193
[2] Romano J (2013) Therapeutic review: colchicine. *Journal of Exotic Pet Medicine* **22(4)**, 405–408

Colestyramine (Cholestyramine)
(Questran*) POM

Formulations: Oral: 4 g powder/sachet.

Action: Ion exchange resin.

Use: In rabbits and susceptible rodents for absorbing toxins produced in the GI tract following the development of overgrowth of Clostridium.

Safety and handling: Normal precautions should be observed.

Contraindications: No information available.

Adverse reactions: Constipation may develop.

Drug interactions: Colestyramine reduces the absorption of digoxin, anticoagulants, diuretics and thyroxine.

DOSES
Mammals: Rabbits: 2 g/animal p.o. syringed gently with 20 ml water q24h; Guinea pigs: 1 g/animal mixed with water p.o. q24h.
Birds, Reptiles, Amphibians, Fish: No information available.

Copper sulphate (Cupric sulphate)
(Proprietary formulations are available)

Formulations: Liquid for immersion.

Action: No information available.

Use: For the treatment of protozoan and monogenean ectoparasites, some fungi and bacteria in fish. It is strongly recommended that a proprietary formulation is used initially to avoid problems related to purity and to enable accurate dosing. Copper has a low therapeutic index and is toxic to gill tissue. It is commonly used to treat diseases in marine aquaria by prolonged immersion but is toxic to invertebrates, elasmobranchs, algae and many plants. Although copper can be used to treat ectoparasites in freshwater fish, other remedies are safer. The solubility of copper is reduced at higher pH and it is absorbed or inactivated by high levels of calcareous materials and organic matter. Free copper ion levels must be maintained between 0.15–0.20 mg/l for the chemical to be effective – this requires monitoring using a commercial test kit then adjusting the dose initially twice daily. A stock solution is made by dissolving 1 gram of copper sulphate pentahydrate ($CuSO_4$ $5H_2O$) in 250 ml distilled water to produce 1 mg copper/ml and enables accurate dosing of the chemical. Copper can be removed using inactivated carbon.

Safety and handling: Normal precautions should be observed.

Contraindications: Do not use in the presence of invertebrates.

Adverse reactions: No information available.

Drug interactions: No information available.

DOSES
Fish: 100 mg/l by immersion for 1–5 minutes; 0.15 mg/l by prolonged immersion until therapeutic effect (at least 10 days); follow the manufacturer's recommendations for proprietary formulations.
Mammals, Birds, Reptiles, Amphibians: No information available.

Corydcepic acid see **Mannitol**

Crisantaspase (Asparaginase, L-Asparginase)
(Asparginase*, Elspar*, Erwinase*) **POM**

Formulations: Injectable: vials of 5,000 or 10,000 IU powder for reconstitution.

Action: Lymphoid tumour cells are not able to synthesize asparagine and are dependent upon supply from the extracellular fluid. Crisantaspase deprives malignant cells of this amino acid, which results in cessation of protein synthesis and cell death.

Use: Main indication is treatment of lymphoid malignancies.

Safety and handling: Cytotoxic drug; see specialist texts for further advice on chemotherapeutic agents. Store in a refrigerator.

Contraindications: Patients with active pancreatitis or a history of pancreatitis. History of anaphylaxis associated with previous administration.

Adverse reactions: Anaphylaxis may follow administration, especially if repeated. Premedication with an antihistamine is recommended before administration. Gastrointestinal disturbances, hepatotoxicity and coagulation deficits may also be observed.

Drug interactions: Administration with or before vincristine may reduce clearance of vincristine and increase toxicity; thus, if used in combination the vincristine should be given 12–24 hours before the enzyme.

DOSES
See Appendix for chemotherapy protocols in ferrets.
Mammals: Ferrets: 10,000 IU/m^2 s.c. weekly for the first 3 weeks as part of a chemotherapeutic protocol; **Guinea pigs:** 10,000 IU/m^2 s.c., i.m. q3wk.
Birds, Reptiles, Amphibians, Fish: No information available.

Cupric sulphate see Copper sulphate

Cyclophosphamide
(Cyclophosphamide*, Endoxana*) **POM**

Formulations: Injectable: 100 mg, 200 mg, 500 mg, 1000 mg powder for reconstitution. **Oral:** 50 mg tablets.

Action: Metabolites crosslink DNA resulting in inhibition of DNA synthesis and function.

Use: Treatment of lymphoproliferative diseases, myeloproliferative disease and immune-mediated diseases. The use of cyclophosphamide in immune-mediated haemolytic anaemia is controversial and therefore it is not recommended as an immunosuppressant in the management of this disease. May have a role in management of certain sarcomas and carcinomas. Use with caution in patients with renal failure; dose reduction may be required. Has been used in treatment of lymphosarcoma in cockatoos and lymphoma in the green iguana.

Safety and handling: Cytotoxic drug; see specialist texts for further advice on chemotherapeutic agents.

Contraindications: No information available.

Adverse reactions: Myelosuppression, with the nadir usually occurring 7–14 days after the start of therapy depending on species;

regular monitoring of WBCs recommended. A metabolite of cyclophosphamide (acrolein) may cause a sterile haemorrhagic cystitis. The cystitis may be persistent. This risk may be reduced by increasing water consumption or by giving furosemide to ensure adequate urine production. Other effects include vomiting, diarrhoea, hepatotoxicity, nephrotoxicity and a reduction in hair growth rate.

Drug interactions: Increased risk of myelosuppression if thiazide diuretics given concomitantly. Absorption of orally administered digoxin may be decreased, may occur several days after dosing. Barbiturates increase cyclophosphamide toxicity due to increased rate of conversion to metabolites. Phenothiazines and chloramphenicol reduce cyclophosphamide efficacy. If administered with doxorubicin there is an increased risk of cardiotoxicity. Insulin requirements are altered by concurrent cyclophosphamide.

DOSES
See Appendix for chemotherapy protocols in ferrets.
Mammals: Ferrets: As part of a multi-drug protocol for lymphoma; Guinea pigs: 300 mg/m^2 i.p. q24h.
Birds: Lymphosarcoma: 200 mg/m^2 intraosseous q7d.
Reptiles: 3 mg/kg i.v. q2wk as part of a chemotherapy protocol in one case report in the green iguana[a].
Amphibians, Fish: No information available.

References
[a] Folland DW, Johnston MS, Thamm DH and Reavill D (2011) Diagnosis and management of lymphoma in a green iguana (*Iguana iguana*). *Journal of the American Veterinary Medical Association* **239(7)**, 985–991

Cyclosporin(e) see Ciclosporin

Cypermethrin
(F10 Germicidal Wound Spray with Insecticide) ESPA

Formulations: Topical: various formulations including benzalkonium chloride 0.4 g polyhexanide 0.03 g and cypermethrin 0.25 g spray; barrier ointment and shampoo formulations.

Action: Acts as a sodium open-channel blocker, resulting in muscular convulsions and death in arthropods.

Use: To repel insects and eliminate fly strike infestations.

Safety and handling: Normal precautions should be observed. May be harmful to aquatic organisms. Do not contaminate aquaria, ponds or waterways.

Contraindications: Do not use in fish or other aquatic organisms.

Adverse reactions: No adverse reactions reported in small mammals if used at dosage regime advised by manufacturer.

Drug interactions: No information available.

DOSES
Mammals: Apply ointment or spray to wound site and repeat if necessary once a week. May need to be re-applied if the animal is exposed to rain.
Fish: Do not use.
Birds, Reptiles, Amphibians: No information available.

Cyproheptadine
(Periactin*) **POM**

Formulations: Oral: 4 mg tablet.

Action: Binds to and blocks the activation of H1 histamine and serotonin receptors.

Use: Management of allergic disease and appetite stimulation. Use with caution in cases with urinary retention, angle-closure glaucoma and pyloroduodenal obstruction. Specific doses for animals have not been determined by pharmokinetic studies and clinical effectiveness has not been established.

Safety and handling: Normal precautions should be observed.

Contraindications: No information available.

Adverse reactions: May cause mild sedation, polyphagia, weight gain. May reduce seizure threshold.

Drug interactions: No information available.

DOSES
Mammals: Ferrets, Chinchillas, Guinea pigs: 0.5 mg p.o. q12h.
Birds, Reptiles, Amphibians, Fish: No information available.

Cyromazine
(Rearguard) **NFA-VPS**

Formulations: Topical: 6% solution in ready-to-use bottle with built-in applicator sponge.

Action: Inhibits larval development by inhibiting the deposition of chitin into the cuticle.

Use: Prevention of blowfly strike in rabbits for up to 10 weeks after application. To be applied in early summer before any flies are seen. Will not kill adult flies or larger maggots already present, but prevents eggs developing into maggots. Bathing the rabbit after application may reduce efficacy so is not recommended.

Safety and handling: Normal precautions should be observed.

Contraindications: Do not use in rabbits less than 10 weeks of age, or pregnant or breeding does. Do not apply to broken skin.

Adverse reactions: Transient inappetence may occur for 24–48h after treatment.

Drug interactions: No information available.

DOSES
Mammals: Apply topically to fur from middle of the back to tip of tail and between back legs q6–10wks.
Birds, Reptiles, Amphibians, Fish: No information available.

Cytarabine (Cytosine arabinoside, Ara-C)
(Cytarabine*, Cytosar-U*) **POM**

Formulations: Injectable: 100 mg, 500 mg powders for reconstitution.

Action: The active nucleotide metabolite ara-CTP is incorporated into DNA and inhibits pyrimidine and DNA synthesis. Cytarabine is therefore S phase-specific.

Use: Management of lymphoma in the ferret.

Safety and handling: Cytotoxic drug; see specialist texts for further advice on chemotherapeutic agents. After reconstitution, store at room temperature and discard after 48 hours or if a slight haze develops.

Contraindications: Do not use if there is evidence of bone marrow suppression or substantial hepatic impairment.

Adverse reactions: Vomiting, diarrhoea, leucopenia. As it is a myelosuppressant, careful haematological monitoring is required. Conjunctivitis, oral ulceration, hepatotoxicity and fever have also been seen.

Drug interactions: Oral absorption of digoxin is decreased. Activity of gentamicin may be antagonized. Simultaneous administration of methotrexate increases the effect of cytarabine.

DOSES
See Appendix for chemotherapy protocols in ferrets.
Mammals: Ferrets: 1 mg/animal p.o., s.c. q24h for 2 days.
Birds, Reptiles, Amphibians, Fish: No information available.

Deferoxamine (Desferrioxamine)
(Desferal*) POM

Formulations: Injectable: 500 mg vial for reconstitution.

Action: Deferoxamine chelates iron, and the complex is excreted in the urine.

Use: To remove iron from the body following poisoning. Also used for haemochromatosis (common in toucans, hornbills and softbills, though unusual in other birds).

Safety and handling: Normal precautions should be observed.

Contraindications: Avoid in severe renal disease.

Adverse reactions: Administration i.m. is painful. Anaphylactic reactions and hypotension may develop if administered rapidly i.v.

Drug interactions: No information available.

DOSES
Birds: Various doses proposed, ranging from 20 mg/kg p.o. q4h to 40 mg/kg i.m. q24h (mynahs) to 100 mg/kg p.o., s.c., i.m. q24h for up to 14 weeks [a,1].
Mammals, Reptiles, Amphibians, Fish: No information available.

References
[a] Dierenfeld E and Phalen DN (2006) A comparison of four regiments for treatment of iron storage disease using the European Starling (*Sturnus vulgaris*) as a model. *Journal of Avian Medicine and Surgery* **20(2)**, 74–79

[1] Sheppard C and Dierenfeld E (2002) Iron storage disease in birds: speculation on etiology and implications for captive husbandry. *Journal of Avian Medicine and Surgery* **16(3)**, 192–197

Delmadinone
(Tardak) POM-V

Formulations: Injectable: 10 mg/ml suspension.

Action: Progestogens suppress FSH and LH production.

Use: In birds it may be useful for behavioural regurgitation or behaviour associated with sexual frustration. Can also be used to assess the effects of chemical castration prior to surgical castration in rats.

Safety and handling: Normal precautions should be observed.

Contraindications: No information available.

Adverse reactions: Possible adverse effects include a transient reduction in fertility and libido, polyuria and polydipsia, an increased appetite, and hair colour change at the site of injection.

Drug interactions: Cortisol response to ACTH stimulation is significantly suppressed after just one dose of delmadinone.

DOSES

Mammals: Rats: 1 mg/animal i.m, s.c.
Birds: 1 mg/kg i.m. once.
Reptiles, Amphibians, Fish: No information available.

Desferrioxamine see Deferoxamine

Deslorelin
(Suprelorin) **POM-V**

Formulations: Implant containing 4.7 mg or 9.4 mg of active product.

Action: Desensitizes GnRH receptors, thereby decreasing release of LH and FSH. This leads to reduction in testosterone and sperm production.

Use: Chemical contraception in susceptible species. In males, there is a 14-day surge in testosterone followed by lowering of levels. Infertility is achieved from 6 weeks up to at least 6 months after initial treatment. Treated male animals should therefore still be kept away from females within the first 6 weeks following initial treatment. Any mating that occurs more than 6 months after the administration of the product may result in pregnancy. Disinfection of the site should be undertaken prior to implantation to avoid introduction of infection. If the hair is long, a small area should be clipped, if required. The product should be implanted subcutaneously in the loose skin on the back between the lower neck and the lumbar area. Avoid injection of the implant into fat, as release of the active substance might be impaired in areas of low vascularization. The biocompatible implant does not require removal. However, should it be necessary to end treatment, implants may be surgically removed. Implants can be located using ultrasonography. Deslorelin implants effectively prevent reproduction and the musky odour of intact male and female ferrets, and are therefore considered a suitable alternative for surgical neutering in these animals. Surgical neutering of ferrets has been implicated as an aetiological factor in the development of hyperadrenocorticism in this species. Deslorelin implants can be given to neutered ferrets to decrease the development or progression of adrenocortical disease. In rabbits, the effects on reproductive behaviour and fertility are considered negligible in males [a], although implants appear to reduce ovarian activity if placed prior to puberty in females [b]. However, the possibility of masking future uterine pathology makes use in rabbits difficult to advise without careful monitoring. The use of the implant in birds and reptiles has been reported for a range of behavioural and reproductive (e.g. excessive egg laying) disorders but with variable effect and duration of action between species. In Quaker parrots and cockatiels, one study showed a 6 month prevention of egg laying using a 4.7 mg implant[c]. In male birds, has been used to counter aggressive behaviour with variable response. Has also been used for management of a Sertoli cell tumour in budgerigars and ovarian neoplasia in cockatiels [d,e].

Safety and handling: Pregnant women should not administer the product.

Contraindications: No information available.

Adverse reactions: Moderate swelling at the implant site may be observed for 14 days. A significant decrease in testicle size will be seen during the treatment period. In very rare cases, a testicle may be able to ascend the inguinal ring.

Drug interactions: No information available.

DOSES

Mammals: Ferrets: 1 implant per animal. The 9.4 mg implant (authorized in males only) lasts approximately 3–4 years. The 4.7 mg implant is not authorized in either sex and lasts approximately 1–2 years. Females will come into oestrus for approximately 2 weeks after implantation; **Guinea pigs:** 1 implant per animal for contraception in females, although appears ineffective in males[f]; **Rats:** 1 implant per animal provides contraceptive and reduced reproductive behaviour effects for >1 year in males and females; **Others:** Effects are variable and depend on the exact pathology, species and sex.

Birds, Reptiles, Amphibians: 1 implant per animal regardless of size, placed subcutaneously. The 9.4 mg implant appears to last longer than the 4.7 mg but duration of either is variable.

Fish: No information available.

References

[a] Goericke-Pesch S, Groeger G and Wehrend A (2015) The effects of a slow release GnRH agonist implant on male rabbits. *Animal Reproduction Science* **152**, 83–89

[b] Geyer A, Daub L, Otzdorff C et al. (2016) Reversible estrous cycle suppression in prepubertal female rabbits treated with slow-release deslorelin implants. *Theriogenology* **85(2)**, 282–287

[c] Petritz OA, Sanchez-Migallon Guzman D, Paul-Murphy J et al. (2013) Evaluation of the efficacy and safety of single administration of 4.7 mg deslorelin acetate implants on egg production and plasma sex hormones in Japanese quail (*Coturnix coturnix japonica*). *American Journal of Veterinary Research* **74(2)**, 316–323

[d] Keller KA, Beaufrère H, Brandão J et al. (2013) Long-term management of ovarian neoplasia in two cockatiels (*Nymphicus hollandicus*). *Journal of Avian Medicine and Surgery* **27(1)**, 44–52

[e] Straub J and Zenker I (2013) First experience in hormonal treatment of sertoli cell tumors in budgerigars (*M. undulates*) with absorbable extended release GnRH chips (Suprelorin®). *1st International Conference on Avian, Herpetological and Exotic Mammal Medicine*. Wiesbaden, pp. 299–301

[f] Forman C, Wehrend A and Goericke-Pesch S (2016) Deslorelin implants are suitable for contraception in female, but not male guinea pigs. *Proceedings of the 8th International Symposium on Canine and Feline Reproduction, Paris*

Dexamethasone

(Aurizon, Dexadreson, Dexafort, Dexa-ject, Rapidexon, Voren, Dexamethasone*, Maxidex*, Maxitrol*) **POM-V**

Formulations: Ophthalmic: 0.1% solution (Maxidex, Maxitrol). Maxitrol also contains polymyxin B and neomycin. **Injectable:** 2 mg/ml solution; 1 mg/ml, 3 mg/ml suspension; 2.5 mg/ml suspension with 7.5 mg/ml prednisolone. **Oral:** 0.5 mg tablet. (1 mg of dexamethasone is equivalent to 1.1 mg of dexamethasone acetate, 1.3 mg of dexamethasone isonicotinate or dexamethasone sodium phosphate, or 1.4 mg of dexamethasone trioxa-undecanoate.)

Action: Alters the transcription of DNA, leading to alterations in cellular metabolism which cause a reduction in inflammatory response.

Use: Anti-inflammatory drug. Also used to prevent and treat anaphylaxis associated with transfusion or chemotherapeutic agents. Anti-inflammatory potency is 7.5 times greater than prednisolone. On a dose basis 0.15 mg dexamethasone is equivalent to 1 mg prednisolone. Dexamethasone has a long duration of action and low mineralocorticoid activity and is particularly suitable for short-term high-dose therapy in conditions where water retention would be a disadvantage. Unsuitable for long-term daily or alternate-day use. Animals on chronic therapy should be tapered off steroids when discontinuing the drug. Use shorter-acting preparations wherever possible in birds and rabbits. The use of long-acting steroids in most cases of shock and spinal injury is of no benefit and may be detrimental. Used for the treatment of shock, trauma and chronic stress in fish.

Safety and handling: Normal precautions should be observed.

Contraindications: Do not use in pregnant animals. Systemic corticosteroids are generally contraindicated in patients with renal disease and diabetes mellitus. Impaired wound healing and delayed recovery from infections may be seen. Topical corticosteroids are contraindicated in ulcerative keratitis.

Adverse reactions: A single dose of dexamethasone or dexamethasone sodium phosphate suppresses adrenal gland function for up to 32 hours. Prolonged use of glucocorticoids suppresses the hypothalamic-pituitary axis (HPA), causing adrenal atrophy, elevated liver enzymes, cutaneous atrophy, weight loss, PU/PD, vomiting and diarrhoea. GI ulceration may develop. Hyperglycaemia and decreased serum T4 values may be seen in patients receiving dexamethasone. Corticosteroids should be used with care in birds as there is a high risk of immunosuppression and side effects, such as hepatopathy and a diabetes mellitus-like syndrome. In rabbits, even small single doses can potentially cause severe adverse reactions. Ferrets are particularly susceptible to GI ulceration, and concurrent gastric protectants may be advisable, especially in stressed animals.

Drug interactions: There is an increased risk of GI ulceration if used concurrently with NSAIDs. The risk of developing hypokalaemia is increased if corticosteroids are administered concomitantly with amphotericin B or potassium-depleting diuretics (furosemide, thiazides). Dexamethasone antagonizes the effect of insulin. Phenobarbital or phenytoin may accelerate the metabolism of glucocorticoids and antifungals (e.g. itraconazole) may decrease it.

DOSES

Mammals: Ophthalmic: Apply small amount of ointment to affected eye(s) q6–24h or 1 drop of solution in affected eye(s) q6–12h. **Ferrets:** 0.5–2.0 mg/kg s.c., i.m., i.v. q24h; 1 mg/kg i.m., i.v. once followed with prednisolone (post adrenalectomy); **Rabbits:** 0.2–0.6 mg/kg s.c., i.m., i.v. q24h; **Guinea pigs:** 0.6 mg/kg i.v., i.m., s.c. q24h (pregnancy toxaemia); **Primates:** 0.5–2 mg/kg i.v., i.m., s.c. once (cerebral oedema); 0.25–1 mg/kg i.v., i.m., s.c. q24h (inflammation); **Sugar gliders:** 0.5–2 mg/kg s.c., i.m., i.v.; **Others:** anti-inflammatory: 0.055–0.2 mg/kg i.m., s.c. q12–24h tapering dose over 3–14 days.

Birds: 2–6 mg/kg i.v., i.m. q12–24h.

Reptiles: Inflammation, non-infectious respiratory disease: 2–4 mg/kg i.m., i.v. q24h for 3 days.

Amphibians: 1.5 mg/kg s.c., i.m. q24h.

Fish: 1–2 mg/kg i.m., intracoelomic or 10 mg/l for 60 minute bath q12–24h.

Dexmedetomidine

(Dexdomitor) **POM-V**

Formulations: Injectable: 0.1 mg/ml, 0.5 mg/ml solution.

Action: Agonist at peripheral and central alpha-2 adrenoreceptors producing dose-dependent sedation, muscle relaxation and analgesia.

Use: To provide sedation and premedication when used alone or in combination with opioid analgesics and may also provide additional analgesia. Dexmedetomidine combined with ketamine can be used to provide a short duration (20–30 min) of surgical anaesthesia. Dexmedetomidine is the pure dextroenantiomer of medetomidine. As the levomedetomidine enantiomer is largely inactive, dexmedetomidine is twice as potent as the racemic mixture (medetomidine). Administration of dexmedetomidine reduces the biological load presented to the animal, resulting in quicker metabolism of concurrently administered anaesthetic drugs and a potentially faster recovery from anaesthesia. Dexmedetomidine is a potent drug that causes marked changes in the cardiovascular system, including an initial peripheral vasoconstriction that results in an increase in blood pressure and a compensatory bradycardia. After 20–30 min vasoconstriction wanes, while blood pressure returns to normal values. Heart rate remains low due to the central sympatholytic effect of alpha-2 agonists. These cardiovascular changes result in a fall in cardiac output; central organ perfusion is well maintained at the expense of redistribution of blood flow away from the peripheral tissues. Respiratory system function is well maintained; respiration rate may fall but is accompanied by an increased depth of respiration. Oxygen supplementation is advisable in all animals that have received dexmedetomidine for sedation. Combining dexmedetomidine with an opioid provides improved analgesia and sedation. Lower doses of dexmedetomidine should be used in combination with other drugs. Reversal of dexmedetomidine sedation or premedication with atipamezole at the end of the procedure shortens the recovery period, which is advantageous. Analgesia should be provided with other classes of drugs before atipamezole. High doses (>10 µg/kg) are associated with greater physiological disturbances than doses of 1–10 µg/kg. Using dexmedetomidine in combination with opioids in the lower dose range can provide good sedation and analgesia with minimal side effects. The lower concentration of dexmedetomidine is designed to increase the accuracy of dosing in smaller species.

Safety and handling: Normal precautions should be observed.

Contraindications: Do not use in animals with cardiovascular or other systemic disease. Use of dexmedetomidine in geriatric patients is not advisable. It should not be used in pregnant animals, nor in animals likely to require or receiving sympathomimetic amines.

Adverse reactions: Causes diuresis by suppressing ADH secretion, a transient increase in blood glucose by decreasing endogenous insulin secretion, and mydriasis and decreased intraocular pressure. Vomiting after i.m. administration is common, so dexmedetomidine should be avoided when vomiting is contraindicated (e.g. foreign body, raised intraocular pressure). Due to effects on blood glucose, use in diabetic animals is not recommended. Spontaneous arousal from deep sedation following stimulation can occur with all alpha-2 agonists, aggressive animals sedated with dexmedetomidine must still be managed with caution.

Drug interactions: No information available.

DOSES
When used for sedation is generally given as part of a combination. See Appendix for sedation protocols in all species.
Mammals: Ferrets: 0.04–0.1 mg/kg s.c., i.m.; **Rabbits:** 0.025–0.05 mg/kg i.v. or 0.05–0.15 mg/kg s.c., i.m.
Birds: Buzzards: 0.1 mg atropine + 25 µg (micrograms)/kg dexmedetomidine i.m.; **Kestrels:** 0.05 mg atropine + 75 µg/kg dexmedetomidine i.m. as induction for isoflurane general anaesthesia [a].
Reptiles: Usually combined with ketamine and/or opioids/midazolam to provide light anaesthesia (**see Appendix**).
Tegus: 0.2 mg/kg (analgesia) [b]; **Ball pythons:** 0.1–0.2 mg/kg (sedation or possible analgesia) [c].
Amphibians, Fish: No information available.

References

[a] Santangelo B, Ferrari D, Di Martino I et al. (2009) Dexmedetomidine chemical restraint of two raptor species undergoing inhalation anaesthesia. *Veterinary Research Communications* **33(1)**, 209–211

[b] Bisetto SP, Melo CF and Carregaro AB (2018) Evaluation of sedative and antinociceptive effects of dexmedetomidine, midazolam and dexmedetomidine– midazolam in tegus (*Salvator merianae*). *Veterinary Anaesthesia and Analgesia* **45(3)**, 320–328

[c] Bunke LG, Sladky KK and Johnson SM (2018) Antinociceptive efficacy and respiratory effects of dexmedetomidine in ball pythons (*Python regius*). *American Journal of Veterinary Research* **79(7)**, 718–726

Dextrose see Glucose

Diazepam
(Dialar*, Diazemuls*, Diazepam Rectubes*, Rimapam*, Stesolid*, Tensium*, Valclair*, Valium*)
POM

Formulations: Injectable: 5 mg/ml emulsion (2 ml ampoules, Diazemuls). **Oral:** 2 mg, 5 mg, 10 mg tablets; 2 mg/5 ml solution. **Rectal:** 2 mg/ml (1.25, 2.5 ml tubes), 4 mg/ml (2.5 ml tubes) solutions; 10 mg suppositories.

Action: Enhances activity of the major inhibitory central nervous system neurotransmitter, gamma-aminobutyric acid (GABA), through binding to the benzodiazepine site of the $GABA_A$ receptor.

Use: Anticonvulsant, anxiolytic and skeletal muscle relaxant (e.g. urethral muscle spasm and tetanus). Diazepam is the drug of choice for the short-term emergency control of severe epileptic seizures and status epilepticus. In guinea pigs it may be used to reduce the excitability associated with extreme pruritus (e.g. with ectoparasitic infestations). It may also be used in combination with ketamine to offset muscle hypertonicity associated with ketamine, and with opioids and/or acepromazine for pre-anaesthetic medication in the critically ill. It provides very poor sedation or even excitation when used alone in healthy animals. Used in birds for the short-term management of feather plucking. Diazepam has a high lipid solubility, which facilitates its oral absorption and rapid central effects. Liver disease will prolong duration of action. In the short term repeated doses of diazepam or a CRI will lead to drug accumulation and prolonged recovery. Flumazenil (a benzodiazepine antagonist) will reverse the effects of diazepam. The development of dependence on benzodiazepines may occur after regular use, even with therapy of only a few weeks, and the dose should be gradually reduced in these cases if the benzodiazepine is being withdrawn.

Safety and handling: Substantial adsorption of diazepam may occur on to some plastics and this may cause a problem when administering diazepam by continuous i.v. infusion. The use of diazepam in PVC infusion bags should be avoided; giving sets should be kept as short as possible and should not contain a cellulose propionate volume-control chamber. If diazepam is given by continuous i.v. infusion the compatible materials include glass, polyolefin, polypropylene and polyethylene.

Contraindications: Benzodiazepines should be avoided in patients with CNS depression, respiratory depression, severe muscle weakness or hepatic impairment (as may worsen hepatic encephalopathy). They are also contraindicated in the long-term treatment of behavioural disorders due to the risks of disinhibition and interference with memory and learning.

Adverse reactions: Sedation, muscle weakness and ataxia are common. Rapid i.v. injection or oral overdose may cause marked paradoxical excitation (including aggression) and elicit signs of pain; i.v. injections should be made slowly (over at least 1 minute for each 5 mg). Intramuscular injection is painful and results in erratic drug absorption. Rectal administration is effective for emergency control of seizures if i.v. access is not possible, but the time to onset is delayed to 5–10 min. The duration of action may be prolonged after repeated doses in rapid succession, in older animals, those with liver dysfunction and those receiving beta-1 antagonists. Chronic dosing leads to a shortened half-life due to activation of the hepatic microsomal enzyme system and tolerance to the drug may develop. The propylene glycol formulation of injectable diazepam can cause thrombophlebitis, therefore the emulsion formulation is preferred for i.v. injection.

Drug interactions: Do not dilute or mix with other agents. Due to extensive metabolism by the hepatic microsomal enzyme system, interactions with other drugs metabolized in this way are common. Cimetidine and omeprazole inhibit metabolism of diazepam and may prolong clearance. Concurrent use of phenobarbital may lead to a decrease in the half-life of diazepam. An enhanced sedative effect may be seen if antihistamines or opioid analgesics are administered with diazepam, and diazepam will reduce the dose requirement of other anaesthetic agents. When given with diazepam the effects of digoxin may be increased. Diazepam may be used in combination with tricyclic antidepressant therapy for the management of more severe behavioural responses.

DOSES
When used for sedation is generally given as part of a combination. See Appendix for sedation protocols in all species.
Mammals: Ferrets: seizures: 2–5 mg/kg i.m. once; urethral sphincter muscle relaxation post urinary catheterization or obstruction: 0.5 mg/kg p.o., i.m., i.v. q6–8h; **Rabbits:** epileptic seizures, pre-anaesthetic sedation, muscle relaxation: 1–5 mg/kg i.v.; **Guinea pigs:** 0.5–5.0 mg/kg i.m. as required; **Chinchillas, Rats, Mice, Hamsters, Gerbils:** 2.5–5 mg/kg i.m., i.p. once; **Primates:** sedation and seizures: 0.5–1 mg/kg p.o., i.m.; **Sugar gliders, Hedgehogs:** sedation and seizures: 0.5–2 mg/kg p.o., s.c., i.m.

Birds: Epileptic seizures: 0.1–1 mg/kg i.v., i.m. once; Appetite stimulant in raptors: 0.2 mg/kg p.o. q24h.
Reptiles: Epileptic seizures: 2.5 mg/kg i.m., i.v.
Amphibians, Fish: No information available.

Diazoxide
(Eudemine*) **POM**

Formulations: Injectable: 15 mg/ml solution. **Oral:** 50 mg tablet.

Action: A diuretic that causes vasodilation and inhibits insulin secretion by blocking calcium mobilization.

Use: Used to manage hypoglycaemia caused by hyperinsulinism due to insulinoma in ferrets. In humans it is also used in the short-term management of acute hypertension.

Safety and handling: Normal precautions should be observed.

Contraindications: No information available.

Adverse reactions: The commonest adverse effects are anorexia, vomiting and diarrhoea. Hypotension, tachycardia, bone marrow suppression, pancreatitis, cataracts and electrolyte and fluid retention may occur. Drug efficacy may diminish over a period of months.

Drug interactions: Phenothiazines and thiazide diuretics may increase the hyperglycaemic activity of diazoxide, whilst alpha-adrenergic blocking agents (e.g. phenoxybenzamine) may antagonize the effects of diazoxide.

DOSES
Mammals: Ferrets: 5–30 mg/kg p.o. q12h.
Birds, Reptiles, Amphibians, Fish: No information available.

Diclofenac
(Voltarol Ophtha*, Voltarol Ophtha Multidose*) **POM**

Formulations: Ophthalmic: 0.1% solution in 5 ml bottle and in single-use vial.

Action: COX inhibitor that produces local anti-inflammatory effects.

Use: Used in cataract surgery to prevent intraoperative miosis and reflex (axonal) miosis caused by ulcerative keratitis. Used to control pain and inflammation associated with corneal surgery and in ulcerative keratitis when topical corticosteroid use is contraindicated.

Safety and handling: Normal precautions should be observed.

Contraindications: No information available.

Adverse reactions: As with other topical NSAIDs, diclofenac may cause local irritation. Topical NSAIDs should be used with caution in ulcerative keratitis as they can delay epithelial healing. Topical NSAIDs, and most specifically diclofenac, have been associated with an increased risk of corneal 'melting' (keratomalacia) in humans, although this has not been reported in the veterinary literature. Topical NSAIDs have the potential to increase intraocular pressure and should be used with caution in animals predisposed to glaucoma. Regular monitoring is advised. Use of systemic formulations has been associated with death in some species of birds.

Drug interactions: Ophthalmic NSAIDs may be used safely with other ophthalmic pharmaceuticals, although concurrent use of drugs which adversely affect the corneal epithelium (e.g. gentamicin) may lead to increased corneal penetration of the NSAID. The concurrent use of topical NSAIDs with topical corticosteroids has been identified as a risk factor in humans for precipitating corneal problems.

DOSES
Mammals: Topically as required (from 1 drop every 30 mins for 2 hours prior to cataract surgery, to 1 drop q4h for general anti-inflammatory effects) [a].
Birds: Not recommended (see note above on adverse reactions).
Reptiles, Amphibians, Fish: No information available.

References
[a] Waterbury L and Flach A (2006) Comparison of ketorolac tromethamine, diclofenac sodium and loteprednol etabonate in an animal model of ocular inflammation. *Journal of Ocular Pharmacology and Therapeutics* **22**, 155–159

Diflubenzuron (Dimilin)
(Aradol, CestoNemEx, Parazin) **ESPA**

Formulations: Immersion: 1 g/l (CestoNemEx), 1.64 g/l (Aradol); 4 g tablet for dissolution in water (Parazin).

Action: Inhibits chitin synthesis during ecdysis (moulting) of exoskeleton in crustacean parasites.

Use: Treatment of crustacean ectoparasites in fish (e.g. *Argulus, Ergasilus, Lernaea*). Only effective during moulting of immature life stages of the parasites, including eggs, but not adults. It is highly toxic to non-target species and must not be used in the presence of invertebrates. It is persistent in the environment. Some formulations may require approval for use from relevant authorities in some countries.

Safety and handling: Normal precautions should be observed.

Contraindications: Do not use in the presence of aquatic invertebrates.

Adverse reactions: No information available.

Drug interactions: No information available.

DOSES

Fish: 0.03 mg/l by prolonged immersion or 0.01 mg/l by prolonged immersion q6d for 3 treatments [1,2]; follow the manufacturer's recommendations for proprietary formulations.

Mammals, Birds, Reptiles, Amphibians: No information available.

References

[1] Noga EJ (2010) *Fish Disease Diagnosis and Treatment, 2nd edn*. Wiley-Blackwell, Oxford

[2] Stoskopf MK (1993) *Fish Medicine*. Saunders, Philadelphia

Digoxin

(Digoxin*, Lanoxin*, Lanoxin PG*) **POM**

Formulations: Oral: 62.5 μg, 125 μg, 250 μg tablets; 50 μg/ml elixir. **Injectable:** 100 μg/ml, 250 μg/ml.

Action: Inhibits Na^+/K^+ ATPase, leading to an increase in intracellular sodium. Sodium is exchanged for calcium, resulting in an increase in intracellular calcium and hence a mild positive inotropic effect. Digoxin slows the heart rate by decreasing the rate of sinoatrial node firing and inhibiting AV nodal conduction. These effects result primarily from parasympathetic activation and sympathetic inhibition, although it may also produce a modest direct depression of nodal tissue. The combination of a slower heart rate and increased force of contraction increases cardiac output in patients with supraventricular tachyarrhythmias. Digoxin improves baroreceptor reflexes that are impaired in heart failure.

Use: Management of heart failure and supraventricular tachyarrhythmias. It is primarily used to control the ventricular rate in cases of heart failure with concurrent atrial fibrillation. Digoxin/diltiazem combination therapy results in more effective rate control than monotherapy. In ferrets and rabbits it is used in the treatment of dilated cardiomyopathy. Serum levels should be checked after 5–7 days, with a sample taken at least 8 hours post-pill. The bioavailability of digoxin varies between the different formulations: i.v. = 100%; tablets = 60%; and elixir = 75%. If toxic effects are seen or the drug is ineffective, serum levels of digoxin should be assessed; the ideal therapeutic level is a trough serum concentration in the region of 1 ng/ml to optimize beneficial effects and minimize toxic side effects, with a suggested range of 0.6–1.2 ng/ml. Decreased dosages or an increase in dosing intervals may be required in geriatric patients, obese animals or those with significant renal dysfunction. The intravenous route is rarely indicated and, if used, should be done very slowly and with extreme care.

Safety and handling: Normal precautions should be observed.

Contraindications: Frequent ventricular arrhythmias or atrioventricular block.

Adverse reactions: Hypokalaemia predisposes to toxicity in all species. Signs of toxicity include anorexia, vomiting, diarrhoea, depression or arrhythmias (e.g. AV block, bigeminy, paroxysmal ventricular or atrial tachycardias with block, and multiform ventricular premature contractions). Lidocaine and phenytoin may be used to control digoxin-associated arrhythmias. Intravenous administration may cause vasoconstriction.

Drug interactions: Antacids, chemotherapy agents (e.g. cyclophosphamide, cytarabine, doxorubicin, vincristine), cimetidine and metoclopramide may decrease digoxin absorption from the GI tract. The following may increase the serum level, decrease the elimination rate or enhance the toxic effects of digoxin: amiodarone, antimuscarinics, diazepam, erythromycin, loop and thiazide diuretics (hypokalaemia), oxytetracycline, quinidine and verapamil. Spironolactone may enhance or decrease the toxic effects of digoxin.

DOSES

Mammals: Ferrets: 5–10 μg (micrograms)/kg p.o. q12–24h; **Rabbits:** 3–30 μg/kg p.o. q24–48h; **Hamsters:** 0.05–0.1 mg/kg p.o. q12–24h; **Primates:** 0.02–0.12 mg/kg i.m., i.v. q12–24h; **Hedgehogs:** 10 μg/kg p.o. q12–24h.

Birds: Raptors: 0.02–0.05 mg/kg p.o. q12h for 2–3 days then reduce to 0.01 mg/kg p.o. q12–24h; **Pigeons, Parrots:** 0.02–0.05 mg/kg p.o. q24h [a,1].

Reptiles, Amphibians, Fish: No information available.

References

[a] Wilson RC, Zenoble RD, Horton Jr CR and Ramsey DT (1989) Single Dose Digoxin Pharmacokinetics in the Quaker Conure (*Myiopsitta monachus*). *Journal of Zoo and Wildlife Medicine* **20(4)**, 432–434

[1] Fitzgerald BC, Dias S and Martorell J (2018) Cardiovascular Drugs in Avian, Small Mammal, and Reptile Medicine. *Veterinary Clinics of North America: Exotic Animal Practice* **21(2)**, 399–442

Diltiazem

(Hypercard, Dilcardia SR*) **POM-V, POM**

Formulations: Oral: 10 mg (Hypercard), 60 mg (generic) tablets. Long-acting preparations authorized for humans, such as Dilcardia SR (60 mg, 90 mg, 120 mg capsules), are available but their pharmacokinetics have been little studied in animals to date.

Action: Inhibits inward movement of calcium ions through slow (l-type) calcium channels in myocardial cells, cardiac conduction tissue and vascular smooth muscle; vascular smooth muscle is more sensitive to diltiazem than myocardial tissues (relative activity of 7:1). Diltiazem causes a reduction in myocardial contractility (negative inotrope, although less effective than verapamil), depressed electrical activity (retarded atrioventricular conduction) and decreases vascular resistance (vasodilation of cardiac vessels and peripheral arteries and arterioles).

Use: Used in ferrets and rabbits as in other species to control supraventricular tachyarrhythmias and for hypertrophic cardiomyopathy. Used to decrease the ventricular rate in atrial fibrillation either as monotherapy or in combination with digoxin. Digoxin/diltiazem combination therapy results in more effective rate control than monotherapy. Diltiazem is preferred to verapamil by many because it has effective antiarrhythmic properties with minimal negative inotropy. Diltiazem is less effective than amlodipine in the management of hypertension. Reduce the dose in patients with hepatic or renal impairment.

Safety and handling: Normal precautions should be observed.

Contraindications: Diltiazem is contraindicated in patients with second- or third-degree AV block, marked hypotension or sick sinus syndrome, and should be used cautiously in patients with systolic dysfunction or acute or decompensated congestive heart failure.

Adverse reactions: No information available.

Drug interactions: If diltiazem is administered concurrently with beta-adrenergic blockers (e.g. propranolol), there may be additive negative inotropic and chronotropic effects. The co-administration of diltiazem and beta-blockers is not recommended. The activity of diltiazem may be adversely affected by calcium salts or vitamin D. There are conflicting data regarding the effect of diltiazem on serum digoxin levels and monitoring of these levels is recommended if the drugs are used concurrently. Cimetidine inhibits the metabolism of diltiazem, thereby increasing plasma concentrations. Diltiazem enhances the effect of theophylline, which may lead to toxicity. It may affect quinidine and ciclosporin concentrations. Diltiazem may displace highly protein-bound agents from plasma proteins. Diltiazem may increase intracellular vincristine levels by inhibiting outflow of the drug from the cell.

DOSES
Mammals: Ferrets: 1.5–7.5 mg/kg p.o. q12h; **Rabbits:** 0.5–1.0 mg/kg p.o. q12–24h.
Birds, Reptiles, Amphibians, Fish: No information available.

Dimercaprol (British anti-lewisite)
(Dimercaprol*) **POM**

Formulations: Injectable: 50 mg/ml solution in peanut oil.

Action: Chelates heavy metals.

Use: Treatment of acute toxicity caused by arsenic, gold, bismuth and mercury, and used as an adjunct (with edetate calcium disodium) in lead poisoning.

Safety and handling: Normal precautions should be observed.

Contraindications: Severe hepatic failure.

Adverse reactions: Intramuscular injections are painful. Dimercaprol—metal complexes are nephrotoxic. This is particularly so with iron, selenium or cadmium; do not use for these metals. Alkalinization of urine during therapy may have protective effects for the kidney.

Drug interactions: Iron salts should not be administered during therapy.

DOSES
Birds: 2.5 mg/kg i.m. q4h for 2 days then q12h until signs resolve[1,2].
Mammals, Reptiles, Amphibians, Fish: No information available.

References
1. De Francisco N, Ruiz Troya JD and Agüera EI (2003) Lead and lead toxicity in domestic and free living birds. *Avian Pathology* **32(1)**, 3–13
2. Richardson JA, Murphy LA, Khan SA and Means C (2001) Managing pet bird toxicoses. *Exotic DVM* **3(1)**, 23–27

Dimethylsulfoxide (DMSO)
(Rimso-50*) **POM**

Formulations: Injectable: 50%, 90% liquid; medical grade only available as a 50% solution, other formulations are available as an industrial solvent. **Topical:** 70%, 90% gel; 70% cream.

Action: The mechanism of action is not well understood. Antioxidant activity has been demonstrated in certain biological settings and is thought to account for the anti-inflammatory activity.

Use: Management of otitis externa and haemorrhagic cystitis induced by cyclophosphamide. Although efficacy is unproven it has been used in the treatment of renal amyloidosis and prior to surgical treatment of pododermatitis (bumblefoot) in birds. In humans, DMSO is authorized for the treatment of interstitial cystitis. DMSO is very rapidly absorbed through the skin following administration by all routes and is distributed throughout the body. Metabolites of DMSO are excreted in the urine and faeces. DMSO is also excreted through the lungs and skin, producing a characteristic sulphuric odour. Humans given DMSO experience a garlic-like taste sensation after administration.

Safety and handling: Should be kept in a tightly closed container because it is very hygroscopic. Gloves should be worn during topical application and the product should be handled with care.

Contraindications: No information available.

Adverse reactions: Adverse effects include local irritation and erythema caused by local histamine release. Intravenous administration of solutions with concentrations >20% may cause haemolysis and diuresis.

Drug interactions: DMSO should not be mixed with other potentially toxic ingredients when applied to the skin because of profound enhancement of systemic absorption.

DOSES

Birds: May be applied topically to lesions (e.g. bumblefoot) as an anti-inflammatory prior to surgery. May be combined with other drugs as a carrying agent.

Mammals, Reptiles, Amphibians, Fish: No information available.

Dimilin see Diflubenzuron

Dinoprost tromethamine
(Prostaglandin F2)
(Enzaprost, Lutalyse) **POM-V**

Formulations: Injectable: 5 mg/ml solution.

Action: Stimulates uterine contraction, causes cervical relaxation and inhibits progesterone production by the corpus luteum.

Use: Used in the termination of pregnancy at any stage of gestation and to stimulate uterine contractions in the treatment of open pyometra. Possesses prokinetic effects on the caecum of the rabbit.

Safety and handling: Pregnant woman and asthmatics should avoid handling this agent.

Contraindications: Do not use for the treatment of closed pyometra as there is a risk of uterine rupture. Do not use in birds if the ureterovaginal sphincter is not dilated.

Adverse reactions: Hypersalivation, panting, tachycardia, vomiting, urination, defecation, transient hyperthermia, locomotor incoordination and mild CNS signs have been reported. Such effects usually diminish within 30 min of drug administration. There is no adverse effect on future fertility. Severe adverse effects have been reported in birds.

Drug interactions: The effect of oxytocin would be potentiated by prostaglandins and inhibited by progestogens.

DOSES

Mammals: Rabbits: 0.2 mg/kg single i.m. injection following 3 days of oral liquid paraffin to assist in emptying impacted caecal contents.
Birds: 0.02–0.1 mg/kg i.m., intracloacal once.
Reptiles, Amphibians, Fish: No information available.

Dinoprostone (Prostaglandin E2)
(Prostin E2*) **POM**

Formulations: Topical: 0.4 mg/ml gel.

Action: Stimulates uterine contraction, causes cervical relaxation and inhibits progesterone production by the corpus luteum.

Use: Used to relax the vagina and induce uterine contractions in egg-bound birds.

Safety and handling: Pregnant women and asthmatics should avoid handling this agent.

Contraindications: No information available.

Adverse reactions: Uterine rupture may occur.

Drug interactions: No information available.

DOSES
Birds: Apply a thin layer of gel to the cloacal mucosa once.
Mammals, Reptiles, Amphibians, Fish: No information available.

Diphenhydramine
(Dreemon*, Nytol*) **P**

Formulations: Oral: 25 mg tablet; 2 mg/ml solution. Other products are available of various concentrations and most contain other active ingredients.

Action: The antihistaminergic (H1) effects are used to reduce pruritus and prevent motion sickness. It is also a mild anxiolytic and sedative.

Use: In birds it is used in the management of allergic rhinitis, hypersensitivity reactions and allergic dermatopathies. In ferrets it is used before vaccination if a previous vaccine reaction has been encountered, or for prevention of sneezing or coughing when these interrupt eating or sleeping. In rabbits it may also be used to reduce possible nausea associated with torticollis. Liquid is very distasteful.

Safety and handling: Normal precautions should be observed.

Contraindications: Urine retention, glaucoma and hyperthyroidism.

Adverse reactions: No information available.

Drug interactions: An increased sedative effect may occur if used with benzodiazepines or other anxiolytics/hypnotics. Avoid the concomitant use of other sedative agents. Diphenhydramine may enhance the effect of adrenaline and partially counteract anticoagulant effects of heparin.

DOSES
Mammals: Ferrets: 0.5–2 mg/kg p.o., s.c. q8–12h for allergic reactions; for preventative management of vaccination reactions, give the high end of the dose range by i.m. injection prior to vaccination; **Rabbits:** 2 mg/kg p.o., s.c., i.m. q12h for torticollis; **Guinea pigs:** 1–5 mg/kg s.c. prn; **Chinchillas, Hamsters, Rats, Mice:** 1–2 mg/kg p.o., s.c. q12h; **Primates:** 5 mg/kg/day p.o., i.m. total dose divided q6–8h.
Birds: 2–4 mg/kg p.o. q12h.
Reptiles, Amphibians, Fish: No information available.

Domperidone
(Domperidone*, Motilium*) **POM**

Formulations: Oral: 10 mg tablet, 1 mg/ml suspension.

Action: A potent antiemetic with a similar mechanism of action to metoclopramide, but with fewer adverse CNS effects as it cannot penetrate the blood–brain barrier. It is gastrokinetic in humans and rabbits.

Use: Treatment of vomiting and reduced gastrointestinal motility. In rabbits, it has a significant prokinetic action on gastric emptying.

Safety and handling: Normal precautions should be observed.

Contraindications: Gastrointestinal obstruction or perforation.

Adverse reactions: No information available.

Drug interactions: No information available.

DOSES
Mammals: Rabbits: 0.5 mg/kg p.o. q12h.
Birds, Reptiles, Amphibians, Fish: No information available.

Dopamine
(Dopamine*) **POM**

Formulations: Injectable: 200 mg in 5 ml vial (40 mg/ml solution), 800 mg in a 5 ml vial (160 mg/ml solution).

Action: Dopamine is an endogenous catecholamine and precursor of noradrenaline, with direct and indirect (via release of noradrenaline) agonist effects on dopaminergic and beta-1 and alpha-1 adrenergic receptors.

Use: Improvement of haemodynamic status. Main indications are treatment of shock following correction of fluid deficiencies, acute heart failure, and support of blood pressure during anaesthesia. Dobutamine is preferred for support of systolic function in patients with heart failure. Dopamine is a potent and short-acting drug, therefore it should be given in low doses by continuous rate infusion, and accurate dosing is important. Dopamine should be diluted in normal saline to an appropriate concentration. At low doses (<10 µg/kg/min) dopamine acts on dopaminergic and beta-1 adrenergic receptors, causing vasodilation, increased force of contraction and heart rate, and resulting in an increase in cardiac output and organ perfusion; systemic vascular resistance remains largely unchanged. At higher doses (>10 µg/kg/min) dopaminergic effects are overridden by the alpha effects, resulting in an increase in systemic vascular resistance and reduced peripheral blood flow. Dopamine has been shown to vasodilate mesenteric blood vessels via DA1 receptors. There may be an improvement in urine output but this may be entirely due to inhibition of proximal tubule sodium ion reabsorption and an improved cardiac output and blood pressure rather than directly improving renal blood flow. The dose of dopamine should be adjusted according to clinical effect, therefore monitoring of arterial blood pressure during administration is advisable. All sympathomimetic drugs have pro-arrhythmic properties, therefore ECG monitoring is advised.

Safety and handling: Solution should be discarded if it becomes discoloured.

Contraindications: Discontinue or reduce the dose of dopamine should cardiac arrhythmias arise.

Adverse reactions: Extravasation of dopamine causes necrosis and sloughing of surrounding tissue due to tissue ischaemia. Should extravasation occur, infiltrate the site with a solution of 5–10 mg phentolamine in 10–15 ml of normal saline using a syringe with a fine needle. Nausea, vomiting, tachyarrhythmias and changes in blood pressure are the most common adverse effects. Hypotension may develop with low doses, and hypertension may occur with high doses. Sudden increases in blood pressure may cause a severe bradycardia. All dopamine-induced arrhythmias are most effectively treated by stopping the infusion.

Drug interactions: Risk of severe hypertension when monoamine oxidase inhibitors, doxapram and oxytocin are used with dopamine. Halothane may increase myocardial sensitivity to catecholamines. The effects of beta-blockers and dopamine are antagonistic.

DOSES
Mammals: Guinea pigs: 0.08 mg/kg i.v. prn.
Birds: 5–10 µg (micrograms)/kg/min to counter isoflurane-induced hypotension. More effective than dobutamine [a].
Reptiles, Amphibians, Fish: No information available.

References
[a] Schnellbacher RW, Da Cunha AF, Beaufrère H et al. (2012) Effects of dopamine and dobutamine on isoflurane-induced hypotension in Hispaniolan Amazon parrots (*Amazona ventralis*). *American Journal of Veterinary Research* **73(7)**, 952–958

Dorzolamide
(CoSopt*, Dorzolamide*, Dorzolamide with Timolol*, Trusopt*) **POM**

Formulations: Ophthalmic drops: 20 mg/ml (2%) (Dorzolamide, Trusopt), 2% dorzolamide + 0.5% timolol (CoSopt, Dorzolamide with Timolol); 5 ml bottle, single-use vials (CoSopt, Trusopt).

Action: Reduces intraocular pressure by reducing the rate of aqueous humour production by inhibiting the formation of bicarbonate ions within the ciliary body epithelium.

Use: In the control of all types of glaucoma, either alone or in combination with other topical drugs. It may be less tolerated than brinzolamide because of its less physiological pH of 5.6. The concurrent use of a topical and a systemic carbonic anhydrase inhibitor is not beneficial as there is no additional decrease in intraocular pressure compared with either route alone.

Safety and handling: Normal precautions should be observed.

Contraindications: Severe hepatic or renal impairment. Dorzolamide/timolol is not the drug of choice in uveitis or anterior lens luxation.

Adverse reactions: Local irritation and blepharitis. Dorzolamide may cause more local irritation than brinzolamide. Dorzolamide/timolol causes miosis.

Drug interactions: No information available.

DOSES
Mammals: Rabbits: 1 drop/eye q8–12h; Rats: 1 drop 1% solution (dilute standard formulation with sterile water) q12h.
Birds: 1 drop/eye q12h [1,2].
Reptiles, Amphibians, Fish: No information available.

References
[1] Fordham M, Rosenthal K, Durham A, Duda L and Komáromy AM (2010) Intraocular osteosarcoma in an Umbrella cockatoo (*Cacatua alba*). *Veterinary Ophthalmology* **13**, 103–108
[2] Jayson S, Guzman DSM, Petritz O, Freeman K and Maggs DJ (2014) Medical management of acute ocular hypertension in a western screech owl (*Megascops kennicottii*). *Journal of Avian Medicine and Surgery* **28(1)**, 38–45

Doxapram
(Dopram-V, Doxapram hydrochloride)
POM-VPS, POM-V, POM

Formulations: Injectable: 20 mg/ml solution. Oral: 20 mg/ml drops.

Action: Stimulates respiration by increasing the sensitivity of aortic and carotid body chemoreceptors to arterial gas tensions.

Use: Stimulates respiration during and after general anaesthesia. In neonatal animals, used to stimulate or initiate respiration after birth, particularly in those delivered by caesarean section. The dose should be adjusted according to the requirements of the situation; adequate but not excessive doses should be used. A patent airway is essential. Must not be used indiscriminately to support respiratory function. Severe respiratory depression should be controlled by tracheal intubation, followed by IPPV and then resolution of the initiating cause. Duration of effect in mammals is 15–20 minutes. Has also been used to aid assessment of laryngeal function under light anaesthesia. Not effective at stimulating respiration in the face of hypoxaemia (pre-oxygenation of hypoventilating neonates is recommended, along with removal of obstructive secretions). Used for the treatment of respiratory depression in fish.

Safety and handling: Protect from light.

Contraindications: Do not use in animals without a patent airway.

Adverse reactions: Overdose can cause excessive hyperventilation, which may be followed by reduced carbon dioxide tension in the blood leading to cerebral vasoconstriction. This could result in cerebral hypoxia in some animals. Doxapram is irritant and may cause a thrombophlebitis, avoid extravasation or repeated i.v. injection into the same vein. Use doxapram injection with caution in neonates because it contains benzyl alcohol which is toxic. Overdosage signs include hypertension, skeletal muscle hyperactivity, tachycardia and generalized CNS excitation including seizures; treatment is supportive using short-acting i.v. barbiturates or propofol and oxygen. Effects in pregnant/lactating animals are not known.

Drug interactions: Hypertension may occur with sympathomimetics. The use of theophylline concurrently with doxapram may cause increased CNS stimulation. As doxapram may stimulate the release of adrenaline, its use within 10 min of the administration of anaesthetic agents that sensitize the myocardium to catecholamines (e.g. halothane) should be avoided. Doxapram is compatible with 5% dextrose or normal saline, but is incompatible with sodium bicarbonate or thiopental. High doses administered during or after anaesthesia with halogenated hydrocarbon anaesthetics, such as halothane, may precipitate cardiac arrhythmias. Doxapram injection should be used with extreme caution in animals that have been sedated with morphine. Administration of doxapram at 10 mg/kg to such animals may be followed by convulsions.

DOSES
Mammals: Ferrets, Rabbits, Chinchillas, Rats, Mice, Hamsters, Gerbils, Hedgehogs: 5–10 mg/kg i.v., i.m., i.p., sublingual once; Guinea pigs: 2–5 mg/kg i.v., s.c., i.p. once; **Primates:** 2 mg/kg i.v.; Sugar gliders: 2 mg/kg i.v. once.
Birds: 5–20 mg/kg i.m., i.v., intratracheal, intraosseous once[1].

Reptiles: 4–12 mg/kg i.m., i.v., p.o. once.
Fish: 5 mg/kg i.v., intracoelomic [2], topically to the gills.
Amphibians: No information available.

References
[1] Lierz M and Korbel R (2012) Anesthesia and analgesia in birds. *Journal of Exotic Pet Medicine* **21(1)**, 44–58
[2] Hadfield C, Whitaker BR and Clayton LA (2007) Emergency and critical care of fish. *Veterinary Clinics of North America: Exotic Animal Practice* **10**, 647–675

Doxepin
(Sinepin*, Sinequan*, Zonalon*) **POM**

Formulations: Oral: 25 mg, 50 mg capsules.

Action: Doxepin blocks noradrenaline and serotonin re-uptake in the brain, resulting in antidepressive activity, while the H1 and H2 blockage result in antipruritic effects. Its metabolite, desmethyldoxepin, is also psychoactive.

Use: Management of pruritus and psychogenic dermatoses where there is a component of anxiety, including compulsive disorders. Data are lacking as to its efficacy at the suggested doses. Used in birds for organophosphate toxicity. When used in birds it is important to monitor for cardiac arrhythmias.

Safety and handling: Normal precautions should be observed.

Contraindications: Hypersensitivity to tricyclic antidepressants, glaucoma, history of seizures or urinary retention and severe liver disease.

Adverse reactions: Sedation, dry mouth, diarrhoea, vomiting, excitability, arrhythmias, hypotension, syncope, increased appetite, weight gain and, less commonly, seizures and bone marrow disorders have been reported in humans.

Drug interactions: Should not be used with monoamine oxidase inhibitors or drugs which are metabolized by cytochrome P450 2D6, e.g. chlorphenamine and cimetidine.

DOSES
Birds: Feather plucking: 1–2 mg/kg p.o. q12h [1]; organophosphate toxicity: 0.2 mg/kg i.m. q4h.
Mammals, Reptiles, Amphibians, Fish: No information available.

References
[1] van Zeeland YRA, Spruit BM, Rodenburg TA *et al.* (2009) Feather damaging behaviour in parrots: a review with consideration of comparative aspects. *Applied Animal Behaviour Science* **121(2)**, 75–95

Doxorubicin (Adriamycin)
(Doxorubicin*) **POM**

Formulations: Injectable: 10 mg, 50 mg powders for reconstitution; 10 mg, 50 mg/vial solutions.

Action: Inhibits DNA synthesis and function.

Use: Treatment of lymphoma in the ferret. Has been used to treat lymphoma in a green iguana. It may be used alone or in combination with other antineoplastic therapies. Premedication with i.v. chlorphenamine or dexamethasone is recommended. Doxorubicin is highly irritant and must be administered via a preplaced i.v. catheter. The reconstituted drug should be administered over a minimum period of 10 min into the side port of a freely running i.v. infusion of 0.9% NaCl. Do not use heparin flush. May need to reduce dose in patients with liver disease. Use with caution in patients previously treated with radiation as can cause radiation recall.

Safety and handling: Potent cytotoxic drug that should only be prepared and administered by trained personnel. See specialist texts for further advice on chemotherapeutic agents. After reconstitution the drug is stable for at least 48h at 4°C. A 1.5% loss of potency may occur after 1 month at 4°C but there is no loss of potency when frozen at −20°C. Filtering through a 0.22 μm filter will ensure adequate sterility of the thawed solution. Store unopened vials under refrigeration.

Contraindications: Do not use in patients with existing cardiac or renal disease.

Adverse reactions: Allergic reactions have been reported; acute anaphylactic reactions should be treated with adrenaline, steroids and fluids. Doxorubicin causes a dose-dependent cumulative cardiotoxicity in dogs (leading to cardiomyopathy and congestive heart failure), and this may be of concern in ferrets. The risk of cardiotoxicity is greatly increased when the cumulative dose is >240 mg/m^2. It may also cause tachycardia and arrhythmias on administration; monitor with ECG and/or echocardiograms. Anorexia, vomiting, severe leucopenia, thrombocytopenia, haemorrhagic gastroenteritis and nephrotoxicity are the major adverse effects. A CBC and platelet count should be monitored whenever therapy is given. If the neutrophil count drops below 3×10^9/l or the platelet count drops below 50×10^9/l, treatment should be suspended. Once the counts have stabilized, doxorubicin can be restarted at the same dose. If haematological toxicity occurs again, or if GI toxicity is recurrent, the dose should be reduced by 10–25%. Extravasation injuries secondary to perivascular administration may be serious, with severe tissue ulceration and necrosis possible. Dexrazoxane can be used to treat extravasation if it occurs. Ice compresses may also be beneficial (applied for 15 min q6h).

Drug interactions: Barbiturates increase plasma clearance of doxorubicin. The agent causes a reduction in serum digoxin levels. Do not mix doxorubicin with other drugs. Doxorubicin is incompatible with dexamethasone, 5-fluorouracil and heparin; concurrent use will lead to precipitate formation.

DOSES

See Appendix for chemotherapy protocols in ferrets.

Mammals: Ferrets: 20 mg/m^2 or 1–2 mg/kg i.v. every 3 weeks for a maximum of 5 doses. Also used as part of a multi-drug protocol for lymphoma.

Birds: 2 mg/kg i.v. infused in normal saline over 20 minutes[a].

Reptiles: 0.26–0.75 mg/kg i.v. reported as part of a successful chemotherapy protocol in a green iguana[1].

Amphibians, Fish: No information available.

References

[a] Gilbert CM, Filippich LJ and Charles BG (2004) Doxorubicin pharmacokinetics following a single-dose infusion to sulphur-crested cockatoos (*Cacatua galerita*). *Australian Veterinary Journal* **82(12)**, 769–772

[1] Folland DW, Johnston MS, Thamm DH and Reavill D (2011) Diagnosis and management of lymphoma in a green iguana (*Iguana iguana*). *Journal of the American Veterinary Medical Association* **239(7)**, 985–991

Doxycycline

(Doxyseptin 300, Karidox, Ornicure, Pulmodox, Ronaxan, Vibramycin*, Vibravenos*) **POM-V**

Formulations: Oral: 20 mg, 100 mg tablets (Ronaxan), 300 mg tablets (Doxyseptin); 260 mg/sachet powder (Ornicure); 100 mg/ml oral solution (Karidox). Injectable: 20 mg/ml long-acting injection (Vibravenos; import on an STC).

Action: Bacteriostatic agent inhibiting protein synthesis at the initiation step by interacting with the 30S ribosomal subunit.

Use: Antibacterial (including spirochaetes such as *Helicobacter* and *Campylobacter*), antirickettsial, antimycoplasmal and antichlamydial activity. It is the drug of choice to treat avian chlamydiosis; treatment may be required for 6 weeks in birds. It is not affected by, and does not affect, renal function as it is excreted in faeces, and is therefore recommended when tetracyclines are indicated in animals with renal impairment. It is preferred by some authors to oxytetracycline for use in birds. Being extremely lipid-soluble, it penetrates well into prostatic fluid and bronchial secretions. Administer with food. Injection is very irritant in birds: must alternate injection sites or divide dose if large volume to inject.

Safety and handling: Normal precautions should be observed.

Contraindications: Do not administer to pregnant animals. Do not administer if there is evidence of oesophagitis or dysphagia.

Adverse reactions: Nausea, vomiting and diarrhoea. Oesophagitis and oesophageal ulceration may develop; administer with food or a water bolus to reduce this risk. Administration during tooth development may lead to discoloration of the teeth, although the risk is less than with other tetracyclines.

Drug interactions: Absorption of doxycycline is reduced by antacids, calcium, magnesium and iron salts, although the effect is less marked than that seen with water-soluble tetracyclines. Phenobarbital and phenytoin may increase its metabolism, thus decreasing plasma levels. Do not use in combination with bactericidal antimicrobials.

DOSES
See Appendix for guidelines on responsible antibacterial use.
Mammals: Rabbits: 2.5–4 mg/kg p.o. q24h; **Rats, Mice:** 5 mg/kg p.o. q12h; **Other rodents:** 2.5 mg/kg p.o. q12h or 70–100 mg/kg s.c., i.m. of the long-acting preparation (Vibravenos); **Primates:** 3–4 mg/kg p.o. q12h; **Hedgehogs:** 2.5–10 mg/kg p.o., s.c., i.m. q12h.
Birds: Raptors: 50 mg/kg p.o. q12h, 100 mg/kg i.m. q7d (Vibravenos); **Parrots:** 15–50 mg/kg p.o. q24h, 1000 mg/kg in soft food/dehulled seed, 75–100 mg/kg i.m. q7d (Vibravenos; lowest dose rate for macaws) [a,b,c,d]; course of treatment with doxycycline for chlamydiosis = 45 days; **Passerines/Pigeons:** 40 mg/kg p.o. q12–24h, 200–500 mg/l in water (soft or deionized water only).
Reptiles: 50 mg/kg i.m. once, then 25 mg/kg i.m. q72h.
Amphibians: 50 mg/kg i.m. q7d.
Fish: No information available.

References
a   Flammer K and Papich M (2005) Assessment of plasma concentrations and effects of injectable doxycycline in three psittacine species. *Journal of Avian Medicine and Surgery* **19(3)**, 216–224
b   Flammer K and Whitt-Smith D (2001) Plasma concentrations of doxycycline in selected psittacine birds when administered in water for potential treatment of *Chlamydophila psittaci* infection. *Journal of Avian Medicine and Surgery* **15(4)**, 276–282
c   Powers LV, Flammer K and Papich M (2000) Preliminary investigation of doxycycline plasma concentrations in Cockatiels (*Nymphicus hollandicus*) after administration by injection or in water or feed. *Journal of Avian Medicine and Surgery* **14(1)**, 23–30
d   Saturation T (2008) Administration of doxycycline in drinking water for treatment of spiral bacterial infection in Cockatiels. *Journal of Zoo and Wildlife Medicine* **39(3)**, 499–501

Edetate calcium disodium (CaEDTA)
(Ledclair*) **POM**

Formulations: Injectable: 200 mg/ml solution.

Action: Heavy metal chelating agent.

Use: Lead and zinc poisoning. Dilute strong solution to a concentration of 10 mg/ml in 5% dextrose before use. Blood lead levels may be confusing, therefore monitor clinical signs during therapy. Measure blood lead levels 2–3 weeks after completion of treatment in order to determine whether a second course is required or if the animal is still being exposed to lead. Ensure there is no lead in the GI tract before administering (e.g. use laxatives) nor any residual heavy metals elsewhere (e.g. powdered zinc in coat or an environmental source).

Safety and handling: Normal precautions should be observed.

Contraindications: Use with caution in patients with impaired renal function.

Adverse reactions: Reversible nephrotoxicity is usually preceded by other clinical signs of toxicity (e.g. depression, vomiting, diarrhoea). Injections are painful.

Drug interactions: No information available.

DOSES
Mammals: Ferrets: 20–30 mg/kg s.c. q12h; **Rabbits:** 27.5 mg/kg s.c. q6h; **Rodents:** 25–30 mg/kg s.c. q6–12h. Repeat treatment for 5 days on, 5 days off until blood lead or zinc levels are normal when measured at the end of the period off treatment.
Birds: 35–50 mg/kg i.m., s.c. q12h for 5 days followed by 2 days of no treatment, then repeat until metal particles are no longer visible on radiographs[a]. 100 mg/kg i.m. weekly has been proposed in zinc toxicosis.
Reptiles: 10–40 mg/kg i.m. q12h.
Amphibians, Fish: No information available.

References
[a] Sears J, Cooke SW, Cooke ZR and Heron TJ (1989) A method for the treatment of lead poisoning in the mute swan (*Cygnus olor*) and its long-term success. *British Veterinary Journal* **145(6)**, 586–595

Emamectin benzoate
(Lice-Solve, Slice) **ESPA, POM-V**

Formulations: Immersion: 10 g, 100 g sachets of powder containing 1.4% emamectin. In food: 2.5 kg pouch of powder containing 5 g emamectin benzoate.

Action: Irreversibly binds to and opens GABA and glutamate-gated channels, leading to flaccid paralysis and death of the parasite.

Use: Treatment of crustacean parasites of fish (*Argulus*, *Ergasilus* spp.). For use in closed water systems. Turn off UV and carbon filters for 24 h after adding the product to the water. Ensure good aeration of the water during treatment. Emamectin rapidly biodegrades in sunlight.

Safety and handling: Normal precautions should be observed. Do not dispose of down drains or in waterways.

Contraindications: Do not use at the same time as other fish or pond treatments. Do not use in ponds containing orfe (*Leuciscus* spp.) or terrapins.

Adverse reactions: No information available.

Drug interactions: No information available.

DOSES

Fish: 56 µg (micrograms)/l by prolonged immersion, repeat after 1 month. **Goldfish:** 0.05 mg/kg bodyweight daily in food for 7 days; **Koi:** 0.005 mg/kg bodyweight daily in food for 7 days[a].

Mammals, Birds, Reptiles, Amphibians: No information available.

References

[a] Hanson SK, Hill JE, Watson CA, Yanong RP and Endris R (2011) Evaluation of emamectin benzoate for the control of experimentally induced infestations of *Argulus* sp. in goldfish and koi carp. *Journal of Aquatic Animal Health* **23(1)**, 30–34

Emodepside
(Profender) **POM-V**

Formulations: Topical: 21.4 mg/ml emodepside with praziquantel solution in spot-on pipettes.

Action: Stimulates presynaptic secretin receptors resulting in paralysis and death of the parasite.

Use: Treatment of roundworms (adult and immature) and tapeworms (adult) including *Toxocara cati*, *Toxascaris leonina*, *Ancylostoma tubaeforme*, *Aelurostrongylus abstrusus*, *Dipylidium caninum*, *Taenia taeniaeformis*, *Echinococcus multilocularis*. Do not shampoo until substance has dried. Treatment of a variety of reptile endoparasites including oxyurids, ascarids, strongylids, trichostrongylids and capillarids.

Safety and handling: Women of child-bearing age should avoid contact with this drug or wear disposable gloves when using it.

Contraindications: Do not use in pregnant mammals. Studies in rabbits and rats suggest it may interfere with fetal development *in utero*.

Adverse reactions: Ingestion may result in salivation or vomiting. Harmful to aquatic animals.

Drug interactions: Possible interaction with P-glycoprotein substrates/inhibitors.

DOSES

Mammals: Rabbits: 0.14 ml/kg topically once (reported for *Trichostrongylus colubriformis*).

Reptiles: <1.12 ml/kg Profender applied topically once (corresponding to 24 mg emodepside and 96 mg praziquantel/kg) [a,b].

Birds, Amphibians, Fish: No information available.

References

[a] Schilliger L, Betremieux O, Rochet J, Krebber R and Schaper R (2009) Absorption and efficacy of a spot-on combination containing emodepside plus praziquantel in reptiles. *Revue de Médecine Vétérinaire* **160(12)**, 557–561

[b] Tang PK, Pellett S, Blake D and Hedley J (2017) Efficacy of a Topical Formulation Containing Emodepside and Praziquantel (Profender®, Bayer) against Nematodes in Captive Tortoises. *Journal of Herpetological Medicine and Surgery* **27(3)**, 116–122

Enalapril
(Enacard) **POM-V**

Formulations: Oral: 1 mg, 2.5 mg, 5 mg, 10 mg, 20 mg tablets.

Action: Angiotensin converting enzyme (ACE) inhibitor. It inhibits conversion of angiotensin I to angiotensin II and inhibits the breakdown of bradykinin. Overall effect is a reduction in preload and afterload via venodilation and arteriodilation, decreased salt and water retention via reduced aldosterone production and inhibition of the angiotensin-aldosterone-mediated cardiac and vascular remodelling. Efferent arteriolar dilation in the kidney can reduce intraglomerular pressure and therefore glomerular filtration. This may decrease proteinuria.

Use: Treatment of congestive heart failure caused by mitral regurgitation or dilated cardiomyopathy. Often used in conjunction with diuretics when heart failure is present as most effective when used in these cases. Can be used in combination with other drugs to treat heart failure (e.g. pimobendan, spironolactone, digoxin). May be beneficial in cases of chronic renal insufficiency, particularly protein-losing nephropathies. May reduce blood pressure in hypertension. ACE inhibitors are more likely to cause or exacerbate prerenal azotaemia in hypotensive animals and those with poor renal perfusion (e.g. acute, oliguric renal failure). Use cautiously if hypotension, hyponatraemia or outflow tract obstruction are present. Regular monitoring of blood pressure, serum creatinine, urea and electrolytes is strongly recommended with ACE inhibitor treatment. Hypotension, azotaemia and hyperkalaemia are all indications to stop or reduce ACE inhibitor treatment in rabbits.

Safety and handling: Normal precautions should be observed.

Contraindications: Do not use in cases of cardiac output failure.

Adverse reactions: Potential adverse effects include hypotension, hyperkalaemia and azotaemia. Monitor blood pressure, serum creatinine and electrolytes when used in cases of heart failure. Dosage should be reduced if there are signs of hypotension (weakness, disorientation). Anorexia, vomiting and diarrhoea are rare. It is not recommended for breeding, pregnant or lactating animals, as safety has not been established. In rabbits, treatment with ACE inhibitors can be associated with an increase in azotaemia and significant hypotension; treatment should start at the lower end of the range.

Drug interactions: Concomitant treatment with potassium-sparing diuretics (e.g. spironolactone) or potassium supplements could result in hyperkalaemia. However, in practice, spironolactone and ACE inhibitors appear safe to use concurrently. There may be an increased risk of nephrotoxicity and decreased clinical efficacy when used with NSAIDs. There is a risk of hypotension with concomitant administration of diuretics, vasodilators (e.g. anaesthetic agents, antihypertensive agents) or negative inotropes (e.g. beta-blockers).

DOSES
Mammals: Ferrets: 0.25–0.5 mg/kg p.o. q24–48h; **Rabbits:** 0.25–0.5 mg/kg p.o. q24–48h; **Rodents:** 0.5–1.0 mg/kg p.o. q24h; **Primates:** 0.3 mg/kg p.o. q24h; **Common marmosets:** 0.5 mg/kg p.o. q48h; **Sugar gliders, Hedgehogs:** 0.5 mg/kg p.o. q24h.
Birds: 1.25 mg/kg p.o. q12h[1].
Reptiles, Amphibians, Fish: No information available.

References
1 Fitzgerald BC, Dias S and Martorell J (2018) Cardiovascular Drugs in Avian, Small Mammal, and Reptile Medicine. *Veterinary Clinics: Exotic Animal Practice* **21(2)**, 399–442

Enilconazole
(Imaverol) **POM-VPS**

Formulations: Topical: 100 mg/ml (10%) liquid.

Action: Inhibition of cytochrome P450-dependent synthesis of ergosterol in fungal cells, causing increased cell wall permeability and allowing leakage of cellular contents.

Use: Fungal infections of the skin and nasal aspergillosis. Has been shown to inhibit zoospores of *Batrachochytrium dendrobatidis in vitro* but there is no information on systemic clinical treatment of amphibians with chytridiomycosis.

Safety and handling: Normal precautions should be observed.

Contraindications: No information available.

Adverse reactions: Hepatotoxic if swallowed. Avoid contact with eyes.

Drug interactions: No information available.

DOSES

Mammals: Rabbits: Dilute 1:50 in water to produce a 2 mg/ml (0.2%) solution. Apply topically to lesions every 1–3 days for 3–4 applications and then check success of therapy with fungal culture; Hamsters: 0.2% rinse topically every 7 days until fungal cultures negative.

Birds: Dilute 1:10 in water and give 0.5 ml/kg/day intratracheally for 7–14 days[a].

Reptiles: Dilute 1:50 in water. Apply topically to lesions every 2–3 days.

Amphibians, Fish: No information available.

References
[a] Perelman B, Smith B, Bronstein D, Gur-Lavie A and Kuttin ES (1992) Use of azole compounds for the treatment of experimental aspergillosis in turkeys. *Avian Pathology* **21(4)**, 591–599

Enrofloxacin

(**Baytril**, **Enrobactin**, **Enrocare**, Enrotab, Enrotron, Enrox, **Enroxil**, Floxabactin, Floxibac, Powerflox, Quinoflox, Xeden, Zobuxa) **POM-V**

Formulations: Injectable: 25 mg/ml, 50 mg/ml, 100 mg/ml solutions. **Oral:** 15 mg, 50 mg, 150 mg, 250 mg tablets; 25 mg/ml solution.

Action: Enrofloxacin is a bactericidal antimicrobial which inhibits bacterial DNA gyrase. The bactericidal action is concentration-dependent, meaning that pulse-dosing regimens may be effective, particularly against Gram-negative bacteria.

Use: Ideally fluoroquinolone use should be reserved for infections where culture and sensitivity testing predicts a clinical response and where first- and second-line antimicrobials would not be effective. Active against *Mycoplasma* and many Gram-positive and Gram-negative organisms, including *Pasteurella*, *Staphylococcus*, *Pseudomonas aeruginosa*, *Klebsiella*, *Escherichia coli*, *Mycobacterium*, *Proteus* and *Salmonella*. Relatively ineffective against obligate anaerobes. Fluoroquinolones are highly lipophilic drugs that attain high concentrations within cells in many tissues and are particularly effective in the management of soft tissue, urogenital (including prostatic) and skin infections. For the treatment of non-tubercular mycobacterial disease, enrofloxacin can be combined with clarithromycin and rifampin. Administration by i.v. route is not authorized but has been used in cases of severe sepsis. If this route is used, administer slowly as the carrier contains potassium. Dilute solution for injection 1 in 4 with water if dosing small mammals orally. Switch to oral medications in birds as soon as possible. Used for the treatment of bacterial disease in fish, particularly those caused by Gram-negative organisms.

Safety and handling: Normal precautions should be observed.

Contraindications: Fluoroquinolones are relatively contraindicated in growing small mammals as cartilage abnormalities have been reported in young mice, rats, guinea pigs and rabbits after administration of fluoroquinolones similar to enrofloxacin.

Adverse reactions: In birds, joint lesions have been induced in nestling pigeons with high doses of enrofloxacin, and in all species, muscle necrosis may be seen following i.m. administration. Enrofloxacin should be used with caution in epileptics until further information is available, as in humans they potentiate CNS adverse effects when administered concurrently with NSAIDs. Excitation and diarrhoea have been reported in Galapagos tortoises.

Drug interactions: Adsorbents and antacids containing cations (Mg^{2+}, Al^{3+}) may bind to fluoroquinolones and prevent their absorption from the GI tract. The absorption of fluoroquinolones may also be inhibited by sucralfate and zinc salts; separate doses of these drugs by at least 2 hours. Fluoroquinolones increase plasma theophylline concentrations. Cimetidine may reduce the clearance of fluoroquinolones and so should be used with caution in combination with these drugs. Efficacy may be reduced due to chelation when used as a bath treatment for fish in hard water with high levels of divalent metal cations (Ca^{2+}, Mg^{2+}).

DOSES
See Appendix for guidelines on responsible antibacterial use.
Mammals: Ferrets: 5–10 mg/kg p.o., s.c., i.m. q12h or 10–20 mg/kg p.o., s.c., i.m. q24h; **Rabbits:** 10–20 mg/kg p.o., s.c., i.v. q24h; **Rodents:** 5–20 mg/kg s.c., p.o. q12–24h; **Primates:** 5 mg/kg p.o., s.c. q12–24h; **Sugar gliders:** 5 mg/kg p.o., s.c., i.m. q12h; **Hedgehogs:** 2.5–10 mg/kg p.o., s.c., i.m. q12h; **Others:** 5–10 mg/kg s.c., p.o. q12h or 20 mg/kg s.c., p.o. q24h.
Birds: 10 mg/kg p.o., i.m. q12h (licensed dose) or 100–200 mg/l drinking water[a].
Reptiles: Variable absorption when given p.o. so i.m. administration may be more appropriate in critically ill animals. **Most species:** 5–10 mg/kg i.m., p.o. q24–48h; **Indian star tortoises:** 5 mg/kg i.m. q12–24h[b]; **Gopher tortoises:** 5 mg/kg i.m. q24–48h; **Hermann's tortoises:** 10 mg/kg intracoelomic; **Red-eared sliders:** 5 mg/kg i.m. or 10 mg/kg p.o., i.m., s.c., intracoelomic q24h or 500 mg/l as a 6–8 h bath q24h[c]; **Savannah monitors:** 10 mg/kg i.m. q5d; **Green iguanas:** 5 mg/kg p.o., i.m. q24h; **Bearded dragons:** 10 mg/kg i.m.[d] Burmese pythons: 10 mg/kg i.m., then q48h; **Pit vipers:** 10 mg/kg i.m. q48–72h. **South American Rattlesnakes:** 10 mg/kg i.m.
Amphibians: 5–10 mg/kg p.o., s.c., i.m. topical application q24h[e].
Fish: 5–10 mg/kg i.m., intracoelomic, p.o. q24–48h for 7 doses or 2.5–5 mg/l by immersion for 5 h q24–48h for 5–7 treatments[f].

References
[a] Flammer K, Aucoin DP and Whitt DA (1991) Intramuscular and oral disposition of enrofloxacin in African grey parrots following single and multiple doses. *Journal of Veterinary Pharmacology and Therapeutics* **14(4)**, 359–366

[b] Raphael BL, Papich M and Cook RA (1994) Pharmacokinetics of enrofloxacin after a single intramuscular injection in Indian star tortoises (*Geochelone elegans*). *Journal of Zoo and Wildlife Medicine* **25**, 88–94

[c] James SB, Calle PP, Raphael BL *et al.* (2003) Comparison of injectable versus oral enrofloxacin pharmacokinetics in red-eared slider turtles (*Trachemys scripta elegans*). *Journal of Herpetological Medicine and Surgery* **13(1)**, 5–10

[d] Salvadori M, Vercelli C, De Vito V *et al.* (2017) Pharmacokinetic and pharmacodynamic evaluations of a 10 mg/kg enrofloxacin intramuscular administration in bearded dragons (*Pogona vitticeps*): a preliminary assessment. *Journal of Veterinary Pharmacology and Therapeutics* **40(1)**, 62–69

[e] Howard AM, Papich MG, Felt SA *et al.* (2010) The pharmacokinetics of enrofloxacin in adult African clawed frogs (*Xenopus laevis*). *Journal of the American Association for Laboratory Animal Science* **49(6)**, 800–804

[f] Lewbart G, Vaden S, Deen J *et al.* (1997) Pharmacokinetics of enrofloxacin in the red pacu (*Colossoma brachypomum*) after intramuscular, oral and bath administration. *Journal of Veterinary Pharmacology and Therapeutics* **20**, 124–128

Epinephrine see Adrenaline
Epoetin alfa, Epoetin beta see Erythropoietin
Equine chorionic gonadotrophin see Serum gonadotrophin

Erythromycin
(Erythrocin, Erythromycin*, Erythroped*) **POM-V, POM**

Formulations: Injectable: 200 mg/ml solution; 1 g/vial powder for reconstitution. Oral: 250 mg, 500 mg tablets/capsules; 25 mg/ml suspension; powder authorized for chickens.

Action: May be bactericidal (time-dependent) or bacteriostatic, depending upon drug concentration and bacterial susceptibility. It binds to the 50S ribosome, inhibiting peptide bond formation.

Use: Has a similar antibacterial spectrum to penicillins. It is active against Gram-positive cocci (some *Staphylococcus* species are resistant), Gram-positive bacilli and some Gram-negative bacilli (*Pasteurella*). Some strains of *Actinomyces*, *Nocardia*, *Chlamydia* and *Rickettsia* are also inhibited by erythromycin. Most of the Enterobacteriaceae (*Pseudomonas*, *Escherichia coli*, *Klebsiella*) are resistant. It is used in hamsters to treat proliferative ileitis (*Lawsonia intracellularis*) and in ferrets to control *Campylobacter* infection, although it may not eliminate intestinal carriage of this organism. Being a lipophilic weak base, it is concentrated in fluids that are more acidic than plasma, including milk, prostatic fluid and intracellular fluid. Resistance to erythromycin can be quite high, particularly in staphylococcal organisms. Erythromycin acts as a GI prokinetic by stimulating motilin receptors. Different esters of erythromycin are available. It is likely that the kinetics and possibly the toxicity will differ, depending on the ester used. Erythromycin's activity is enhanced in an alkaline pH. As the base is acid-labile it should be administered on an empty stomach. Used for the treatment of bacterial diseases in fish where practical.

Safety and handling: Normal precautions should be observed.

Contraindications: In humans the erythromycin estolate salt has been implicated in causing cholestatic hepatitis. Although not demonstrated in veterinary medicine, this salt should be avoided in animals with hepatic dysfunction. Avoid oral administration in small herbivores (e.g. rabbits).

Adverse reactions: Care should be taken in cases of hepatic or renal impairment. Avoid oral administration in small herbivores (e.g. rabbits), as can cause fatal enterotoxaemia. Its use as a prokinetic in these species is not advised. Use as a immersion treatment for fish may be harmful to biological filtration systems and is not advised.

Drug interactions: Erythromycin may enhance the absorption of digoxin from the GI tract and increase serum levels of cisapride, methylprednisolone, theophylline and terfenadine. The interactions with cisapride and terfenadine proved particularly significant in human medicine, leading to fatal or near-fatal arrhythmias in some patients receiving both drugs. Erythromycin should not be used in combination with other macrolide, lincosamide or chloramphenicol antimicrobials as antagonism may occur.

DOSES
See Appendix for guidelines on responsible antibacterial use.
Mammals: Ferrets: 10 mg/kg p.o. q6h; **Hamsters, Rats, Mice:** 20 mg/kg p.o. q12h or 0.13 mg/ml drinking water; **Primates:** 75 mg/kg p.o. q12h; **Hedgehogs:** 10 mg/kg p.o., i.m. q12h.
Birds: 20 mg/kg i.m., s.c. q8h; 60 mg/kg p.o. q12h or 125 mg/l of drinking water; 200 mg/kg soft feed.
Fish: 10–20 mg/kg i.m. q24h for 1–3 treatments or 100–200 mg/kg p.o. q24h for 7–21 days.
Reptiles, Amphibians: No information available.

Erythropoietin (Epoetin alfa, Epoetin beta)
(Eprex*, Neorecormon*) **POM**

Formulations: Injectable: 1000 IU, 2000 IU, 5000 IU powders for reconstitution; 2000 IU/ml, 4000 IU/ml, 10,000 IU/ml, 40,000 IU/ml solutions. Eprex is epoetin alfa. Neorecormon is epoetin beta.

Action: Stimulates division and differentiation of red blood cells.

Use: Recombinant human erythropoietin (r-HuEPO) is predominantly used to treat anaemia associated with chronic renal failure, although it is also used to treat anaemic human patients with cancer and rheumatoid arthritis. Erythropoietin is not indicated in conditions where high serum concentrations of the hormone already exist (e.g. haemolytic anaemia, anaemia due to blood loss), where the anaemia is due to iron deficiency or where systemic hypertension is present. Monitoring and/or supplementation of iron may be necessary, especially if response to treatment is poor. Darbepoetin may be a better choice in many cases.

Safety and handling: Normal precautions should be observed.

Contraindications: Conditions where high serum concentrations of erythropoietin already exist.

Adverse reactions: Local and systemic allergic reactions may rarely develop (skin rash at the injection site, pyrexia, arthralgia and mucocutaneous ulcers).

Drug interactions: No information available.

DOSES
Mammals: Ferrets, Rabbits: epoetin alfa: 50–150 IU/kg i.m., s.c. q48–72h; Primates: 50–100 IU/kg s.c., i.v. 3 times a week. Once desired PCV reached, administer q7d for at least 4 weeks for maintenance.
Birds, Reptiles, Amphibians, Fish: No information available.

Ethylene glycol monophenyl ether see Phenoxyethanol

Eugenol (Isoeugenol, Oil of clove) (Koi calm) ESPA

Formulations: Immersion: Oil for dissolution in water.

Action: Produces anaesthesia by impeding peripheral nerve signal transmission to the CNS.

Use: For the sedation, immobilization, anaesthesia and euthanasia of fish. Ideally, the drug should be used in water from the tank or pond of origin to minimize problems due to changes in water chemistry. Over-the-counter preparations contain about 1 g eugenol per ml but are poorly soluble in water and must be made into a stock solution (e.g. 1:10 with 95% ethanol produces 100 mg/ml) for more accurate dosing. The anaesthetic solution should be used on the day of preparation and be well aerated during use. Food should be withheld from fish for 12–24 h before anaesthesia to reduce the risk of regurgitation. The stage of anaesthesia reached is determined by the concentration used and the duration of exposure since absorption continues throughout the period of immersion. Different species vary in their response and may require different concentrations. It is recommended to use the lower dose rates to test the selected drug concentration and exposure time with a small group before medicating large numbers. Fish may retain some movement during anaesthesia, making it less desirable to use during surgery. Anaesthetized fish should be returned to clean water from their normal environment to allow recovery. For euthanasia, use 5–10 times the normal anaesthetic dose and keep the fish in the solution for at least 60 minutes after respiration ceases.

Safety and handling: Normal precautions should be observed.

Contraindications: No information available.

Adverse reactions: Cardiorespiratory depression and death have been noted in some tropical marine fish (e.g. tangs, surgeonfish).

Drug interactions: No information available.

DOSES

Amphibians: Leopard frogs: 255 mg/l results in variable degree of sedation [a]; **African clawed frogs:** 350 mg/l resulted in anaesthesia after 5–10 minutes immersion [b]; **Tiger salmanders:** 450 mg/l resulted in anaesthesia in ~10 minutes in 80% of animals [c].

Fish: Anaesthesia: 40–120 mg/l by immersion; Euthanasia: 500–1000 mg/ml by immersion or undiluted 10 drops/l (whisk to thoroughly mix with water) by immersion [1]. Follow manufacturer's recommendations for proprietary formulations.

Mammals, Birds, Reptiles: No information available.

References

[a] Lafortune M, Mitchell MA and Smith JA (2001) Evaluation of Medetomidine, Clove Oil and Propofol for Anesthesia of Leopard Frogs, *Rana pipiens*. *Journal of Herpetological Medicine and Surgery* **11(4)**, 13–18

[b] Guénette SA, Hélie P, Beaudry F and Vachon P (2007) Eugenol for anesthesia of African clawed frogs (*Xenopus laevis*). *Veterinary Anaesthesia and Analgesia* **34(3)**, 164–170

[c] Mitchell MA, Riggs SM, Singleton CB, Diaz-Figueroa O and Hale LK (2009) Evaluating the clinical and cardiopulmonary effects of clove oil and propofol in tiger salamanders (*Ambystoma tigrinum*). *Journal of Exotic Pet Medicine* **18(1)**, 50–56

[1] Sneddon LU (2012) Clinical anaesthesia and analgesia in fish. *Journal of Exotic Pet Medicine* **21**, 32–43

Famciclovir
(Famvir*) **POM**

Formulations: Oral: 125 mg, 250 mg tablet.

Action: Inhibits viral replication (viral DNA polymerase); depends on viral thymidine kinase for phosphorylation.

Use: Famciclovir is a pro-drug for penciclovir, which is closely related to aciclovir. Famciclovir is virostatic and is unable to eradicate latent viral infection. Has been used experimentally in ducks to control hepatitis B virus infection.

Safety and handling: Normal precautions should be observed.

Contraindications: No information available.

Adverse reactions: Little information available. A dose of 90 mg/kg caused no changes in liver enzymes (single dose) but adversely affected the conjunctival goblet cell density and therefore the quality of the tear film in cats.

Drug interactions: No information available.

DOSES
Birds: Ducklings: 10 mg/kg p.o. q24h [a].
Reptiles: 10–30 mg/kg p.o. q24h used to manage ranavirus outbreak in Eastern box turtles [b].
Mammals, Amphibians, Fish: No information available.

References
[a] Lin E, Luscombe C, Colledge D, Wang YY and Locarnini S (1998) Long-term therapy with the guanine nucleoside analog penciclovir controls chronic duck hepatitis B virus infection in vivo. Antimicrobial Agents and Chemotherapy **42(8)**, 2132–2137
[b] Sim RR, Allender MC, Crawford LK et al. (2016) Ranavirus epizootic in captive eastern box turtles (Terrapene carolina carolina) with concurrent herpesvirus and mycoplasma infection: management and monitoring. Journal of Zoo and Wildlife Medicine **47(1)**, 256–270

Famotidine
(Pepcid*) **POM**

Formulations: Oral: 20 mg, 40 mg tablets.

Action: Potent histamine (H2) receptor antagonist blocking histamine-induced gastric acid secretion. It is many times more potent than cimetidine, but has poorer oral bioavailability (37%).

Use: Management of gastric and duodenal ulcers, idiopathic, uraemic or drug-related erosive gastritis, oesophagitis, and hypersecretory conditions secondary to gastrinoma, mast cell neoplasia or short bowel syndrome. Reduction of vomiting due to gastric ulceration is typically achieved in about 2 weeks. However, animals should be treated for at least 2 weeks after the remission of clinical signs, so a minimum treatment duration of 28 days is recommended. Currently cimetidine is the only antiulcer drug with a veterinary market authorization. Has little effect on GI motility in humans.

Safety and handling: Normal precautions should be observed.

Contraindications: No information available.

Adverse reactions: In humans famotidine has fewer side effects than cimetidine.

Drug interactions: Famotidine is devoid of many of the interactions of the H2 related antagonist cimetidine.

DOSES
Mammals: Ferrets: 0.25–0.5 mg/kg p.o., i.v., s.c. q24h; **Rabbits:** 0.5 mg/kg p.o., s.c., i.v. q12h; **Guinea pigs:** 0.4 mg/kg p.o., s.c. q24h; Chinchillas: 0.5 mg/kg s.c. q24h; **Primates:** 0.5–0.8 mg/kg p.o. q24h. ***Birds, Reptiles, Amphibians, Fish:*** No information available.

Febantel see Pyrantel

Fenbendazole
(Bob Martin Easy to Use Wormer, Granofen, **Lapizole**, **Panacur**, Zerofen) **NFA-VPS, ESPA**

Formulations: Oral: 222 mg/g granules (22%); 20 mg/ml oral suspension (2%); 25 mg/ml oral suspension (2.5%); 100 mg/ml oral suspension (10%); 187.5 mg/g oral paste (18.75%).

Action: Inhibits fumarate reductase system of parasites thereby blocking the citric acid cycle and also reduces glucose absorption by the parasite.

Use: Treatment of oxyurids, ascarids (including larval stages), hookworms, whipworms, tapeworms (*Taenia*), *Oslerus osleri*, *Aelurostrongylus abstrusus*, *Angiostrongylus vasorum*, *Capillaria aerophila*, *Ollulanus tricuspis*, *Physaloptera rara* and *Paragonimus kellicotti* infections. Fenbendazole has 100% efficacy in clearing *Giardia* cysts. It is used in rabbits for the treatment of *Encephalitozoon cuniculi*. Unlike some other benzimidazoles, fenbendazole is safe to use in pregnant animals. Used for the treatment of non-encysted gastrointestinal nematodes, some cestodes (*Bothriocephalus*) and external monogenean parasites in fish.

Safety and handling: Normal precautions should be observed.

Contraindications: No information available.

Adverse reactions: Birds, especially vultures and storks, and some raptors, are more sensitive to adverse reactions affecting bone marrow, intestinal and liver functions. In pigeons and doves, mortality of 50% has occurred at doses of 20 mg/kg p.o. given on 3 consecutive days. Vomiting, depression and death within 96 h are recorded in some raptors. Feather damage has also been reported in pigeons. Has been associated with profound leucopenia in *Testudo hermanni* following two courses of 50 mg/kg fenbendazole given daily for 5 days per course. Avoid in reptiles with suspected septicaemia. Some species of fish (e.g. discus) may react adversely to some formulations of fenbendazole by immersion. The sudden death of a large burden of nematodes may cause tissue damage or intestinal blockage.

Drug interactions: No information available.

DOSES

Mammals: Rabbits: *E. cuniculi:* 20 mg/kg p.o. q24h for 28 days[a]; Oxyuriasis: 50 ppm (50 mg/kg) in feed for 5 days[b]; **Primates:** 50 mg/kg p.o. q24h for 3 days; **Sugar gliders:** 20–50 mg/kg p.o. q24h for 3 days, repeat in 14 days; **Hedgehogs:** 10–30 mg/kg p.o. q24h for 5 days; **Other small mammals:** 20–50 mg/kg p.o. q24h for 5 consecutive days; the higher end of the range is suggested for giardiasis only.

Birds:
- Nematodes[c]: 20–100 mg/kg p.o., administer 2 doses separated by 10 days; capillariasis: 25 mg/kg p.o. q24h for 5 consecutive days; **Pigeons:** 16 mg/kg p.o. once, repeat after 10 days if necessary or 10–20 mg/kg p.o. q24h for 3 days, repeat after 2 weeks; **Passerines:** 20 mg/kg p.o. q24h for 3 doses. Not advisable to give more than 50 mg/kg in unfamiliar species.
- Giardiasis: 50 mg/kg p.o. q24h for 3 doses[d].

Reptiles:
- Nematodes: 50–100 mg/kg p.o., per cloaca once or 20–25 mg/kg p.o., per cloaca q24h over 3–5 day course[e]; Repeated doses have been advised but may be unnecessary as complete effect may not be seen until 31 days post-treatment[f].
- Giardiasis and flagellates: 50 mg/kg p.o. q24h for 3–5 days.

Amphibians: 100 mg/kg p.o., repeat in 2 weeks.

Fish: External monogenean parasites: 25 mg/l by immersion for 12 h; Gastrointestinal nematodes: 50 mg/kg p.o. q24h for 2 days, repeat in 14 days.

References
[a] Suter C, Müller-Doblies UU, Hatt JM and Deplazes P (2001) Prevention and treatment of *Encephalitozoon cuniculi* infection in rabbits with fenbendazole. *Veterinary Record* **148(15)**, 478–480

[b] Düwel D and Brech K (1981) Control of oxyuriasis in rabbits by fenbendazole. *Laboratory Animal* **15(2)**, 101–105

[c] Lawrence K (1983) Efficacy of fenbendazole against nematodes of captive birds. *Veterinary Record* **112**, 433–434

[d] Yazwinski TA, Andrews P, Holtzen H et al. (1986) Dose-titration of fenbendazole in the treatment of poultry nematodiasis. *Avian Diseases* **30(4)**, 716–718

[e] Holt PE (1982) Efficacy of fenbendazole against the nematodes of reptiles. *Veterinary Record* **110**, 302–304

[f] Giannetto S, Brianti E, Poglayen G et al. (2007) Efficacy of oxfendazole and fenbendazole against tortoise (*Testudo hermanni*) oxyurids. *Parasitology Research* **100**, 1069–1073

Fentanyl

(Fentadon, Durogesic*, Fentanyl*, Fentora*, Sublimaze*) **POM-V CD SCHEDULE 2, POM CD SCHEDULE 2**

Formulations: Oral: 100 µg, 200 µg, 400 µg, 600 µg, 800 µg tablets. **Injectable:** 50 µg/ml solution. **Transdermal:** 12.5 µg/h, 25 µg/h, 50 µg/h, 75 µg/h, 100 µg/h patches.

Action: Synthetic pure mu (OP3) receptor agonist.

Use: Very potent opioid analgesic (50 times more potent than morphine) used to provide profound intraoperative analgesia. Can also be used at low dose rates for postoperative analgesia. Use of potent opioids during anaesthesia contributes to a balanced anaesthesia technique, therefore the dose of other concurrently administered anaesthetic agents should be reduced. Fentanyl has a rapid onset of action after i.v. administration and short duration of action (10–20 min depending on dose). After prolonged administration (>4 hours) or high doses its duration of action is significantly prolonged as the tissues become saturated. It can be used intraoperatively to provide analgesia by intermittent bolus doses or by a continuous rate infusion. Postoperatively fentanyl can be given by continuous rate infusion to provide analgesia, doses at the low end of the dose range should be used and respiratory function monitored. Its clearance is similar to morphine whilst its elimination half-life is longer, reflecting its higher lipid solubility and volume of distribution.

Safety and handling: Veterinary surgeons must undergo training in order to become authorized to prescribe transdermal fentanyl and receive the drug from veterinary wholesalers. The transdermal solution of fentanyl is very concentrated with the potential to cause opioid overdose (associated with respiratory depression) if absorbed systemically by humans (e.g. through contact with the skin or mucosal surfaces such as the eyes and mouth). Personal protective clothing consisting of latex or nitrile gloves, eye protection and suitable protective clothing must be worn when handling the product. Following application to the skin, the site must not be touched for at least 5 min until the solution is dry. It is advisable to wear gloves when handling animals to which transdermal fentanyl has been applied for up to 72 hours following application or to wash hands immediately after handling the animal in this time window. Owners should be advised that children <15 kg body weight should not be allowed to come into contact with animals treated with transdermal fentanyl until 72 hours after application. The manufacturer provides information to give to the owner at the time of discharge, detailing the effects of the drug and the risks of human exposure. Other animals should not be allowed to come into contact with the site of application on treated animals for 72 hours following application. If animals are sent home with transdermal fentanyl patches the owners must be warned about the dangers of patch ingestion by humans or other animals.

Contraindications: No information available.

Adverse reactions: Intraoperative administration is likely to cause respiratory depression, therefore, respiration should be monitored and facilities must be available to provide positive pressure ventilation. Rapid i.v. injection can cause severe bradycardia, even asystole, therefore the drug should be given slowly. A reduction in heart rate is likely whenever fentanyl is given, atropine can be administered to counter bradycardia if necessary. Apart from the effects on heart rate, fentanyl has limited other effects on cardiovascular function when used at clinical dose rates.

Drug interactions: Fentanyl can be used to reduce the dose requirement for other anaesthetic drugs in patients with cardiovascular instability or systemic disease.

DOSES
Mammals: Ferrets: 10–30 μg (micrograms)/kg/h i.v. CRI, reduce to 1.25–5 μg/kg/h for postoperative analgesia; **Rabbits:** 7.5 μg/kg q20min; 30–100 μg/kg/h by CRI during anaesthesia; **Primates:** 5–10 μg/kg i.v. or 25 μg/kg/h CRI [a].

Birds: Red-tailed hawks: 20 μg (micrograms) bolus i.v. followed by 0.2–0.5 μg/kg/min i.v. infusion reduced isoflurane requirement without effect on heart rate or blood pressure [b]; **White (umbrella) cockatoos:** 0.02 mg/kg i.m. produced no analgesia but was well tolerated; 0.2 mg/kg produced some analgesia but signs of hyperactivity in some birds in first 15–30 min after administration [c].

Reptiles: 12 μg (micrograms)/h transdermal fentanyl patch results in plasma concentrations above analgesic threshold in mammals, when tested in ball pythons [d] and prehensile-tailed skinks [e]. Analgesic efficacy not established, although anecdotally may be useful in snakes.

Amphibians, Fish: No information available.

References
[a] Valverde CR, Mama KR, Kollias-Baker C, Steffey EP and Baggot JD (2000) Pharmacokinetics and cardiopulmonary effects of fentanyl in isoflurane-anaesthetized rhesus monkeys (*Macaca mulatta*). *American Journal of Veterinary Research* **61(8)**, 931–934

[b] Pavez JC, Hawkins MG, Pascoe PJ, Knych HKD and Kass PH (2011) Effect of fentanyl target controlled infusions on isoflurane minimum anaesthetic concentration and cardiovascular function in red tailed hawks (*Buteo jamaicensis*). *Veterinary Anaesthesia and Analgesia* **38(4)**, 344–351

[c] Hoppes S, Flammer K, Hoersch K, Papich M and Paul-Murphy J (2003) Disposition and analgesic effects of fentanyl in white cockatoos (*Cacatua alba*). *Journal of Avian Medicine and Surgery* **17(3)**, 124–131

[d] Kharbush RJ, Gutwillig A, Hartzler KE *et al.* (2017) Antinociceptive and respiratory effects following application of transdermal fentanyl patches and assessment of brain μ-opioid receptor mRNA expression in ball pythons. *American Journal of Veterinary Research* **78(7)**, 785–795

[e] Gamble KC (2008) Plasma fentanyl concentrations achieved after transdermal fentanyl patch application in prehensile-tailed skinks, *Corucia zebrata*. *Journal of Herpetological Medicine and Surgery* **18(3)**, 81–85

Fentanyl/Fluanisone
(Hypnorm) **POM-V CD SCHEDULE 2**

Formulations: Injectable: 0.2 mg/ml fentanyl with 10 mg/ml fluanisone.

Action: Fentanyl is a pure mu opioid agonist and fluanisone is a butyrophenone; the combination produces neuroleptanalgesia.

Use: Licensed for use in rabbits, guinea pigs, mice and rats. Sedation and analgesia for restraint and to allow minor procedures to be carried out in mice, rats, rabbits, guinea pigs and primates. Combined with a benzodiazepine it can be used to produce anaesthesia with muscle relaxation for surgery. It can be used for premedication prior to induction of anaesthesia with propofol or alfaxalone in rabbits. Fentanyl/fluanisone produces a long duration of sedation and analgesia in small mammals (30–60 min), the duration of action is dependent on dose and varies between species. When used in combination with a benzodiazepine to produce anaesthesia, the lowest end of the dose range of fentanyl/fluanisone should be used. Hypnorm is miscible with midazolam at appropriate dilutions, enabling a single injection to produce anaesthesia. Duration of anaesthesia is approximately 20–40 min, although recovery can be very prolonged. Various dose regimens for different species have been published. Prolonged respiratory depression in the recovery period can be avoided by the administration of a partial mu agonist (buprenorphine) at the end of the procedure. This will reverse respiratory depression induced by fentanyl and provide continued analgesia. Small mammals should be weighed before drug administration, accurate dosing is imperative to prevent overdose. Oxygen supplementation via a face mask is recommended during sedation and anaesthesia of all animals.

Safety and handling: Normal precautions should be observed.

Contraindications: Animals with pre-existing respiratory compromise.

Adverse reactions: Respiratory depression can occur when given in high doses, particularly during the recovery period. Administration of buprenorphine in the recovery period can ameliorate respiratory depression and sedation, and provide ongoing analgesia. Measures should be taken to maintain normothermia during the sedation/anaesthesia and recovery period.

Drug interactions: No information available.

DOSES
When used for sedation is generally given as part of a combination. See Appendix for sedation protocols in all species.
Mammals: Rabbits: 0.1–0.5 ml/kg i.m.; **Guinea pigs:** 0.5–1 ml/kg i.m.; **Rats:** 0.2–0.5 ml/kg i.m., i.p.; **Mice:** 0.1–0.5 ml/kg i.p.; **Primates:** 0.1–0.3 ml/kg i.m. Doses at the highest 50% of these ranges are associated with extremely long recoveries and potentially

hypothermia. Reversal with partial or complete opioid antagonists may be required in such cases. Doses for sick animals should start at the lowest end of the range.

Birds, Reptiles, Amphibians, Fish: No information available.

Finasteride

(Proscar*) **POM**

Formulations: Oral: 5 mg tablet.

Action: Competitively inhibits dihydrotestosterone (DHT) production within the prostate. DHT is the main hormonal stimulus for the development of benign prostatic hyperplasia.

Use: Treatment of benign prostatic hyperplasia associated with adrenal gland disease.

Safety and handling: Women of child-bearing age should avoid handling crushed or broken tablets as finasteride is potentially teratogenic.

Contraindications: Do not use in breeding ferrets.

Adverse reactions: Secreted into semen and causes fetal anomalies.

Drug interactions: No information available.

DOSES
Mammals: Ferrets: 5 mg/kg p.o. q24h.
Birds, Reptiles, Amphibians, Fish: No information available.

Fipronil

(**Amflee Combo Spot-on Solution for Cats and Ferrets, Bob Martin Clear Plus Spot-on Solution for Cats and Ferrets**, Certifect, Effipro, Eliminall, Felevox, **Fiproclear Combo Spot-on Solution,** Fipronil, Fiprospot, **Fleanil Duo Spot-on Solution for Cats and Ferrets, Frontline Combo Spot On Cat, Frontline Plus Spot On Cat, Fyperix Combo Spot-on Solution for Cats and Ferrets, PrestiGon Combo Spot-on Solution for Cats and Ferrets**) **NFA-VPS, POM-V**

Formulations: Topical: 10% w/v fipronil spot-on pipettes in a wide range of sizes (Effipro, Frontline); with S-methoprene (Frontline Combo); with S-methoprene and amitraz (Certifect). Also 0.25% w/v fipronil spray in alcohol base (Effipro and Frontline sprays) in a range of sizes.

Action: Fipronil interacts with ligand-gated (GABA) chloride channels, blocking pre- and postsynaptic transfer of chloride ions, resulting in death of parasites on contact.

Use: Treatment of fleas, lice and ticks in mammals and birds. Treatment of mites and ticks in reptiles. Has been used to treat *Hirstiella* mites in green iguanas, but still needs further safety evaluation in other species. Beware of use in juvenile reptiles and immediately after skin slough due to increased permeability of skin and associated toxicity. Treatment of the environment is also recommended. Care with overuse of alcohol-based spray in birds[a].

Safety and handling: Normal precautions should be observed.

Contraindications: Do not use in rabbits. Beware of use in debilitated reptiles, those which have recently shed their skin and in small species where overdosage and toxicity may occur. May be harmful to aquatic organisms.

Adverse reactions: Local pruritus or alopecia may occur at the site of application.

Drug interactions: A low dose of amitraz has been shown to have a synergistic effect on the speed of tick kill, thus reducing the risk of transmission for tick-borne pathogens.

DOSES
Mammals: Ferrets: spray 3–6 ml/kg (6–12 pumps/kg 100 ml application) q30–60d; One spot-on pipette of 0.5 ml/animal (50 mg fipronil, 60 mg *S*-methoprene) applied topically to back of neck; Rodents: 7.5 mg/kg topically (15 pumps/kg 100 ml application) q30–60d. **Other mammals:** apply lightly q14d.
Birds: Use spray form q30–60d. Apply to cotton wool and dab behind head, under wings and at base of tail (raptors/parrots) or lightly under each wing (pigeons/passerines).
Reptiles: Spray on to cloth first then wipe over surface of reptile q7–14d until negative for ectoparasites.
Amphibians, Fish: Not indicated.

References
[a] Kitulagodage M, Astheimer LB and Buttemer WA (2008) Diacetone alcohol, a dispersant solvent, contributes to acute toxicity of a fipronil-based insecticide in a passerine bird. *Ecotoxicology and Enviromental Safety* **71(2)**, 597–600

Florfenicol
(Florocol, Nuflor) POM-V

Formulations: Injectable: 300 mg/ml, 450 mg/ml solution. Oral: 500 mg/g powder.

Action: Bacteriostatic antimicrobial that acts by binding to the 50S ribosomal subunit of susceptible bacteria, preventing bacterial protein synthesis.

Use: Treatment of bacterial diseases in fish.

Safety and handling: Normal precautions should be observed.

Contraindications: No information available.

Adverse reactions: No information available.

Drug interactions: No information available.

DOSES

Fish: 25–50 mg/kg i.m., intracoelomic q24h or 5–50 mg/kg p.o. q24h for 10 days [a,b].

Mammals, Birds, Reptiles, Amphibians: No information available.

References

[a] Yanong RP, Curtis EW, Simmons R *et al.* (2005) Pharmacokinetic studies of florfenicol in koi carp and threespot gourami *Trichogaster trichopterus* after oral and intramuscular treatment. *Journal of Aquatic Animal Health* **17(2)**, 129–137

[b] Lewbart G, Papich MG and Whitt-Smith D (2005) Pharmacokinetics of florfenicol in the red pacu (*Piaractus brachypomum*) after single dose intramuscular injection. *Journal of Veterinary Pharmacology and Therapeutics* **28**, 317–319

Flubendazole
(Anti Fluke &Wormer, Flubenol, Flukasol Suspension, Fluke-M) **ESPA**

Formulations: Immersion: 5% powder (Fluke-M); <0.8% liquid (Flukasol Suspension), 1% liquid (Anti Fluke & Wormer).

Action: Benzimidazoles bind to a structural protein of the parasite microtubules, important organelles involved in major cell processes, causing paralysis, death and expulsion of the parasites.

Use: Treatment of monogenetic trematode ectoparasites (e.g. skin and gill flukes) and internal nematodes in fish. Used to kill snails and hydra in aquaria. Flubendazole has a low solubility but a high potency.

Safety and handling: Normal precautions should be observed.

Contraindications: No information available.

Adverse reactions: No information available.

Drug interactions: No information available.

DOSES

Fish: 2 mg/l by prolonged immersion once and change 30% of water after 6 days. Follow manufacturer's recommendations for proprietary formulations.

Mammals, Birds, Reptiles, Amphibians: No information available.

Flucloxacillin

(Floxapen*, Flucloxacillin*) **POM**

Formulations: Injectable: Flucloxacillin sodium: 250 mg, 500 mg, 1 g powders for reconstitution. **Oral:** Flucloxacillin sodium: 250 mg or 500 mg capsules; powder for reconstitution with water giving a final concentration of 125 mg/5 ml, 250 mg/5 ml. Formulations of flucloxacillin with ampicillin are available (Co-fluampicil, Magnapen).

Action: Beta-lactamase-resistant, narrow-spectrum beta-lactam antibiotic. It binds to penicillin-binding proteins, decreasing bacterial cell wall strength and rigidity, and affecting cell division, growth and septum formation. Flucloxacillin is bactericidal and works in a time-dependent fashion.

Use: Stable in gastric acid so can be given orally but food significantly reduces its bioavailability. It is less active than penicillin G or V against *Streptococcus* and obligate anaerobic bacteria, and is indicated for the treatment of infections caused by beta-lactamase-producing *Staphylococcus*. Patients with significant renal or hepatic dysfunction may need dosage adjustment. The amount of sodium in flucloxacillin sodium may be clinically important for patients on restricted sodium intakes. Although flucloxacillin is absorbed from the GI tract, food has a significant inhibitory effect on its bioavailability; doses must be given on an empty stomach therefore limiting potential use in rabbits and rodents. As flucloxacillin kills in a time-dependent fashion, dosing regimens should be designed to maintain tissue concentrations above the MIC throughout the interdosing interval. Use with care in hepatic disease or hepatic impairment.

Safety and handling: Normal precautions should be observed.

Contraindications: Do not administer to animals with a history of sensitivity to beta-lactam antimicrobials. Use of penicillins should be avoided in rabbits, other small herbivores, hamsters and gerbils especially via the oral route.

Adverse reactions: Nausea, diarrhoea and skin rashes are the commonest adverse effects. Cholestatic hepatitis has been reported in humans. Avoid oral administration in small herbivores (e.g. rabbits), hamsters and gerbils as penicillins can cause fatal enterotoxaemia.

Drug interactions: Avoid the concomitant use of bacteriostatic antibiotics. The aminoglycosides (e.g. gentamicin) may inactivate penicillins when mixed together in parenteral solutions. A synergistic effect is seen when beta-lactam and aminoglycoside antimicrobials are used concurrently.

DOSES

See Appendix for guidelines on responsible antibacterial use.
Mammals: Rats: 200 mg/kg s.c. q8h [a].
Birds, Reptiles, Amphibians, Fish: No information available.

References

[a] Gisby J, Beale AS, Bryant JE and Toseland CD (1994) Staphylococcal osteomyelitis – a comparison of co-amoxiclav with clindamycin and flucloxacillin in an experimental rat model. *Journal of Antimicrobial Chemotherapy* **34(5)**, 755–764

Fluconazole
(Diflucan*, Fluconazole*) **POM**

Formulations: Oral: 50 mg, 150 mg, 200 mg capsules; 40 mg/ml suspension. Injectable: 2 mg/ml solution.

Action: Inhibition of the synthesis of ergosterol in fungal cell membranes, thus causing increased cell wall permeability and allowing leakage of cellular contents.

Use: Effective against *Blastomyces*, *Candida*, *Cryptococcus*, *Coccidioides*, *Histoplasma* and *Microsporum canis* infections and variably effective against *Aspergillus* and *Penicillium* infections. Has been used for treatment of dermatophytosis in green iguanas. In amphibians, it prolonged survival in frogs with chytridiomycosis but did not prevent mortality. It attains therapeutic concentrations in the CNS and respiratory tract. It is excreted by the kidney, producing high concentrations in urine. Reduce dose in animals with renal impairment and liver disease. This drug should be used until clinical signs have resolved and the organism is no longer present; this may take up to 2 months in some cases.

Safety and handling: Normal precautions should be observed.

Contraindications: Do not use in pregnant/lactating animals.

Adverse reactions: Adverse effects may include nausea and diarrhoea. May be hepatotoxic. May cause vomiting in birds.

Drug interactions: Fluconazole (due to inhibition of cytochrome P450-dependent liver enzymes) may increase plasma theophylline concentrations. In humans, fluconazole has led to terfenadine toxicity when the two drugs were administered together. Fluconazole increases ciclosporin blood levels.

DOSES
Mammals: Rabbits: 25–43 mg/kg i.v. infusion (slow) q12h; 37.5 mg/kg p.o. q12h for *Aspergillus* keratitis; 5 mg/kg p.o. q24h for cryptococcal meningitis.
Birds: 10–20 mg/kg p.o. q24–48h [a].
Reptiles: 5 mg/kg p.o. q24h (iguanas with dermatophytosis).
Amphibians: 60 mg/kg p.o. q24h. Baths at 25 mg/l prolonged survival in frogs with chytridiomycosis but did not prevent mortality [b].
Fish: No information available.

References
[a] Flammer K and Papich M (2006) Pharmacokinetics of fluconazole after oral administration of single and multiple doses in African grey parrots. *American Journal of Veterinary Research* **67(3)**, 417–422
[b] Berger L, Speare R, Marantelli G and Skerratt LF (2009) A zoospore inhibition technique to evaluate the activity of antifungal compounds against *Batrachochytrium dendrobatidis* and unsuccessful treatment of experimentally infected green tree frogs (*Litoria caerulae*) by fluconazole and benzalkonium chloride. *Research in Veterinary Science* **87(1)**, 106–110

Fludrocortisone
(Florinef*) **POM**

Formulations: Oral: 0.1 mg tablets.

Action: Aldosterone analogue that increases potassium excretion and sodium retention but which also has some glucocorticoid properties.

Use: Treatment of adrenocortical insufficiency (post-adrenalectomy). Fludrocortisone is about 125 times more potent as a mineralocorticoid than is hydrocortisone but it is also about 12 times more potent as a glucocorticoid (and therefore about 3 times more potent than prednisolone). Monitor sodium and potassium concentrations separately (not just the ratio) 4–6 hours post-pill. Supplemental doses of prednisolone may be required at times of metabolic or physical stress.

Safety and handling: Normal precautions should be observed.

Contraindications: No information available.

Adverse reactions: Hypertension, oedema (including cerebral oedema) and hypokalaemia with overdosages. Long-term overdose may result in clinical signs of hypercortisolism.

Drug interactions: Hypokalaemia may develop if fludrocortisone is administered concomitantly with amphotericin B or potassium-depleting diuretics (furosemide, thiazides).

DOSES
Mammals: Ferrets: post-adrenalectomy: 0.05–0.1 mg/kg p.o. q24h.
Birds, Reptiles, Amphibians, Fish: No information available.

Flumazenil
(Flumazenil*) **POM**

Formulations: Injectable: 0.1 mg/ml

Action: Benzodiazepine antagonist.

Use: For the complete or partial reversal of the central sedative effects of benzodiazepines.

Safety and handling: Normal precautions should be observed.

Contraindications: No information available.

Adverse reactions: In humans, palpitations have been reported following rapid injection.

Drug interactions: No information available.

DOSES
Mammals: Rabbits: 0.01–0.1 mg/kg i.m., i.v.; **Chinchillas:** 0.1 mg/kg s.c. [a]; **Primates:** 0.02 mg/kg i.v.

Birds: Most species: 0.02–0.1 mg/kg i.m., i.v.; **Amazon parrots:** 0.05 mg/kg intranasally [b]; **Parakeets:** 0.13 mg/kg intranasally [c]; **Canaries:** 0.25–0.31 mg/kg intranasally [d]; **Zebra finches:** 0.3 mg/kg i.m. [e]

Reptiles: 0.05 mg/kg i.m., s.c., i.v.

Amphibians, Fish: No information available.

References

[a] Henke J, Baumgartner C, Röltgen I, Eberspächer E and Erhardt W (2004) Anaesthesia with midazolam/medetomidine/fentanyl in chinchillas (*Chinchilla lanigera*) compared to anaesthesia with xylazine/ketamine and medetomidine/ketamine. *Journal of Veterinary Medicine Series A* **51(5)**, 259–264

[b] Mans C, Guzman DSM, Lahner LL, Paul-Murphy J and Sladky KK (2012) Sedation and physiologic response to manual restraint after intranasal administration of midazolam in Hispaniolan Amazon parrots (*Amazona ventralis*). *Journal of Avian Medicine and Surgery* **26(3)**, 130–140

[c] Vesal N and Eskandari MH (2006) Sedative effects of midazolam and xylazine with or without ketamine and detomidine alone following intranasal administration in Ring-necked Parakeets. *Journal of the American Veterinary Medical Association* **228(3)**, 383–388

[d] Vesal N and Zare P (2006) Clinical evaluation of intranasal benzodiazepines, α2-agonists and their antagonists in canaries. *Veterinary Anaesthesia and Analgesia* **33(3)**, 143–148

[e] Prather JF (2012) Rapid and reliable sedation induced by diazepam and antagonized by flumazenil in zebra finches (*Taeniopygia guttata*). *Journal of Avian Medicine and Surgery* **26(2)**, 76–85

Fluoxetine
(Reconcile, Prozac*) **POM-V, POM**

Formulations: Oral: 8 mg, 16 mg, 20 mg, 32 mg, 64 mg tablets; 4 mg/ml liquid. Liquid formulation and some tablet sizes are available in the UK but not under veterinary authorization. Veterinary formulation (Reconcile) only available in certain European regions (not the UK).

Action: Fluoxetine and its primary metabolite norfluoxetine block serotonin re-uptake in the brain, resulting in antidepressive activity and a raising in motor activity thresholds. It also has minor noradrenaline re-uptake inhibition properties.

Use: Has been used to control feather picking and other compulsive type behaviours in psittacines but relapse following discontinuation of therapy is common. Should be used with a specifically constructed behaviour modification plan and with caution.

Safety and handling: Normal precautions should be observed.

Contraindications: Known sensitivity to fluoxetine or other SSRIs, history of seizures.

Adverse reactions: Common reactions include lethargy, decreased appetite and vomiting, which may result in minor weight loss. Trembling, restlessness and other GI disturbances may also occur and must be distinguished from a paradoxical increase in anxiety which has been reported in some cases. Owners should be warned of a potential increase in aggression in response to medication.

Drug interactions: Fluoxetine should not be used within 2 weeks of treatment with an MAOI (e.g. selegiline) and an MAOI should not be used within 6 weeks of treatment with fluoxetine. Fluoxetine, like other SSRIs, antagonizes the effects of anticonvulsants and so is not recommended for use with epileptic patients or in association with other agents which lower seizure threshold, e.g. phenothiazines. Caution is warranted if fluoxetine is used concomitantly with aspirin or other anticoagulants since the risk of increased bleeding in the case of tissue trauma may be increased.

DOSES
Mammals: Rats: 1–1.5 mg/kg p.o. q24h; *Primates:* 0.45–2.0 mg/kg p.o. q24h[a]; *Sugar gliders:* 2–5 mg/kg p.o. q12h.
Birds: 1–4 mg/kg p.o. q24h.
Reptiles, Amphibians, Fish: No information available.

References
[a] Fontenot MB, Musso MW, McFatter RM and Anderson GM (2009) Dose finding study of fluoxetine and venlafaxine for the treatment of self-injurious and stereotypic behaviour in rhesus macaques (*Macaca mulatta*). *Journal of the American Association for Laboratory Animal Science* **48(2)**, 176–184

Flurbiprofen
(Ocufen*) **POM**

Formulations: Ophthalmic: 0.03% solution in single-use vials.

Action: Inhibits prostaglandin synthesis producing an anti-inflammatory and analgesic action. Prostaglandins also play a role in the miosis produced during intraocular surgery by constricting the iris sphincter independently of cholinergic mechanisms.

Use: Before cataract surgery. It is also useful for anterior uveitis and ulcerative keratitis when topical corticosteroids are contraindicated. Topical NSAIDs have the potential to increase intraocular pressure and should be used with caution in animals predisposed to glaucoma.

Safety and handling: Normal precautions should be observed.

Contraindications: No information available.

Adverse reactions: As with other topical NSAIDs, flurbiprofen may cause local irritation. Topical NSAIDs can be used in ulcerative keratitis but with caution as they can delay epithelial healing. Topical NSAIDs have been associated with an increased risk of corneal 'melting' (keratomalacia) in humans, although this has not been reported in the veterinary literature. Regular monitoring is advised.

Drug interactions: Ophthalmic NSAIDs may be used safely with other ophthalmic pharmaceuticals, although concurrent use of drugs which adversely affect the corneal epithelium (e.g. gentamicin) may lead to increased corneal penetration of the NSAID. The concurrent use of topical NSAIDs with topical corticosteroids has been identified as a risk factor in humans for precipitating corneal problems.

DOSES
Mammals, Birds, Reptiles: 1 drop per eye q6–12h depending on severity of inflammation. 1 drop q30min for 4 doses preoperatively (presurgical protocols vary widely).
Amphibians, Fish: No information available.

Fluticasone
(Flixotide*) **POM**

Formulations: Inhalational: 50 µg, 125 µg, 250 µg metered inhalations (Evohaler).

Action: Binds to specific nuclear receptors and affects gene transcription such that many aspects of inflammation are suppressed.

Use: Used as an inhaled corticosteroid in the management of inflammatory airway disease. Administer via commercially available chambers and masks specifically designed for veterinary use. Not useful for acute bronchospasm (and cases of fluticasone-induced bronchospasm have been reported in humans).

Safety and handling: Normal precautions should be observed.

Contraindications: No information available.

Adverse reactions: Inhaled steroids are known to suppress the hypothalamic-pituitary-adrenal axis, although they are considered generally safer than systemic steroids.

Drug interactions: No information available.

DOSES
Mammals: Rabbits: 50–250 µg (micrograms)/animal q12–24h via feline spacer chamber administration.
Birds, Reptiles, Amphibians, Fish: No information available.

Formaldehyde (Formalin, Formol, Methanediol, Methanol)
(FMG Mixture, Formaldehyde 30% Solution, Protoban) **ESPA**

Formulations: Immersion: proprietary formulations are available (Formaldehyde 30% Solution); also available in combination with malachite green (FMG Mixture, Protoban).

Action: A biocide causing cell death by cross-linking with proteins.

Use: Treatment of protozoan and some monogenetic ectoparasites of fish. It has some effect on fungal infections of fish eggs (water mould) but little activity against most bacteria. Formalin is an aqueous solution of 37–40% formaldehyde gas (= 100% formalin);

diluted solutions are described according to the content of formalin, not formaldehyde. It is strongly recommended that a proprietary formulation is used initially to avoid problems related to purity and to enable accurate dosing. Dilute the measured dose 1:100 before adding to the fish tank or pond. Formalin can be irritating to the gills and chemically removes dissolved oxygen from the water, thus extra aeration must be provided. Do not use in water >27°C. It is usually supplied with 12–15% methanol to stabilize the solution and prevent the formation of paraformaldehyde, which appears as a white precipitate and is toxic to fish. Toxicity is increased at higher temperatures, low pH and low water hardness. Formaldehyde is toxic to some species of elasmobranchs (e.g. sharks, rays), plants and algae. Considered to have a synergistic effect with malachite green against protozoan ectoparasites.

Safety and handling: Formalin must be handled with care; wear protective gloves and use a respirator. It is volatile and irritating, carcinogenic and may cause contact hypersensitivity to skin and airways. Use in well-ventilated areas. Should be stored in dark bottles above 4°C to prevent paraformaldehyde formation.

Contraindications: Do not mix with potassium permanganate.

Adverse reactions: Fish gasping at the surface in water with low dissolved oxygen.

Drug interactions: No information available.

DOSES
Fish: All doses based on full strength formalin (= 37% formaldehyde): 0.125–0.25 ml/l by immersion for 30–60 min q24h for 2–3 days or 0.015–0.025 ml/l by prolonged immersion q48h for 3 treatments; follow the manufacturer's recommendations for proprietary formulations.
Mammals, Birds, Reptiles, Amphibians: No information available.

Formalin see **Formaldehyde**
Formol see **Formaldehyde**

Framycetin
(Canaural) **POM-V**

Formulations: Topical: 5 mg/g suspension (Canaural also contains fusidic acid, nystatin and prednisolone).

Action: Aminoglycosides inhibit bacterial protein synthesis and require an oxygen-rich environment to be effective, thus they are ineffective in low-oxygen sites (abscesses, exudates), making all obligate anaerobic bacteria resistant. They are bactericidal and their mechanism of killing is concentration-dependent, leading to a marked post-antibiotic effect, allowing pulse-dosing regimens which may limit toxicity.

Use: Treatment of aural infections. Framycetin is particularly effective against Gram-negative bacteria, although the combination preparation Canaural has a broad spectrum of activity.

Safety and handling: Normal precautions should be observed.

Contraindications: Do not use in animals with a perforated tympanum. Do not use in conjunction with other products known to be ototoxic. Corticosteroid-free preparations are preferred in pregnant animals and rabbits to avoid the systemic effects of corticosteroids.

Adverse reactions: Aminoglycosides are potentially ototoxic, and ataxia, deafness and nystagmus may be observed where drops have been administered with a perforated tympanum. Local irritation.

Drug interactions: No information available.

DOSES
See Appendix for guidelines on responsible antibacterial use.

Mammals: Widely used anecdotally for the treatment of otitis externa in several species and for parasitic otitis (*Otodectes*) in the ferret at a dose of 2–10 drops per ear q12h.

Birds, Reptiles, Amphibians, Fish: No information available.

Fresh water (dechlorinated) (Tap water, Reverse osmosis water)

Formulations: Liquid.

Action: Enters the cell of marine protozoan ectoparasites causing them to expand rapidly by osmotic pressure until they rupture. Monogenean trematodes are thought to release their hold and drop off, but not all die and some will recover if not removed from the environment.

Use: Treatment of skin and gill disease due to infestation with marine protozoan ectoparasites and monogenean trematodes. Prepare the treatment bath by increasing the water temperature to match that of the aquarium. Add sodium bicarbonate to increase the pH to match that of the aquarium, using a digital pH meter to confirm the result. If necessary, add one part sea water from the aquarium to five parts fresh water to produce a hyposaline solution and reduce the physiological stress on sensitive fish species. Initially, start with shorter bath treatment times and increase as necessary.

Safety and handling: None.

Contraindications: Severely infested fish with marked clinical signs may react badly to the osmotic stress but may tolerate and respond better to hyposalinity treatment (see above).

Adverse reactions: Carefully monitor the reactions of individual fish, which may vary differently to the immediate osmotic shock. Some species (e.g. angelfish) will lose orientation and lie on their sides temporarily, before recovering. If this initial loss of balance persists, then remove and return the fish to the aquarium.

Drug interactions: No information available.

DOSES
Fish: Immersion for 3–15 minutes, repeat weekly prn [1,2].
Mammals, Birds, Reptiles, Amphibians: No information available.

References
[1] Herwig N (1979) *Handbook of drugs and chemicals used in the treatment of fish diseases*. Charles C Thomas, Springfield, Illinois
[2] Noga EJ (2010) *Fish Disease – Diagnosis and Treatment, 2nd edn*. Wiley-Blackwell, Oxford

Furosemide (Frusemide)
(Dimazon, Frusecare, Frusedale, Frusol*) **POM-V, POM**

Formulations: Injectable: 50 mg/ml solution. **Oral:** 20 mg, 40 mg, 1 g tablets; 40 mg/5 ml oral solution.

Action: Loop diuretic, inhibiting the $Na^+/K^+/Cl^-$ cotransporter in the thick ascending limb of the loop of Henle. The net effect is a loss of sodium, potassium, chloride and water in the urine. It also increases excretion of calcium, magnesium and hydrogen as well as renal blood flow and glomerular filtration rate. Transient venodilation may occur following i.v. administration and in some species, bronchodilation may occur; the exact mechanism for both is unclear. Although the majority of avian nephrons lack a Loop of Henle, furosemide still appears effective in birds; however, the mechanism of action is not well understood. The exact mechanism of action in reptiles is also unclear, although it does appear to have a diuretic effect.

Use: Management of congestive heart failure (acute and chronic), non-cardiogenic oedema, hypercalcuric nephropathy, acute renal failure, hyperkalaemia and hypertension. Use with caution in patients with severe electrolyte depletion, hepatic failure and diabetes mellitus.

Safety and handling: Normal precautions should be observed.

Contraindications: Dehydration and anuria. Do not use in dehydrated or hyperuricaemic birds.

Adverse reactions: Hypokalaemia, hypochloraemia, hypocalcaemia, hypomagnesaemia and hyponatraemia; dehydration, polyuria/polydipsia and prerenal azotaemia occur readily. A marked reduction in cardiac output can occur in animals with severe pulmonary disease, low-output heart failure, hypertrophic cardiomyopathy, pericardial or myocardial disorders, cardiac tamponade and severe hypertension. Other adverse effects include ototoxicity, GI disturbances, leucopenia, anaemia, weakness and restlessness.

Drug interactions: Nephrotoxicity/ototoxicity associated with aminoglycosides may be potentiated when furosemide is also used. Furosemide may induce hypokalaemia, thereby increasing the risk of digoxin toxicity. Increased risk of hypokalaemia if furosemide given with acetazolamide, corticosteroids, thiazides and theophylline. Concurrent administration of NSAIDs with furosemide may decrease efficacy and may predispose to nephrotoxicity, particularly in patients with poor renal perfusion. Furosemide may inhibit the muscle relaxation qualities of tubocurarine, but increase the effects of suxamethonium.

DOSES
Mammals: **Ferrets:** 1–4 mg/kg i.v., i.m., p.o. q8–12h; **Rabbits:** 1–4 mg/kg i.v., i.m. q4–6h initially; maintenance doses are often 1–2 mg/kg p.o. q8–24h; **Rodents:** 1–4 mg/kg s.c., i.m. q4–6h or 5–10 mg/kg s.c., i.m. q12h; **Primates:** 1–4 mg/kg p.o., s.c. q12h, **Sugar gliders:** 1–5 mg/kg p.o., i.m., s.c. q6–12h; **Hedgehogs:** 2.5–5 mg/kg p.o., i.m., s.c. q8h.

Birds: 0.1–6.0 mg/kg i.m., s.c., i.v. q6–24h [1,2].

Reptiles: 5 mg/kg i.m. q24h [a].

Amphibians: Not indicated.

Fish: No information available.

References
[a] Parkinson LA and Mans C (2018) Effects of furosemide administration to water-deprived inland bearded dragons (*Pogona vitticeps*). *American Journal of Veterinary Research* **79(11)**, 1204–1208

[1] Watson M (2011) Furosemide. *Journal of Exotic Pet Medicine* **20(1)**, 60–63

[2] Fitzgerald BC, Dias S and Martorell J (2018) Cardiovascular Drugs in Avian, Small Mammal, and Reptile Medicine. *Veterinary Clinics: Exotic Animal Practice* **21(2)**, 399–442

Fusidic acid
(Canaural, Fuciderm, Isathal) POM-V

Formulations: Topical: 5 mg/g fusidate suspension (Canaural also contains framycetin, nystatin and prednisolone); 0.5% fusidic acid + 0.1% betamethasone cream (Fuciderm); 1% fusidic acid viscous solution (Isathal).

Action: Inhibits bacterial protein synthesis.

Use: Active against Gram-positive bacteria, particularly *Staphylococcus pseudintermedius*. It is used topically in the management of staphylococcal infections of the conjunctiva, skin or ear. Fusidic acid is able to penetrate skin and penetrate the cornea gaining access to the anterior chamber of the eye. The carbomer gel vehicle in the ocular preparation may also be efficacious as a surface lubricant.

Safety and handling: Avoid contamination of the container on application.

Contraindications: Corticosteroid-free preparations are preferred in pregnant animals, birds and rabbits to avoid the systemic effects of corticosteroids.

Adverse reactions: No information available.

Drug interactions: No information available.

DOSES
See Appendix for guidelines on responsible antibacterial use.

Mammals: Rabbits: 1 drop per eye q12–24h (Isathal); **Other mammals:** 1 drop per eye q12–24h as necessary (unlicensed).

Birds: Skin: apply a thin layer q24h; Ophthalmic: 1 drop per affected eye q12–24h.

Reptiles, Amphibians, Fish: No information available.

Gabapentin (Gabapentinum)
(Neurontin*) **POM-V CD SCHEDULE 3**

Formulations: Oral: 100 mg, 300 mg, 400 mg capsules; 600 mg, 800 mg film-coated tablets; 50 mg/ml solution.

Action: Gabapentin is an analogue of the neurotransmitter gamma-aminobutyric acid (GABA). The precise mechanism of action of gabapentin is unknown; however, it has been suggested that it mediates its anticonvulsive effect by increasing synaptic levels of GABA in the CNS, most likely through increased synthesis of GABA. Gabapentin has also been demonstrated to decrease the influx of calcium ions into neurons via a specific subunit of voltage-dependent calcium channels. It is believed that some of the therapeutic effect of gabapentin is mediated through binding to these channels. Gabapentin does not interact with sodium-dependent channels and demonstrates no affinity for the common neurotransmitter receptors, including benzodiazepine, glutamate, glycine and dopamine. The mode of action of the analgesic effect of gabapentin is unknown.

Use: Adjunctive therapy in the treatment of seizures refractory to treatment with conventional therapy. Also treatment of neuropathic pain, particularly if insensitive to opioid analgesics. After multiple dosing, peak plasma concentrations of gabapentin are usually achieved within 2 hours of a dose and steady state achieved within 1–2 days. Gabapentin therapy should only be withdrawn slowly. Monitoring of serum levels in human patients does not appear useful. Use with caution in patients with renal impairment, behavioural abnormalities or severe hepatic disease.

Safety and handling: Normal precautions should be observed.

Contraindications: No information available.

Adverse reactions: The most commonly reported adverse effect is mild sedation and ataxia. False-positive readings have been reported with some urinary protein tests in human patients taking gabapentin. Hepatic toxicity has been reported as a rare side effect in human patients.

Drug interactions: The absorption of gabapentin from the GI tract is reduced by antacids containing aluminium with magnesium; it is recommended that gabapentin is taken at least 2 hours after the administration of such an antacid. Cimetidine has been reported to reduce the renal clearance of gabapentin but the product information does not consider this to be of clinical importance.

DOSES
Mammals: Ferrets: 3–5 mg/kg p.o. q8h; **Rabbits:** 2–5 mg/kg p.o. q8h; Rats: 30 mg/kg p.o. q8h; Hamsters: 50 mg/kg p.o. q24h.
Birds: 10–11 mg/kg p.o. q8–24h[a]; **Amazon parrots:** 15 mg/kg p.o. q8h[b].
Reptiles, Amphibians, Fish: No information available.

References

[a] Yaw TJ, Zaffarano BA, Gall A *et al.* (2015) Pharmacokinetic properties of a single administration of oral gabapentin in the great horned owl (*Bubo virginianus*). *Journal of Zoo and Wildlife Medicine* **46(3)**, 547–552.

[b] Baine K, Jones MP, Cox S and Martín-Jiménez T (2015) Pharmacokinetics of compounded intravenous and oral gabapentin in Hispaniolan Amazon parrots (*Amazona ventralis*). *Journal of Avian Medicine and Surgery* **29(3)**, 165–173

Gentamicin

(Clinagel Vet, Easotic, Genta, Otomax, **Tiacil**, Genticin*) **POM-V, POM**

Formulations: Injectable: 40 mg/ml solution for i.v., i.m., s.c. injection (human preparation), 100 mg/ml solution for i.v., i.m., s.c. injection (Genta). **Ophthalmic/aural solution:** 0.5% solution (Tiacil); 0.3% ophthalmic gel (Clinagel). Gentamicin is a component of some topical ear preparations.

Action: Aminoglycosides inhibit bacterial protein synthesis and require an oxygen-rich environment to be effective, thus they are ineffective in low-oxygen sites (abscesses, exudates), making all obligate anaerobic bacteria resistant. They are bactericidal and their mechanism of killing is concentration-dependent, leading to a marked post-antibiotic effect, allowing pulse-dosing regimens which may limit toxicity.

Use: Active against Gram-negative bacteria, but some staphylococcal and streptococcal (*Streptococcus faecalis*) species are also sensitive. All obligate anaerobic bacteria and many haemolytic streptococci are resistant. Use in domestic animals is limited by nephrotoxicity and, more rarely, ototoxicity and neuromuscular blockade. Microbial resistance is a concern, although many bacteria resistant to gentamicin may be susceptible to amikacin. Consider specific glomerular filtration rate measurements to assess risk prior to initiating therapy. The trough serum level should be allowed to fall below 2 µg/ml. When used for 'blind' therapy of undiagnosed serious infections, gentamicin is usually given in conjunction with a penicillin and/or metronidazole. Aminoglycosides are more active in an alkaline environment. Geriatric animals or those with reduced renal function should only be given this drug systemically when absolutely necessary, although the move to dosing q24h should reduce the likelihood of nephrotoxicity. Use with caution in rabbits, birds and reptiles. Fluid therapy is essential during treatment of reptiles; monitor uric acid levels in birds and reptiles. Used for the treatment of bacterial disease in fish.

Safety and handling: Normal precautions should be observed.

Contraindications: Do not use the aural preparation if the tympanum is perforated. Do not use in conjunction with other drugs considered to be nephrotoxic. Avoid oral administration in small herbivores (e.g. rabbits).

Adverse reactions: Gentamicin delays epithelial healing of corneal ulcers and may cause local irritation. Nephrotoxicity and ototoxicity are potential side effects. Cellular casts in urine sediment are an early sign of impending nephrotoxicity; however, urine must be examined immediately to detect their presence and their absence is not a guarantee of safety. Serum creatinine levels rise later and fatal acute renal failure may be inevitable when they do. Gentamicin should not be used during pregnancy. In rabbits and other small herbivores, oral administration (including in impregnated beads) can cause fatal enterotoxaemia. Known nephrotoxicity in some aglomerular species of fish (e.g. toadfish) and toxicity to sensory hair cells of the fish ear.

Drug interactions: Avoid concurrent use of other nephrotoxic, ototoxic or neurotoxic agents (e.g. amphotericin B, furosemide). Increase monitoring and adjust dosages when these drugs must be used together. Aminoglycosides may be chemically inactivated by beta-lactam antibiotics (e.g. penicillins, cephalosporins) or heparin when mixed *in vitro*. The effect of non-depolarizing muscle relaxants (e.g. atracurium, pancuronium, vecuronium) may be enhanced by aminoglycosides. Synergism may occur when aminoglycosides are used with beta-lactam antimicrobials. Activity may be reduced if used in conjunction with bacteriostatic antimicrobials.

DOSES

See Appendix for guidelines on responsible antibacterial use.

Mammals: Ophthalmic: 1 drop per eye q6–8h. Severe ocular infections may require dosing q1–2h. A fortified topical solution (100 mg gentamicin in 5 ml of 0.3% solution, making 14.3 mg/ml) can be used. Otic: 1–3 drops (depending on weight of the animal) in affected ear or apply ointment to affected area q12h. **Ferrets:** 2–5 mg/kg i.v. (over 30 min), i.m., s.c. q12–24h; topically q6–8h; **Rabbits:** 4–8 mg/kg s.c., i.m., i.v. q24h; can be incorporated into antibiotic-impregnated beads (1 g/20 g methylmethacrylate) in surgical sites (e.g. in rabbits following abscess debridement), beads may require surgical removal at a later date; **Guinea pigs:** 6 mg/kg s.c. q24h; **Rats, Mice:** 4–20 mg/kg i.m. q12–24h; **Other rodents:** 2–5 mg/kg s.c., i.m. q12–24h; **Primates:** 2–4 mg/kg i.m., i.v. q12h; **Sugar gliders:** 1.5–2.5 mg/kg s.c., i.m. q12h; **Hedgehogs:** 2 mg/kg s.c., i.m. q8h. Ensure adequate renal function and hydration status before use. **All species:** nebulize 50 mg in 10 ml saline for 15 min q8–12h.

Birds: 2–10 mg/kg i.v., i.m. q6–12h; topically q6–8h; nebulize 50 mg in 10 ml saline for 15 min q8–12h [a].

Reptiles: Chelonians: 2–4 mg/kg i.m. q72h [b]; may also be nebulized at dilution of 10–20 mg gentamicin in 15 ml saline for 15–20 min q8–12h for respiratory tract infections in chelonians and lizards; **Most snakes:** 2.5 mg/kg i.m. q72h; **Blood pythons:** 2.5 mg/kg i.m. once, then 1.5 mg/kg i.m. q96h [c].

Amphibians: 3 mg/kg i.m. q24h; 1 mg/ml solution as 8 h bath q24–48h; 2 mg/ml dilution topically q6–8h for ocular disease [d].

Fish: 2.5–3 mg/kg i.m. q2–3d.

References

[a] Ramsey EC and Vulliet R (1993) Pharmacokinetic properties of gentamicin and amikacin in the cockatiel. *Avian Diseases* **37(2)**, 628–634

[b] Beck K, Loomis M, Lewbart GL *et al.* (1995) Preliminary comparison of plasma concentrations of gentamicin injected into the cranial and caudal limb musculature of the Eastern box turtle (*Terrapene carolina carolina*). *Journal of Zoo and Wildlife Medicine* **26(2)**, 265–268

[c] Hilf M, Swanson D, Wagner R and Yu VL (1991) A new dosing schedule for gentamicin in blood pythons (*Python curtus*): a pharmacokinetic study. *Research in Veterinary Science* **50(2)**, 127–130

[d] Teare JA, Wallace RS and Bush M (1991) Pharmacology of gentamicin in the leopard frog (*Rana pipiens*). *Proceedings of the Annual Conference of the American Association of Zoo Veterinarians*, pp. 128–131

Glucose (Dextrose)
(Aqupharm, 50% Glucose for injection, Vetivex)
POM-V, POM-VPS, POM

Formulations: Injectable: sodium chloride 0.9% w/v, glucose monohydrate 5.5% w/v (Aqupharm No. 3 and Vetivex 3), sodium chloride 0.18% w/v, glucose monohydrate 4.4% w/v (Aqupharm No. 18 and Vetivex 6), other electrolyte solutions with glucose for i.v. use: Glucose 40% and 50% w/v.

Action: Source of energy for cellular metabolism. Osmotic agent.

Use: Dilute glucose solutions are used for fluid replacement (primarily where intracellular and interstitial losses have occurred). Concentrated glucose solutions are used parenterally as an energy source or in the treatment of hypoglycaemia. Patients requiring parenteral nutritional support will require mixtures comprising combinations of amino acids, glucose solutions and fat. **See also Amino acid solutions** for use in parenteral nutrition. Solutions containing >5% glucose are hypertonic and irritant if given other than i.v. The 50% solutions contain 1.7 kcal/ml (8.4 kJ/ml) glucose and are extremely hypertonic (2525 mOsm/l). Use with caution in patients with insulin resistance and diabetes mellitus.

Safety and handling: Multi-use vials of 5% glucose or higher rapidly support bacterial growth and strict aseptic technique is required, single patient use is advised.

Contraindications: No information available.

Adverse reactions: 10–50% solutions are irritant and hyperosmolar; administer through a jugular catheter or dilute appropriately. Glucose infusions may produce severe hypophosphataemia in some patients with prolonged starvation. If glucose loading produces signs of hyperglycaemia, insulin may be added to correct it. See comments under **Amino acid solutions** for use in parenteral nutrition solutions.

Drug interactions: No information available.

DOSES

Mammals:

- Fluid therapy: Fluid requirements depend on the degree of dehydration and ongoing losses.
- Parenteral nutrition: The amount required will be governed by the animal's physiological status, the parenteral nutrition admixture and its ability to tolerate high blood glucose levels. Generally, glucose is used to supply 40–60% of the energy requirement. Seek specialist advice before giving parenteral nutrition. **See Amino acid solutions.**
- Hypoglycaemia: 0.1–2 ml 50% dextrose i.v. slowly over 10 min. Note that to meet minimum needs for maintenance 1 ml/kg/h of 50% glucose is needed.

Birds: Hypoglycaemia: 50–100 mg/kg i.v. as slow bolus.

Reptiles: 50 mg/kg dextrose administered as a 5–10% solution by dilution in crystalloids given by i.v. slowly.

Amphibians, Fish: No information available.

Glutamine
(Dipeptiven*) **POM, GSL**

Formulations: Parenteral: N(2)-L-alanyl-L-glutamine (POM). Oral: 500 mg powder or tablet (GSL).

Action: Conditionally essential amino acid required for energy synthesis in the enterocytes. Supplementation in patients with stress starvation is believed to have beneficial effects on intestinal cell proliferation and for prevention of mucosal atrophy.

Use: GI protectant in stress starvation (i.e. when nutritional support by any route is indicated) and to enhance GI healing in patients with severe GI epithelium damage, such as that caused by parvovirus enteritis. Use with caution in cases with epilepsy or liver disease.

Safety and handling: Normal precautions should be observed.

Contraindications: Avoid in patients with acute hepatic encephalopathy as it is partially metabolized to ammonia and glutamate.

Adverse reactions: May have CNS effects at high doses.

Drug interactions: Glutamine may antagonize the effects of lactulose in patients with hepatic encephalopathy and could potentially affect the efficacy of antiseizure medications.

DOSES

Mammals: Ferrets: 0.5 g/kg p.o. in divided doses daily.

Birds, Reptiles, Amphibians, Fish: No information available.

Glyceryl trinitrate (Nitroglycerin(e))
(Glyceryl trinitrate*, Nitrocine*, Percutol*, Sustac*)
POM

Formulations: Topical: 2% ointment to be applied to skin (Percutol). **Oral:** 2.6 mg, 6.4 mg modified-release tablets (Sustac). **Injectable:** 1 mg/ml, 5 mg/ml solutions (Glyceryl trinitrate, Nitrocine).

Action: Systemic vasodilator. Although a potent coronary vasodilator, its major benefit in small animals follows from a reduction in venous return as a consequence of venodilation. A decrease in venous return reduces left ventricular filling pressures.

Use: Short-term management of cardiogenic oedema (particularly acute pulmonary oedema) in animals with congestive heart failure. It is normally only used for 1–2 days. Its efficacy is debatable. Rotate application sites; suggested sites include the thorax, groin and inside the ears. Rub ointment well into the skin.

Safety and handling: Owners should be cautioned to avoid contact with areas where the ointment has been applied and to wear non-permeable gloves when applying.

Contraindications: Hypotension, hypovolaemia, cerebral haemorrhage, head trauma.

Adverse reactions: Hypotension (reduce dose), tachycardia and a rash at the site of application. Tachyphylaxis can occur. Headaches are common in humans and may be an adverse effect in animals also.

Drug interactions: Concurrent use of ACE inhibitors, anaesthetics, beta-blockers, calcium-channel blockers, corticosteroids and diuretics may enhance the hypotensive effect. NSAIDs may antagonize its hypotensive effects.

DOSES
Mammals: Ferrets: 1–3 mm topically to the skin q12–24h; Rodents: 3 mm topically q6–12h.
Birds, Reptiles, Amphibians, Fish: No information available.

Glycopyrronium (Glycopyrrolate)
(Robinul*) **POM**

Formulations: Injectable: 200 µg/ml solution.

Action: Blocks the action of acetylcholine at muscarinic receptors at the terminal ends of the parasympathetic nervous system, reversing parasympathetic effects. Its quaternary structure prevents it from crossing the blood–brain barrier and so it is devoid of central effects.

Use: Potent antisialagogue agent and has been used preoperatively to decrease oral and bronchial secretions. It is also used to inhibit vagal efferent activity and manage bradycardias caused by the administration of potent opioid drugs. Glycopyrronium is used with long-acting anticholinesterase drugs (e.g. neostigmine, pyridostigmine) during antagonism of neuromuscular block. Glycopyrronium is longer acting than atropine. Routine administration of glycopyrronium prior to anaesthesia as part of premedication is no longer recommended. It causes a reduction in oral and bronchial secretions by decreasing the water content, therefore secretions become more sticky. Administration of potent opioids in the perioperative period can promote bradyarrhythmias but it is better to monitor heart rate and give glycopyrronium to manage a low heart rate if necessary. Administration of very low doses of glycopyrronium i.v. can cause exacerbation of bradyarrhythmias due to a vagal stimulatory effect; giving another dose i.v. will usually cause an increase in heart rate. Glycopyrronium is devoid of central effects and therefore does not cause mydriasis. Glycopyrronium is preferred over atropine in rabbits due to the variable and unpredictable effects of atropine in this species.

Safety and handling: Normal precautions should be observed.

Contraindications: No information available.

Adverse reactions: Tachycardias following overdose of glycopyrronium are usually transient and do not require management. Ventricular arrhythmias may be treated with lidocaine if severe. The incidence of adverse effects is lower than that seen with atropine.

Drug interactions: When mixed with alkaline drugs (e.g. barbiturates) a precipitate may form. Antimuscarinics may enhance the actions of sympathomimetics and thiazide diuretics. The following may enhance the activity of glycopyrronium: antihistamines, quinidine, pethidine, benzodiazepines and phenothiazines. Combining glycopyrronium and alpha-2 adrenergic agonists is not recommended.

DOSES
Mammals: Rabbits: 10–20 µg (micrograms)/kg i.v., i.m. once; may be used in place of the largely ineffective atropine in this species; **Rodents:** 10–20 µg/kg i.v., i.m. once; **Primates:** 5–10 µg/kg i.m. once; **Sugar gliders:** 10–20 µg/kg s.c., i.m., i.v. once; **Hedgehogs:** 10–20 µg/kg s.c., i.m. once.
Birds: Premedication: 10–30 µg (micrograms)/kg i.m., i.v. once[1].
Reptiles: 10 µg (micrograms)/kg i.m., i.v., s.c. once. May be ineffective in green iguanas[a].
Amphibians, Fish: No information available.

References
[a] Pace L and Mader DR (2002) Atropine and glycopyrrolate, route of administration and response in the green iguana (*Iguana iguana*). *Proceedings of the Association of Reptilian and Amphibian Veterinarians* p. 79

[1] Lierz M and Rüdiger K (2012) Anesthesia and analgesia in birds. *Journal of Exotic Pet Medicine* **21(1)**, 44–58

Haemoglobin glutamer
(Oxyglobin) **POM-V**

Formulations: Injectable: 130 mg/ml solution in 60 ml and 125 ml oxygen-impermeable delivery bags.

Action: An ultrapurified, polymerized haemoglobin of bovine origin in modified Ringer's lactate solution which can carry oxygen.

Use: Provides oxygen-carrying capacity for anaemic animals. Because there is no red cell membrane, pre-treatment compatibility testing is not required. The effect of repeated dosing is unknown. It is isosmotic to blood and has a lower viscosity. Use with caution in animals with advanced heart disease or renal impairment (oliguria/anuria) as it can cause volume overload.

Safety and handling: It has a long shelf-life (>2 years) but once the overwrap is removed, the solution must be used within 24 hours, even if stored in a refrigerator, as it has no preservative and slow oxygenation results in methaemoglobin formation.

Contraindications: Not to be used in animals with fluid overload, overhydration or at risk of congestive heart failure. Should not be used in animals previously treated with oxyglobin.

Adverse reactions: Rapid administration to normovolaemic animals could result in hypervolaemia. The solution causes a discoloration of plasma (red, brown) and mucous membranes, sclera, urine and skin (yellow, brown or red). Vomiting, diarrhoea and fever have been reported. There is an increase in plasma total protein and haemoglobin that can artefactually change derived red cell indices on blood screens. Haemoglobinuria is expected and significant urine discoloration can interfere with other colorimetric changes on dipsticks. The package insert contains notes of known interferences with clinical chemistry analysers. Ideally obtain all diagnostic blood and urine samples before administration. The main complication of administration to small mammals is volume overload, leading to pulmonary oedema and pleural effusions; partly due to its potent colloid osmotic effects (slightly better than those of hetastarch) but probably also due to its nitric oxide-scavenging properties leading to vasoconstriction.

Drug interactions: Avoid concomitant administration with other plasma-volume expanders. The manufacturer states that no other medications should be added to the infusion line whilst oxyglobin is being administered. No specific interactions are yet reported.

DOSES

Mammals: 2 ml/kg i.v., intraosseously as a bolus over approximately 10–15 min followed by 0.2–0.4 ml/kg/h CRI.

Birds: 30 ml/kg i.v., intraosseously divided over 24 hours.

Reptiles: 1–2 ml/kg i.v., intraosseously as a slow bolus injection prn [1].

Amphibians, Fish: No information available.

References

[1] Lichtenberger M (2004) Transfusion medicine in exotic pets. *Clinical Techniques in Small Animal Practice* **19(2)**, 88–95

Haloperidol
(Haldol*, Halkid*, Haloperidol*) **POM**

Formulations: Oral: 200 μg/ml, 1 mg/ml, 2 mg/ml solution.
Injectable: 5 mg/ml.

Action: A potent central dopamine type 2 receptor antagonist. Also has antagonistic activity against alpha-1 adrenergic, histaminergic and cholinergic receptors.

Use: Used for the management of compulsive disorders such as feather plucking and self-mutilation in birds. Should be used in association with a behaviour modification plan.

Safety and handling: Normal precautions should be observed.

Contraindications: Avoid in patients with a known hypersensitivity to butyrophenones, those with hypokalaemia, cardiac disease or a history of seizures.

Adverse reactions: Potential extra-pyramidal side effects.

Drug interactions: Should not be used with monoamine oxidase inhibitors (e.g. selegiline), tramadol, beta-blockers, or drugs that prolong the QT interval. Concurrent administration with itraconazole may require a reduction in haloperidol dosage.

DOSES
Mammals: Primates: 0.03−0.05 mg/kg i.m. q12h.
Birds: 0.1−0.9 mg/kg p.o. q12−24h, 1−2 mg/kg i.m. q14−21d.
Reptiles: Boids: 0.5−10 mg/kg i.m. q7−14d.
Fish: 0.5 mg/kg i.m.
Amphibians: No information available.

Heparin (low molecular weight)
(Dalteparin, Enoxaparin)
(Clexane (enoxaparin)*, Fragmin (dalteparin)*) **POM**

Formulations: Injectable: 2,500 IU/ml, 100,000 IU/ml ampoules (dalteparin); 25,000 IU/ml multidose vial plus various pre-filled syringes at concentrations of 12,500 IU/ml and 25,000 IU/ml (dalteparin); pre-filled syringes of 100 mg/ml (enoxaparin). 100 mg enoxaparin is equivalent to 10,000 IU of anti-Factor Xa activity.

Action: Low molecular weight heparin (LMWH) is an anticoagulant that inhibits factor Xa and thrombin. When compared with unfractionated heparin (UFH), LMWH has reduced anti-IIa activity relative to anti-Xa activity (ratio of anti-Xa to anti-IIa is 2−4:1 compared with UFH 1:1). Thus, at therapeutic doses, LMWH has minimal effect on APTT. Therapeutic monitoring of LMWH is by anti-Xa activity (but this may not be practical).

Use: Treatment of thromboembolic complications and hypercoagulable syndromes (e.g. pulmonary thromboembolism, disseminated intravascular coagulation (DIC)) in mammals, although there is no information available in exotic pets. LMWH is also used in the treatment of myocardial infarction, atrial fibrillation, deep vein thrombosis and pulmonary thromboembolism in humans. Its use in DIC is controversial as no beneficial effect has been shown in controlled clinical trials in humans. LMWH is no longer used to try to prevent DIC. May be helpful for treatment of PTFE toxicosis in birds.

Safety and handling: Normal precautions should be observed.

Contraindications: Bleeding disorders or severe renal dysfunction.

Adverse reactions: If an overdosage occurs protamine can be used as an antidote. Heparin should not be administered i.m. as it may result in haematoma formation. Its use in DIC may worsen haemorrhage especially if the patient is thrombocytopenic. Heparin induced thrombocytopenia syndrome is a serious concern in human patients.

Drug interactions: Use with caution with other drugs that can cause changes in coagulation status (e.g. aspirin, NSAIDs). Heparin may antagonize ACTH, corticosteroids or insulin. Heparin may increase plasma levels of diazepam. The actions of heparin may be partially counteracted by antihistamines, digoxin and tetracyclines. Do not mix other drugs in the same syringe as heparin.

DOSES
Birds: PTFE toxicosis: 300 IU/kg i.v. once.
Mammals, Reptiles, Amphibians, Fish: No information available.

Heparin (unfractionated) (UFH)
(Heparin*, Hepsal*) **POM**

Formulations: Injectable: 1,000–25,000 IU/ml solutions; 10 IU/ml in saline, 100 IU/ml in saline.

Action: Heparin is an anticoagulant that exerts its effects primarily by enhancing the binding of antithrombin III (AT III) to factors IIa, IXa, Xa, XIa and XIIa; it is only effective if adequate AT III is present. The AT III/clotting factor complex is subsequently removed by the liver. Heparin inactivates thrombin and blocks the conversion of fibrinogen to fibrin. The inhibition of factor XII activation prevents the formation of stable fibrin clots. Heparin does not significantly change the concentrations of clotting factors, nor does it lyse pre-existing clots.

Use: Treatment of DIC and thromboembolic disease (**see Heparin (low molecular weight) (LMWH)**). Therapy must be carefully monitored as the activity of UFH is somewhat less predictable than LMWH. In veterinary medicine it is mainly used to maintain the patency of catheters/cannulae.

Safety and handling: Normal precautions should be observed.

Contraindications: Major bleeding disorders, increased risk of haemorrhage, thrombocytopenia.

Adverse reactions: If an overdosage occurs protamine can be used as an antidote. Heparin should not be administered i.m. as it may result in haematoma formation. Its use in DIC may worsen haemorrhage especially if the patient is thrombocytopenic. Heparin induced thrombocytopenia syndrome is a serious concern in human patients.

Drug interactions: Use with caution with other drugs that can cause changes in coagulation status (e.g. aspirin, NSAIDs). Heparin may antagonize ACTH, corticosteroids and insulin. Heparin may increase plasma levels of diazepam. The actions of heparin may be partially counteracted by antihistamines, digoxin and tetracyclines. Do not mix other drugs in the same syringe as heparin.

DOSES
Mammals: Catheter maintenance: 1250 IU in 100 ml water for injection.
Birds, Reptiles, Amphibians, Fish: No information available.

Human chorionic gonadotrophin see Chorionic gonadotrophin

Hyaluronate
(Hyabak*, Hylo-Care*, Hylo-Forte*, Hylo-Tear*, Oxyal*, Vismed Multi*) **P**

Formulations: Ophthalmic: 0.1%, 0.15%, 0.18%, 0.3%, 0.4% solution in 10 ml bottle.

Action: Viscoelastic fluid with mucomimetic properties. Sodium hyaluronate is also available in different formulations as a viscoelastic for intraocular surgery.

Use: Used as a tear replacement and is beneficial for the management of quantitative (keratoconjunctivitis sicca (KCS) or dry eye) and qualitative tear film disorders. It has longer corneal contact time than the aqueous tear substitutes.

Safety and handling: Normal precautions should be observed.

Contraindications: No information available.

Adverse reactions: It is tolerated well and ocular irritation is unusual.

Drug interactions: No information available.

DOSES

Mammals: 1 drop per eye q4–6h, although it can be used hourly if required.
Birds, Reptiles, Amphibians, Fish: No information available.

Hydralazine

(Apresoline*, Hydralazine*) **POM**

Formulations: Injectable: 20 mg powder for reconstitution and slow i.v. infusion; **Oral:** 25 mg, 50 mg tablets.

Action: Hydralazine acts chiefly on arteriolar smooth muscle causing vasodilation; it is able to decrease systemic vascular resistance to about 50% of the baseline value. The effects of hydralazine are to reduce afterload and increase heart rate, stroke volume and cardiac output.

Use: Afterload reducer as adjunctive therapy of congestive heart failure secondary to severe or refractory mitral value insufficiency. It can be used to treat systemic hypertension. Hospitalization with frequent monitoring of blood pressure is advised during its use. It is not typically used as a first-line drug in hypertension. As hydralazine may cause sodium and water retention, concomitant use of diuretic therapy is often necessary. Give with food if possible.

Safety and handling: Normal precautions should be observed.

Contraindications: Hypovolaemia, hypotension, renal impairment or cerebral bleeding.

Adverse reactions: Reflex tachycardia, severe hypotension (monitor and adjust doses as necessary), anorexia and vomiting in susceptible species.

Drug interactions: The hypotensive effects of hydralazine may be enhanced by ACE inhibitors (e.g. enalapril), anaesthetics, beta blockers (e.g. propranolol), calcium-channel blockers (e.g. diltiazem, verapamil), corticosteroids, diuretics and NSAIDs. Sympathomimetics (e.g. phenylpropanolamine) may cause tachycardia. The pressor response to adrenaline may be reduced.

DOSES

Mammals: Guinea pigs: 1 mg/kg i.v. prn.
Birds, Reptiles, Amphibians, Fish: No information available.

Hydrochlorothiazide
(Co-amilozide*, Moduret*, Moduretic*) **POM**

Formulations: Oral: 25 mg hydrochlorothiazide + 2.5 mg amiloride, 50 mg hydrochlorothiazide + 5 mg amiloride tablets.

Action: Thiazide diuretic that inhibits reabsorption of sodium and chloride in the distal convoluted tubule, resulting in sodium, chloride and water loss in the urine. It also causes excretion of potassium, magnesium and bicarbonate. It is formulated with a potassium-sparing diuretic (amiloride).

Use: Additional therapy for congestive heart failure when the clinical signs have become refractory to furosemide. However, furosemide therapy should still be continued when using hydrochlorthiazide. It may also be used in the prevention of calcium oxalate urolithiasis. Thiazides have antihypertensive effects, although the exact mechanism is unclear.

Safety and handling: Normal precautions should be observed.

Contraindications: Renal impairment, as it tends to reduce glomerular filtration rate.

Adverse reactions: Hyperglycaemia, hypokalaemia, hyponatraemia, hypochloraemia and volume contraction. It enhances the effects of the renin-angiotensin-aldosterone system in heart failure.

Drug interactions: Increased possibility of hypokalaemia developing if thiazides are used concomitantly with corticosteroids or loop diuretics (furosemide). Thiazide-induced hypokalaemia may increase the risk of digoxin toxicity. Thus, concomitant use of potassium-sparing diuretics (e.g. spironolactone) or potassium supplementation may be necessary during prolonged administration. The concurrent administration of vitamin D or calcium salts with thiazides may exacerbate hypercalcaemia.

DOSES
Reptiles: 1 mg/kg p.o. q24–72h.
Mammals, Birds, Amphibians, Fish: No information available.

Hydrocortisone
(Efcortesol*, Solu-cortef*) **POM**

Formulations: Topical: 0.5%, 1% creams, 1% solution (Hydrocortisone). Injectable: 25 mg/ml solution; 100 mg, 500 mg powders for reconstitution (Solu-cortef). Oral: 10 mg, 20 mg tablets (Hydrocortisone).

Action: Alters the transcription of DNA, leading to alterations in cellular metabolism. It has both glucocorticoid and mineralocorticoid activity.

Use: Topical anti-inflammatory drug also used in the management of hypoadrenocorticism. It has only a quarter of the glucocorticoid potency of prednisolone and one thirtieth that of dexamethasone. On a dose basis 4 mg of hydrocortisone is equivalent to 1 mg prednisolone. Animals on chronic therapy should be tapered off steroids when discontinuing the drug (even following topical administration). The use of steroids in most cases of shock or spinal cord injury is of no benefit and may be detrimental.

Safety and handling: Wear gloves when applying topically as the cream is absorbed through skin.

Contraindications: Do not use in pregnant animals. Systemic corticosteroids are generally contraindicated in patients with renal disease and diabetes mellitus.

Adverse reactions: Catabolic effects of glucocorticoids lead to weight loss and cutaneous atrophy. Iatrogenic hyperadrenocorticism may develop (PU/PD, elevated liver enzymes). Vomiting and diarrhoea, or GI ulceration may develop. Glucocorticoids may increase urine glucose levels and decrease serum T3 and T4 values. Prolonged use of glucocorticoids suppresses the hypothalamic-pituitary axis and causes adrenal atrophy. Impaired wound healing and delayed recovery from infections may be seen. Corticosteroids should be used with care in birds as there is a high risk of immunosuppression and side effects, such as hepatopathy and a diabetes mellitus-like syndrome. In rabbits, even small single doses can potentially cause severe adverse reactions. Ferrets are particularly susceptible to GI ulceration, and concurrent gastric protectants may be advisable, especially in stressed animals.

Drug interactions: Increased risk of GI ulceration if used concurrently with NSAIDs. Glucocorticoids antagonize the effect of insulin. Antiepileptic drugs (phenobarbital) may accelerate the metabolism of corticosteroids and antifungals (e.g. itraconazole) may decrease it. There is an increased risk of hypokalaemia when corticosteroids are used with acetazolamide, amphotericin and potassium-depleting diuretics (furosemide, thiazides).

DOSES
Mammals: Ferrets: 25–40 mg/kg i.v. (shock).
Birds, Reptiles, Amphibians, Fish: No information available.

Hydroxyzine
(Atarax*, Ucerax*) **POM**

Formulations: Oral: 10 mg, 25 mg tablets; 2 mg/ml syrup.

Action: Binds to H1 histamine receptors preventing histamine from binding. Hydroxyzine is metabolized to cetirizine.

Use: Used in feather plucking in birds. Use with caution in cases with urinary retention, angle-closure glaucoma and pyloroduodenal obstruction.

Safety and handling: Normal precautions should be observed.

Contraindications: No information available.

Adverse reactions: May cause mild sedation. May reduce seizure threshold.

Drug interactions: No information available.

DOSES
Mammals: Ferrets, Rabbits: 2 mg/kg p.o. q8–12h.
Birds: 2.2 mg/kg p.o. q8h [a].
Reptiles, Amphibians, Fish: No information available.

References
[a] Krinsley M (1993) Use of Derm Caps liquid and hydroxyzine HCl for the treatment of feather picking. *Journal of the Association of Avian Veterinarians* **7**, 221

Hyoscine see **Butylscopolamine**

Hypromellose
(Hypromellose*, Isopto*, Tears Naturale*) **P**

Formulations: Ophthalmic: 0.3%, 0.5%, 1% solutions in 10 ml dropper bottle, 0.32% (single-use vial). Large variety of other formulations also available.

Action: Cellulose based tear substitute (lacrimomimetic).

Use: Lubrication of dry eyes. In cases of keratoconjunctivitis (KCS or dry eye) it will improve ocular surface lubrication, tear retention and patient comfort while lacrostimulation therapy (e.g. topical ciclosporin) is initiated. It may also be used as a vehicle base for compounding ophthalmic drugs. Patient compliance is poor if used >q4h, consider using a longer acting tear replacement.

Safety and handling: Normal precautions should be observed.

Contraindications: No information available.

Adverse reactions: No information available.

Drug interactions: No information available.

DOSES
Mammals: 1 drop per eye q1h during anaesthesia.
Birds, Reptiles, Amphibians, Fish: No information available.

Imepitoin

(Pexion) **POM-V**

Formulations: Oral: 100 mg, 400 mg tablets.

Action: Imepitoin inhibits seizures via potentiation of the $GABA_A$ receptor-mediated inhibitory effects on the neurons. Imepitoin also has a weak calcium-channel blocking effect, which may contribute to its anticonvulsive properties.

Use: For the management of epileptic seizures due to idiopathic epilepsy in dogs. The choice of initial medication is guided by patient requirements: imepitoin has a more rapid onset of action than phenobarbital (a steady state does not need to be achieved), does not require the determination of serum concentrations and has a less severe adverse effect profile; however, phenobarbital is less expensive and more efficacious.

Safety and handling: Normal precautions should be observed.

Contraindications: The medication should not be used with severely impaired liver, kidney or heart function.

Adverse reactions: The most frequent adverse effect reported is sedation. Other adverse effects are generally mild and transient and include polyphagia, hyperactivity, polyuria, polydipsia, somnolence, hypersalivation, emesis, ataxia, apathy, diarrhoea, prolapsed nictitating membrane, decreased sight and sensitivity to sound.

Drug interactions: Imepitoin has been used in combination with phenobarbital in a small number of cases and no harmful clinical interactions were reported.

DOSES

Mammals: Mice: experimental doses have been reported of 25–60 mg/kg p.o., i.p.
Birds, Reptiles, Amphibians, Fish: No information available.

Imidacloprid

(**Advantage**, Advantix, **Advocate**, Bob Martin Double Action Dewormer, **Moxiclear**, **Prinovox**) **POM-V, AVM-GSL**

Formulations: Topical: 100 mg/ml imidacloprid either as sole agent or else in combination with moxidectin or permethrin (e.g. Advantix, Advocate, Prinovox and others) in spot-on pipettes of various sizes. Numerous GSL and non-authorized formulations.

Action: Binds to postsynaptic nicotinic receptors resulting in paralysis and death of fleas and their larvae.

Use: Treatment and prevention of flea infestation and prevention of heartworm disease in ferrets. Treatment and prevention of flea infestations in rabbits. For the treatment of flea infestations the additional use of an approved insect growth regulator is recommended and the product should be applied every 4 weeks to all in-contact rabbits. Has been used in lizards for the treatment of mites.

Safety and handling: Many combinations contain products that are dangerous to aquatic organisms and birds.

Contraindications: No information available.

Adverse reactions: Transient pruritus and erythema at the site of application may occur.

Drug interactions: No information available.

DOSES
Mammals: Ferrets: 0.4 ml pipette q30d; **Rabbits:** 0.4 ml, 0.8 ml pipettes (use the smaller size in rabbits <4 kg) or 0.125 ml/kg imidacloprid/permethrin formulation for fur mites (*Leporacus* spp.); **Rabbits, Guinea pigs:** 0.1 ml/kg imidacloprid/permethrin formulation; **Rodents:** 20 mg/kg (equivalent to 0.2 ml/kg).
Reptiles: Bearded dragons, Frillneck lizards: 0.2 ml/kg topically q14d for 3 treatments.
Birds, Amphibians, Fish: No information available.

Imidapril
(Prilium) **POM-V**

Formulations: Oral: 75 mg, 150 mg, 300 mg powders for reconstitution.

Action: Angiotensin converting enzyme (ACE) inhibitor. It inhibits conversion of angiotensin I to angiotensin II and inhibits the breakdown of bradykinin. Overall effect is a reduction in preload and afterload via venodilation and arteriodilation, decreased salt and water retention via reduced aldosterone production and inhibition of the angiotensin-aldosterone-mediated cardiac and vascular remodelling. Efferent arteriolar dilation in the kidney can reduce intraglomerular pressure and therefore glomerular filtration. This may decrease proteinuria.

Use: Treatment of congestive heart failure caused by mitral regurgitation or dilated cardiomyopathy. Often used in conjunction with diuretics when heart failure is present as most effective when used in these cases. Can be used in combination with other drugs to treat heart failure (e.g. pimobendan, spironolactone, digoxin). May be beneficial in cases of chronic renal insufficiency, particularly protein-losing nephropathies. May reduce blood pressure in hypertension. ACE inhibitors are more likely to cause or exacerbate prerenal azotaemia in hypotensive animals and those with poor renal perfusion (e.g. acute, oliguric renal failure). Use cautiously if hypotension, hyponatraemia or outflow tract obstruction are present. Regular monitoring of blood pressure, serum creatinine, urea and electrolytes is strongly recommended with ACE inhibitor treatment.

Safety and handling: Normal precautions should be observed.

Contraindications: Do not use in animals with acute renal failure, congenital heart disease, haemodynamically relevant stenoses (e.g. aortic stenosis), obstructive hypertrophic cardiomyopathy or hypovolaemia.

Adverse reactions: Potential adverse effects include hypotension, hyperkalaemia and azotaemia. Monitor blood pressure, serum creatinine and electrolytes when used in cases of heart failure. Dosage should be reduced if there are signs of hypotension (weakness, disorientation). Anorexia, vomiting and diarrhoea are rare.

Drug interactions: Concomitant use of potassium-sparing diuretics (e.g. spironolactone) or potassium supplements could result in hyperkalaemia. However, in practice, spironolactone and ACE inhibitors appear safe to use concurrently. There may be an increased risk of nephrotoxicity and decreased clinical efficacy when used with NSAIDs. There is a risk of hypotension with concomitant administration of diuretics, vasodilators (e.g. anaesthetic agents, antihypertensive agents) or negative inotropes (e.g. beta-blockers).

DOSES

Mammals: Anecdotally this product has been used in rates for protein-losing nephropathy at 0.25 mg/kg p.o. q24h. The liquid formulation makes it easier to accurately titrate doses.

Birds, Reptiles, Amphibians, Fish: No information available.

Insulin

(Caninsulin, Prozinc, Actrapid*, Humulin*, Hypurin*, Insulatard*, Lantus*) **POM-V, POM**

Formulations: Injectable: 40 IU/ml, 100 IU/ml suspensions (for s.c. injection) or 100 IU/ml solutions (for s.c., i.v. or i.m. injection). There are many preparations (including soluble) authorized for use in humans; however, veterinary authorized preparations (lente and PZI), when available, are preferential for both legal and medical reasons.

Action: Binds to specific receptors on the cell surface which then stimulate the formation of glycogen from glucose, lipid from free fatty acids, protein from amino acids and many other metabolic effects.

Use: Treatment of insulin-dependent diabetes mellitus (IDDM) and occasionally as adjunctive therapy in the management of hyperkalaemia associated with urinary tract obstruction. There are various formulations of insulins from various species (see table). Neutral (soluble) insulin is the normal crystalline form. Lente insulins rely on different concentrations of zinc and size of zinc-insulin crystals to provide different durations of activity. Glargine insulin (Lantus) is a pH sensitive, long-acting formulation that precipitates at the site of injection. Hyperkalaemia associated with hypoadrenocorticism is often associated with hypoglycaemia and insulin should be avoided in those cases.

Trade name	Species of insulin	Types available
Actrapid*	Human	Neutral
Caninsulin	Porcine	Lente
Lantus*	Human	Glargine
Humulin*	Human	Neutral, Isophane (NPH)
Hypurin*	Bovine	Neutral, Isophane, Lente, PZI
	Porcine	Neutral, Isophane
Insulatard*	Human or porcine	Isophane
Prozinc	Human	PZI

* = Not authorized for veterinary use.

Safety and handling: Normal precautions should be observed.

Contraindications: Hypoglycaemia.

Adverse reactions: Overdosage results in hypoglycaemia and hypokalaemia.

Drug interactions: Corticosteroids, ciclosporin, thiazide diuretics and thyroid hormones may antagonize the hypoglycaemic effects of insulin. Anabolic steroids, beta-adrenergic blockers (e.g. propranolol), phenylbutazone, salicylates and tetracycline may increase insulin's effect. Administer with caution and monitor patients closely if digoxin is given concurrently. Beta-adrenergic agonists, such as terbutaline, may prevent or lessen insulin-induced hypoglycaemia in humans.

DOSES
Mammals: Ferrets: 0.5–1.0 IU/animal s.c. q12h (lente) or 0.1 IU/animal s.c. q24h (ultralente); **Guinea pigs:** 1–2 IU/kg s.c. q12h; Chinchillas: 1 IU/kg s.c. q12h; **Rats:** 1–3 IU/animal s.c. q12h; Hamsters, Gerbils: 2 IU/animal s.c. q12h; **Primates:** Initially 0.25–0.5 IU/kg/day s.c. (NPH or lente insulin).
Reptiles: Chelonians, Snakes: 1–5 IU/kg i.m. q24–72h; **Lizards:** 5–10 IU/kg i.m. q24–72h; adjust doses according to serial glucose measurement.
Birds, Amphibians, Fish: No information available.

Iodophor see Povidone–iodine

Iron salts (Ferrous sulphate, Ferrous fumarate, Ferrous gluconate, Iron dextran) (Gleptrosil, CosmoFer*, Diafer*, Monofer*, Venofer*) POM-VPS, POM, GSL

Formulations: Injectable: 50 mg/ml iron dextran (CosmoFer), 50 mg/ml iron (III) isomaltoside (Monofer), 100 mg/ml iron (III) isomaltoside (Monofer), 200 mg/ml iron dextran (Gleptosil and several other formulations licensed for pigs), 20 mg/ml iron sucrose (Venofer). **Oral:** 200 mg $FeSO_4$ tablet (ferrous sulphate), ferrous gluconate and other formulations in variable tablet and liquid preparations; ferrous fumarate preparations also typically contain folic acid.

Action: Essential for oxygen-binding in haemoglobin, electron transport chain and oxidative phosphorylation, and other oxidative reactions in metabolism.

Use: Treatment of iron deficiency anaemia and conditions where red blood cell synthesis is high and iron stores are depleted. The oral route should be used if possible. Iron absorption is complex and dependent in part on physiological demand, diet composition, current iron stores and dose. Valid reasons for administering iron parenterally are failure of oral therapy due to severe GI adverse effects, continuing severe blood loss, iron malabsorption, or a non-compliant patient. Modified-release preparations should be avoided as they are ineffective. In most species, iron is absorbed in the duodenum (but there is no specific information in exotic pets) and the release of iron from modified-release preparations occurs lower down the GI tract. Absorption is enhanced if administered 1 hour before or several hours after feeding. Reduce dosage if GI side effects occur.

Safety and handling: Normal precautions should be observed.

Contraindications: Severe infection or inflammation, intolerance to the oral preparation, any anaemia other than iron deficiency anaemia, presence of GI ulcers. Also contraindicated in patients with hepatic, renal (particularly pyelonephritis) or cardiac disease, and untreated urinary tract infections.

Adverse reactions: Parenteral iron may cause arrhythmias, anaphylaxis, shunting of iron to reticuloendothelial stores and iron overload. Oral iron may cause nausea, vomiting, constipation and diarrhoea. The faeces of animals treated with oral iron may be dark in appearance. High doses may be teratogenic and embryotoxic (injectable iron dextran).

Drug interactions: Chloramphenicol can delay the response to iron dextran and its concurrent use should be avoided. Oral preparations bind to tetracyclines and penicillamine causing a decrease in efficacy. Antacids, milk and eggs significantly decrease the bioavailability of oral iron.

DOSES
Mammals: 10 mg/kg i.m. of iron dextran once weekly or prn.
Birds: 10 mg/kg i.m. of iron dextran prn [a].
Reptiles, Amphibians, Fish: No information available.

References
[a] Ros JH, Todd B, Tell LA, Ramsey EC and Fowler ME (1992) Treatment of anemic birds with iron dextran therapy: homologous and heterologous blood transfusions. *Tijdschrift voor diergeneeskunde* **117(Suppl. 1)**, 22–23

Isoeugenol see **Eugenol**

Isoflurane
(Isocare, Isofane, IsoFlo, Isoflurane Vet, Iso-vet, Vetflurane) POM-V

Formulations: Inhalational: 250 ml bottle of liquid isoflurane.

Action: Halogenated ethyl methyl ether and structural isomer of enflurane. The mechanism of action of volatile anaesthetic agents is not fully understood.

Use: Induction and maintenance of anaesthesia. Isoflurane is potent and highly volatile so should only be delivered from a suitable calibrated vaporizer. It is less soluble in blood than halothane but more soluble than sevoflurane, therefore induction and recovery from anaesthesia are quicker than halothane but slower than sevoflurane. The concentration of isoflurane required to maintain anaesthesia depends on the other drugs used in the anaesthesia protocol; the concentration should be adjusted according to clinical assessment of anaesthetic depth. MAC approximately 1.2–1.7% in most species. Isoflurane has a pungent smell and induction of anaesthesia using chambers or masks may be less well tolerated compared with sevoflurane. In amphibians, isoflurane can be delivered by bubbling the solution through water, intubation or by direct application to the skin. In fish, isoflurane is added direct to the water by spraying through a fine hypodermic needle positioned under the water surface but control of the anaesthetic concentration is difficult due to its relative insolubility.

Safety and handling: Measures should be adopted to prevent contamination of the environment with isoflurane during anaesthesia and when handling the agent.

Contraindications: Avoid gaseous induction in rabbits and chelonians as they can breath-hold and develop serious complications.

Adverse reactions: Isoflurane causes dose-dependent hypotension by causing vasodilation, particularly in skeletal muscle. This adverse effect does not wane with time. Isoflurane is a more potent respiratory depressant than halothane, respiratory depression is dose-dependent. Isoflurane does not sensitize the myocardium to catecholamines to the extent that halothane does, but can generate arrhythmias in certain conditions. Isoflurane is not metabolized by the liver (0.2%) and has less effect on liver blood flow compared with halothane. In ferrets, isoflurane can cause marked depression in haematological parameters (especially haematocrit, RBC count, Hb concentration) rapidly after induction, so care should be taken in interpreting blood results if isoflurane is used for restraint, or in anaemic or debilitated ferrets. In American green tree frogs, the use of compounded topical isoflurane jelly has been associated with fatalites, so use is to be avoided in this species [a].

Drug interactions: Opioid agonists, benzodiazepines and N_2O reduce the concentration of isoflurane required to achieve surgical anaesthesia.

DOSES

Mammals: Ferrets, Rabbits, Primates, Sugar gliders, Hedgehogs: 3–5% isoflurane concentration is required to induce anaesthesia in unpremedicated patients, 1.5–3.0% is required for maintenance. The expired concentration required to maintain surgical anaesthesia in 50% of rabbits is 2.05%. **Rodents:** 2–5% for induction, 0.25–4.0% for maintenance.

Birds: 3–5% isoflurane concentration is required to induce anaesthesia in unpremedicated patients [b,c], 1.5–2.5% in 100% oxygen for maintenance. Administration of other anaesthetic agents and opioid analgesics reduces the dose requirement of isoflurane, therefore the dose should be adjusted according to individual requirement.

Reptiles: Lizards, Snakes: 3–5% in 100% oxygen for induction [d], 1.8–4% in 100% oxygen for maintenance [e].

Amphibians: 3–5% in 100% oxygen for induction, 1–2% in 100% oxygen for maintenance or 0.28 ml/100 ml water in bath (closed container), bubbled through water to effect or 0.007–0.015 ml/g topically (closed container), remove excess after induction or mixture of 3 ml isoflurane, 3.5 ml KY jelly and 1.5 ml water applied at 0.025–0.035 ml/g (closed container), remove excess after induction [f].

Fish: 0.4–0.75 ml/l for induction, 0.25–0.4 ml/l for maintenance (add to water).

References

[a] Zec S, Clark-Price SC, Coleman DA and Mitchell MA (2014) Loss and Return of Righting Reflex in American Green Tree Frogs (*Hyla cinerea*) after Topical Application of Compounded Sevoflurane or Isoflurane Jelly: A Pilot Study. *Journal of Herpetological Medicine and Surgery* **24(3)**, 72–76

[b] Curro TG, Brunson DB and Paul-Murphy J (1994) Determination of the ED50 of isoflurane and evaluation of the isoflurane-sparing effect of butorphanol in cockatoos (*Cacatua* spp.). *Veterinary Surgery* **23(5)**, 429–433

[c] Ludders JW, Mitchell GS and Rhode J (1990) Minimal anesthetic concentration and cardiopulmonary dose response of isoflurane in ducks. *Veterinary Surgery* **19(4)**, 304–307

[d] Bertelsen MF, Mosley C, Crawshaw GJ, Dyson D and Smith DA (2005) Inhalation anesthesia in Dumeril's monitor (*Varanus dumerili*) with isoflurane, sevoflurane, and nitrous oxide: effects of inspired gases on induction and recovery. *Journal of Zoo and Wildlife Medicine* **36(1)**, 62–69

[e] Barter LS, Hawkins MG, Brosnan RJ, Antognini JF and Pypendop BH (2006) Median effective dose of isoflurane, sevoflurane, and desflurane in green iguanas. *American Journal of Veterinary Research* **67(3)**, 392–397

[f] Stetter MD, Rahael B, Indiviglio F et al. (1999) Isoflurane anaesthesia in amphibians: comparison of five application methods. *Proceedings of the Annual Conference of the American Association of Zoo Veterinarians*, pp. 255–257

Itraconazole

(**Fungitraxx**, Itrafungol, Sporanox*) **POM, POM-V**

Formulations: Oral: 100 mg capsule, 10 mg/ml oral solution.

Action: Triazole antifungal agent that inhibits the cytochrome systems involved in the synthesis of ergosterol in fungal cell membranes, causing increased cell wall permeability and allowing leakage of cellular contents.

Use: Treatment of aspergillosis, candidiasis, blastomycosis, coccidioidomycosis, cryptococcosis, sporotrichosis, histoplasmosis, a variety of dermatomycoses and *Malassezia*. It is widely distributed in the body, although low concentrations are found in tissues with low protein contents, e.g. CSF, ocular fluid and saliva. Itraconazole extends the activity of methylprednisolone. Treatment of chytridiomycisis in amphibians. Treatment of systemic mycosis in fish.

Safety and handling: Normal precautions should be observed.

Contraindications: Pregnancy. Avoid use if liver disease is present.

Adverse reactions: Vomiting, diarrhoea, anorexia, salivation, depression and apathy, abdominal pain, hepatic toxicosis, drug eruption, ulcerative dermatitis and limb oedema have been reported. It has a narrow safety margin in birds and should be discontinued if emesis or anorexia occurs. Avoid or use with great care in in Grey Parrots as it is not well tolerated.

Drug interactions: In humans, antifungal imidazoles and triazoles inhibit the metabolism of antihistamines (particularly terfenadine), oral hypoglycaemics, antiepileptics and glucocorticoids. Antacids, omeprazole, H2 antagonists and adsorbents may reduce the absorption of itraconazole. Plasma concentrations of ciclosporin, digoxin, benzodiazepines, glucocorticoids and vincristine may be increased by itraconazole.

DOSES

Mammals: Ferrets: dermatophytosis: 15 mg/kg p.o. q24h; **Rabbits:** dermatophytosis: 10 mg/kg p.o. q24h for 15 days; pulmonary aspergillosis: 20–40 mg/kg p.o. q24h; **Rodents:** 2.5–10 mg/kg p.o. q24h; **Mice:** blastomycosis: 50–150 mg/kg p.o. q24h; **Primates:** 10 mg/kg p.o. q24h (gastroenteritis), 5–10 mg/kg p.o. q12h (dermatophytosis); **Sugar gliders, Hedgehogs:** 5–10 mg/kg p.o. q24h.

Birds:
- Candidiasis: 10 mg/kg p.o. q24h for 14 days.
- Aspergillosis treatment: 5–10 mg/kg p.o. q12–24h[a,b] for 8 weeks, repeat course if fungal elements still remain; **Raptors:** doses of up to 20 mg/kg p.o. q12–24h may be used; **Grey Parrots:** avoid or use with great care and only at lowest dose and longest

interval (voriconazole at 12–18 mg/kg p.o. q12h or terbinafine more advisable).

- Aspergillosis prophylaxis: 10–20 mg/kg p.o. q24h in susceptible species (e.g. Gyrs and their hybrids, Goshawks, Snowy Owls, Golden Eagles) during stressful events (e.g. manning) where drug therapy should be started 5 days before the stressful event starts.

Reptiles: 5–10 mg/kg p.o. q24h (most species). Metabolically scaled doses have been suggested for the treatment of *Aspergillus* infections [c]; **Spiny lizard:** 23.5 mg/kg p.o. q24h for 3 days (pharmacokinetic study maintained systemic itraconazole levels for a further 6 days) [d].

Amphibians: 0.0025% bath (2.50 ml aqueous itraconazole (1% Sporanox oral solution) to 1 l amphibian Ringer's solution); 5 minute bath daily for 6 days has been shown to be the lowest effective treatment concentration for chytridiomycosis. Do not use with larvae [e,f].

Fish: 1–5 mg/kg p.o. q24h for 1–7 days.

References

[a] Jones MP, Orosz SE, Cox SK and Frazier DL (2000) Pharmacokinetic disposition of itraconazole in red-tailed hawks (*Buteo jamaicensis*). *Journal of Avian Medicine and Surgery* **14(1)**, 15–22

[b] Orosz SE (1996) Pharmacokinetic properties of itraconazole in blue-fronted Amazon parrots (*Amazona aestiva aestiva*). *Journal of Avian Medicine and Surgery* **10(3)**, 168–173

[c] Girling SJ and Fraser MA (2009) Treatment of *Aspergillus* species infection in reptiles with itraconazole at metabolically scaled doses. *Veterinary Record* **165(2)**, 52–54

[d] Gamble KC, Alvarado TP and Bennett CL (1997) Itraconazole plasma and tissue concentrations in the spiny lizard (*Sceloporus* spp.) following once daily dosing. *Journal of Zoo and Wildlife Medicine* **28(1)**, 89–93

[e] Brannelly LA (2014) Reduced itraconazole concentration and durations are successful in treating *Batrachochytrium dendrobatidis* infection in amphibians. *Journal of Visualized Experiments* **85**, e51166. doi: 10.3791/51166

[f] Brannelly LA, Richards-Zawacki CL and Pessier AP (2012) Clinical trials with itraconazole as a treatment for chytrid fungal infections in amphibians. *Diseases of Aquatic Organisms* **101(2)**, 95–104

Ivermectin

(Alstomec, Animec, Bimectin, Ivomec, Panomec, Qualimec, Qualimintic, Virbamec, **Xeno 450, Xeno 50-mini, Xeno 200 spray**) **POM-V, POM-VPS, ESPA**

Formulations: Injectable: 1% w/v solution. **Topical:** 100 µg/g, 800 µg/g spot-on tubes; 1 µg/ml, 10 µg/ml drops; 200 µg/ml spray (Xeno).

Action: Interacts with GABA and glutamate-gated channels leading to flaccid paralysis of parasites.

Use: Prevention and treatment of internal and external parasites in mammals, birds and reptiles (except chelonians).

Safety and handling: Normal precautions should be observed.

Contraindications: Highly toxic to many species of fish and other aquatic organisms. Do not use in chelonians as can result in neurotoxicity and death. Indigo snakes and skinks have also been suggested to be sensitive to ivermectin so administration to these species is not recommended.

Adverse reactions: Neurotoxicity may be seen if it crosses mammalian blood–brain barrier.

Drug interactions: Dose adjustments may be required when administered concurrently with other therapeutic agents transported by P-glycoprotein.

DOSES

Mammals: Most species: 0.2–0.5 mg/kg s.c., p.o. q7–14d; **Ferrets, Rabbits, Guinea pigs:** apply 450 µg (micrograms)/kg (1 tube Xeno 450) topically; **Ferrets, Small rodents <800 g:** 50 µg/250 g (15 drops Xeno 50-mini) q7–14d; **Primates, Sugar gliders, Hedgehogs:** 0.2–0.4 mg/kg s.c., p.o., repeat at 14 and 28 days (acariasis, nematodes).

Birds: 200 µg (micrograms)/kg i.m., s.c., p.o. q7–14d [a]; **Raptors:** capillariasis: 0.5–1 mg/kg i.m., p.o. q7–14d; *Serratospiculum:* 1 mg/kg p.o., i.m. q7–14d (moxidectin or doramectin may be given at same dose rates); **Passerines, Small psittacids:** systemic dosing as above or 0.2 mg/kg applied topically to skin using 0.02% solution (in propylene glycol) q7–14d; **Pigeons:** 0.5 ml applied topically to bare skin using 0.02% solution q7–14d; **Ornamental birds:** mites and lice: 1 drop/50 g body weight weekly for 3 weeks.

Reptiles: 0.2 mg/kg s.c., p.o. once, repeat in 10–14 days until negative for parasites; may use as environmental control for snake mites (*Ophionyssus natricis*) at dilution of 5 mg/l water sprayed in tank q7–10d (if pre-mix ivermectin with propylene glycol this facilitates mixing with water). Do not use in chelonians.

Amphibians: 0.2–0.4 mg/kg p.o. q14d or 2 mg/kg topically, repeat in 14–21 days or 10 mg/l for 60 minute bath, repeat in 14 days.

Fish: Do not use.

References

[a] Lierz M (2001) Evaluation of the dosage of ivermectin in falcons. *Veterinary Record* **148(19)**, 596–600

Kaolin
(Kaogel VP, Prokolin) **AVM-GSL, general sale**

Formulations: Oral: Kaogel VP: aqueous suspension containing Kaolin Light. Combination products with pectin, magnesium trisilicate, aluminium hydroxide and phosphate, bismuth salts, calcium carbonate or tincture of morphine are also available.

Action: Adsorbent antidiarrhoeal agent with possible antisecretory effect.

Use: Treatment of diarrhoea of non-specific origin. Although stool consistency may improve, studies do not show that fluid balance is corrected or that the duration of morbidity is shortened.

Safety and handling: Normal precautions should be observed.

Contraindications: Intestinal obstruction or perforation.

Adverse reactions: No information available, but the use of kaolin is not advisable in rabbits, guinea pigs and chinchillas due to the risk of decreasing GI motility.

Drug interactions: May decrease the absorption of lincomycin, trimethoprim and sulphonamides.

DOSES
Mammals: Ferrets, Hamsters: 1–2 ml/kg kaolin/pectin p.o. q2–6h; Primates: 0.5–1 ml/kg kaolin/pectin p.o. q2–6h.
Birds: Kaolin/pectin mixture: 15 ml/kg p.o. once.
Reptiles, Amphibians, Fish: No information available.

Ketamine
(**Anaestamine**, Anesketin, Ketamidor, **Ketaset injection**, Ketavet, Narketan-10, Nimatek, Vetalar-V) **POM-V CD SCHEDULE 2**

Formulations: Injectable: 100 mg/ml solution.

Action: Antagonizes the excitatory neurotransmitter glutamate at N-methyl-D-aspartate (NMDA) receptors in the CNS. It interacts with opioid receptors in a complex fashion, antagonizing mu receptors, whilst showing agonist actions at delta and kappa receptors. It does not interact with GABA receptors.

Use: Provision of chemical restraint or dissociative anaesthesia. Ketamine may also provide profound visceral and somatic analgesia and inhibits central sensitization through NMDA receptor blockade and is used to provide perioperative analgesia as an adjunctive agent, although optimal doses to provide analgesia have not been elucidated. Dissociative anaesthesia is associated with mild stimulation of cardiac output and blood pressure, modest respiratory depression and the preservation of cranial nerve reflexes. For example, the eyes remain open during anaesthesia and should be protected using a bland ophthalmic ointment. Used alone at doses adequate to provide general anaesthesia ketamine causes skeletal muscle hypertonicity and movement may occur that is unrelated to surgical stimulation. These effects are normally controlled by the co-administration of alpha-2 adrenergic agonists and/or benzodiazepines. When ketamine is combined with alpha-2 agonists (such as medetomidine or dexmedetomidine) reversal of the alpha-2 agonist should be delayed until 45 min after ketamine administration. In fish, ketamine does not induce a surgical plane of anaesthesia on its own and has been used in combination with medetomidine. Elasmobranchs (sharks and rays) are more susceptible to the effects of ketamine than bony fish.

Safety and handling: Normal precautions should be observed.

Contraindications: Not recommended for animals whose eyes are at risk of perforation or who have raised intraocular pressure.

Adverse reactions: Cardiovascular depression, rather than stimulation, and arrhythmias may arise in animals with a high sympathetic nervous system tone (e.g. animals in shock or severe cardiovascular disease). Tachycardia can also arise after administration of high doses i.v. Respiratory depression may be marked in some animals. Ketamine may result in spacey, abnormal behaviour for 1–2 hours during recovery. Prolonged administration of ketamine by infusion may result in drug accumulation and prolong recovery. Intramuscular injection may be painful.

Drug interactions: No information available.

DOSES
When used for sedation is generally given as part of a combination. See Appendix for sedation protocols in all species.
Mammals:
- Ferrets: 10–30 mg/kg i.m., s.c. alone gives immobilization and some analgesia but there is poor muscle relaxation and prolonged recovery. For general anaesthesia, sedate first and then induce with isoflurane or sevoflurane. Alternatively, combinations of ketamine (10–15 mg/kg) with medetomidine (0.08–0.1 mg/kg i.m., s.c.) or dexmedetomidine (0.04–0.05 mg/ kg i.m., s.c.) will provide a short period of heavy sedation or general anaesthesia in most ferrets. The duration and depth of anaesthesia is increased by the addition of butorphanol at 0.2–0.4 mg/kg i.m., s.c. or buprenorphine at 0.02 mg/kg i.m., s.c. which also provides analgesia. For perioperative/postoperative analgesia: 0.3–1.2 mg/kg/h CRI following 2–5 mg/kg i.v. loading dose. For postoperative analgesia: 0.1–0.4 mg/kg/h CRI.
- Rabbits: 15–30 mg/kg i.m., s.c. alone gives moderate to heavy sedation with some analgesia but there is poor muscle relaxation and prolonged recovery. Alternatively, 5 mg/kg i.v. or 10–15 mg/kg i.m., s.c. in combination with medetomidine (0.05–0.1 mg/kg i.v., 0.1–0.3 mg/kg s.c., i.m.) or

dexmedetomidine (0.025–0.05 mg/kg i.v. or 0.05–0.15 mg/kg s.c., i.m.) and butorphanol (0.1–0.5 mg/kg i.v., s.c., i.m.) or buprenorphine (0.02–0.05 mg/kg i.m., i.v., s.c.) will give a short duration of heavy sedation or anaesthesia in most rabbits. Intravenous combinations are ideally given incrementally to effect. Intraoperatively: May be used as infusion of 10 μg (micrograms)/kg/min; postoperatively: 2–5 μg/kg/min; both preceded by a 250–500 μg/kg loading dose.

- **Guinea pigs:** 10–50 mg/kg i.m., s.c. will provide immobilization, with little muscle relaxation and some analgesia, however it is suggested to use the lower end of the dose range to sedate first and then induce with isoflurane or sevoflurane; alternatively, a combination of ketamine (3–5 mg/kg i.m., s.c.) with medetomidine (0.10 mg/kg i.m., s.c.) or dexmedetomidine (0.05 mg/kg i.m., s.c.) will provide a short period of anaesthesia.

- **Other rodents and small mammals:** 10–50 mg/kg i.m., s.c. will provide immobilization, however it is suggested to use the lower end of the dose range and to induce anaesthesia with isoflurane or sevoflurane or use in combination with other agents (e.g. 5 mg/kg i.m., i.v., s.c. ketamine with 0.05–0.1 mg/kg i.m., i.v. medetomidine).

Birds: Largely superseded by gaseous anaesthesia [a].

Reptiles: Variable sedation and poor muscle relaxation if used alone. Prolonged recovery at higher dose rates. Usually combined with alpha-2 agonists and/or opioids/midazolam to provide deep sedation/light anaesthesia. **Chelonians:** 20–60 mg/kg i.m., i.v. [b]; **Lizards:** 25–60 mg/kg i.m., i.v.; **Snakes:** 20–80 mg/kg i.m., i.v.; all doses given alone. Lower doses are recommended in debilitated reptiles.

Amphibians: 50–150 mg/kg s.c., i.m. alone has long induction and recovery times. It is suggested to use 20–40 mg/kg i.m. in combination with diazepam at 0.2–0.4 mg/kg i.m.

Fish: 66–88 mg/kg i.m. alone or 1–2 mg/kg i.m. ketamine in combination with 0.05–0.1 mg/kg i.m. medetomidine, reversed with 0.2 mg/kg i.m. atipamezole.

References

[a] Redig PT and Duke GE (1976) Intravenously administered ketamine HCl and diazepam for anesthesia of raptors. *Journal of the American Veterinary Medical Association* **169(9)**, 886–888

[b] Holz P and Holz RM (1994) Evaluation of ketamine, ketamine/xylazine and ketamine/midazolam anesthesia in red-eared sliders (*Trachemys scripta elegans*). *Journal of Zoo and Wildlife Medicine* **25(4)**, 531–537

Ketoprofen
(Ketofen) **POM-V**

Formulations: Injectable: 1% solution. Oral: 5 mg, 20 mg tablets.

Action: COX-1 inhibition reduces the production of prostaglandins, while lipoxygenase enzyme inhibition has a potent effect on the vascular and cellular phases of inflammation. It has antipyretic, analgesic and anti-inflammatory effects.

Use: Relief of acute pain from musculoskeletal disorders and other painful disorders. Management of chronic pain. Ketoprofen is not COX-2 selective and is not recommended for preoperative administration. Do not administer perioperatively until the animal is fully recovered from anaesthesia and normotensive. Liver disease will prolong the metabolism of ketoprofen, leading to the potential for drug accumulation and overdose with repeated dosing. Administration of ketoprofen to animals with renal disease must be carefully evaluated. Ketoprofen has shown no significant analgesic effect in chain dogfish or koi, although it had some anti-inflammatory activity in koi that reduced muscle damage. It has also shown a significant reduction in the minimum anaesthetic concentration in goldfish.

Safety and handling: Normal precautions should be observed.

Contraindications: Do not give to dehydrated, hypovolaemic or hypotensive patients or those with GI disease or blood clotting problems. Do not give to pregnant animals or animals <6 weeks of age. Do not use in vultures.

Adverse reactions: GI signs may occur in all animals after NSAID administration. Stop therapy if this persists beyond 1–2 days. Some animals develop signs with one NSAID and not another. A 1–2-week wash-out period should be allowed before starting another NSAID after cessation of therapy. Stop therapy immediately if GI bleeding is suspected. There is a small risk that NSAIDs may precipitate cardiac failure in humans and this risk in animals is unknown.

Drug interactions: Do not administer concurrently or within 24 hours of other NSAIDs and glucocorticoids. Do not administer with other potentially nephrotoxic agents, e.g. aminoglycosides.

DOSES
Mammals: **Ferrets:** 1–3 mg/kg p.o., s.c., i.m. q24h; **Rabbits:** 1–3 mg/kg i.m., s.c. q24h; **Hamsters, Gerbils, Rats:** Up to 5 mg/kg p.o., i.m., s.c. q24h; **Other rodents:** 1–3 mg/kg s.c., i.m. q12–24h.
Birds: 1–5 mg/kg i.m. q8–24h[a]. Do not use in vultures[b].
Reptiles: **Green iguanas:** 2 mg/kg i.v. q24h, longer dosing intervals have been suggested based on pharmacokinetic data; **Bearded dragons:** 2 mg/kg i.m.[c]
Fish: 0.5–2 mg/kg i.m.[d,e,1]
Amphibians: No information available.

References
[a] Graham JE, Kollias-Baker C, Craigmill AL, Thomasy SM and Tell LA (2005) Pharmacokinetics of ketoprofen in Japanese quail (*Coturnix japonica*). *Journal of Veterinary Pharmacology and Therapeutics* **28(4)**, 399–402

[b] Naidoo V, Wolter K, Cromarty D *et al.* (2010) Toxicity of non-steroidal anti-inflammatory drugs to Gyps vultures: a new threat from ketoprofen. *Biology Letters* **6(3)**, 339–341

[c] Greenacre CB, Massi K and Schumacher J (2008) Comparative antinociception of various opioid and non-steroidal anti-inflammatory medications *versus* saline in the Bearded dragon (*Pogona vitticeps*) using electrostimulation. *Proceedings of the Association of Reptilian and Amphibian Veterinarians* pp. 87–88

[d] Harms CA, Lewbart GA, Swanson CR, Kishimori JM and Boylan SM (2005) Behavioral and clinical pathology changes in koi carp (*Cyprinus carpio*) subjected to anesthesia and surgery with and without intra-operative analgesics. *Comparative Medicine* **55(3)**, 221–226

e Ward JL, McCartney SP, Chinnadurai SK and Posner LP (2012) Development of a minimum-anesthetic-concentration depression model to study the effects of various analgesics in goldfish (*Carassius auratus*). *Journal of Zoo and Wildlife Medicine* **43(2)**, 214–222

1 Chatigny F, Creighton CM and Stevens ED (2018) Updated review of fish analgesia. *Journal of the American Association for Laboratory Animal Science* **57(1)**, 5–12

Ketorolac
(Acular*) **POM**

Formulations: Ophthalmic: 0.5% drops in 5 ml bottle.

Action: COX inhibitor that reduces the production of prostaglandins and therefore reduces inflammation.

Use: Treatment of anterior uveitis and ulcerative keratitis when topical corticosteroids are contraindicated. Topical NSAIDs have the potential to increase intraocular pressure and should be used with caution in animals predisposed to glaucoma.

Safety and handling: Normal precautions should be observed.

Contraindications: No information available.

Adverse reactions: As with other topical NSAIDs, ketorolac trometamol may cause local irritation. Topical NSAIDs can be used in ulcerative keratitis but with caution as they can delay epithelial healing. Topical NSAIDs have been associated with an increased risk of corneal 'melting' (keratomalacia) in humans, although this has not been reported in the veterinary literature. Regular monitoring is advised.

Drug interactions: Ophthalmic NSAIDs may be used safely with other ophthalmic pharmaceuticals although concurrent use of drugs which adversely affect the corneal epithelium (e.g. gentamicin) may lead to increased corneal penetration of the NSAID. The concurrent use of topical NSAIDs with topical corticosteroids has been identified as a risk factor in humans for precipitating corneal problems.

DOSES
Mammals: 1 drop per eye q6–24h depending on severity of inflammation.
Birds: 1 drop per eye q12h.
Reptiles, Amphibians, Fish: No information available.

Lactulose
(Duphalac*, Lactugal*, Lactulose*, Laevolac*) **P**

Formulations: Oral: 3.3 g/5 ml lactulose in a syrup base. Lactugal is equivalent to 62–74% w/v of lactulose.

Action: Metabolized by colonic bacteria resulting in the formation of low molecular weight organic acids (lactic, formic, acetic acids). These acids increase osmotic pressure, causing a laxative effect, acidifying colonic contents and thereby trapping ammonia as ammonium ions, which are then expelled with the faeces.

Use: Used to reduce blood ammonia levels in patients with hepatic encephalopathy and to treat constipation. Reduce the dose if diarrhoea develops. Some animals do not like the taste of lactulose. An alternative is lactitol (β-galactosidosorbitol) as a powder to add to food (500 mg/kg/day in 3 or 4 doses, adjusted to produce two or three soft stools per day), although its efficacy in the management of hepatic encephalopathy has not been extensively evaluated.

Safety and handling: Normal precautions should be observed.

Contraindications: Do not administer orally to severely encephalopathic animals at risk of inhalation.

Adverse reactions: Excessive doses cause flatulence, diarrhoea, cramping and dehydration.

Drug interactions: Synergy may occur when lactulose is used with oral antibiotics (e.g. neomycin). Do not use lactulose with other laxatives. Oral antacids may reduce the colonic acidification efficacy of lactulose. Lactulose syrup contains some free lactose and galactose, and so may alter insulin requirements in diabetic patients.

DOSES
Mammals: Ferrets: 0.15–0.75 ml/kg p.o. q12h; **Rodents:** 0.5 ml/kg p.o. q12h.
Birds: Appetite stimulant, hepatic encephalopathy: 0.2–1 ml/kg p.o. q8–12h.
Reptiles: 0.5 ml/kg p.o. q24h.
Amphibians, Fish: No information available.

Latanoprost
(Latanoprost*, Xalatan*) **POM**

Formulations: Ophthalmic: 50 µg/ml (0.005%) solution in 2.5 ml bottle (or 0.2 ml vials).

Action: Agonist for receptors specific for prostaglandin F. It reduces intraocular pressure by increasing outflow.

Use: Management of primary glaucoma and is useful in the emergency management of acute primary glaucoma (superseding mannitol, acetazolamide and dichlorphenamide). Often used in conjunction with other topical antiglaucoma drugs such as carbonic anhydrase inhibitors. Latanoprost may be useful in the management of lens subluxation despite being contraindicated in anterior lens luxation. Latanoprost has comparable activity to travatoprost.

Safety and handling: Store in refrigerator until opened (then at room temperature).

Contraindications: Uveitis and anterior lens luxation.

Adverse reactions: Miosis, conjunctival hyperaemia and mild irritation may develop. Increased iridal pigmentation has been noted in humans.

Drug interactions: Do not use in conjunction with thiomersal-containing preparations.

DOSES
Mammals: Rabbits: 1 drop per eye q8–24h.
Birds, Reptiles, Amphibians, Fish: No information available.

Levamisole
(Chanaverm, Levacide) **POM-VPS**

Formulations: Injectable: 7.5% solution. Oral: 7.5% oral solution.

Action: Imidazothiazoles act by interfering with parasite nerve transmission causing muscular spasm and rapid expulsion from the host.

Use: Treatment of nematodes, particularly lungworm, in hedgehogs. Not recommended in birds as low therapeutic index and severe toxicity reported in some species. Treatment of non-encysted gastrointestinal nematodes in fish (e.g. *Camallanus*) and some immunostimulatory effects have been reported in some species. Limited efficacy against nematode eggs, therefore repeat treatment after 3 weeks.

Safety and handling: Normal precautions should be observed.

Contraindications: No information available.

Adverse reactions: May cause sterility in zebrafish. May cause anorexia at higher doses.

Drug interactions: No information available.

DOSES
Mammals: Primates: 7.5 mg/kg s.c., repeat after 14 days if necessay; Hedgehogs: 10 mg/kg s.c. repeated in 48h, repeat after 14 days if necessary.
Birds: Not recommended.
Amphibians: 6.5–13.5 mg/kg applied topically, repeat in 10 days[a].

Fish: 2.5–10 mg/kg p.o. (in feed) q24h for 7 days or 1–2 mg/l by immersion for 24 hours or 50 mg/l by immersion for 2 hours. Follow manufacturer's recommendations for proprietary formulations.

Reptiles: No information available.

References

a Bianchi CM, Johnson CB, Howard LL and Crump P (2014) Efficacy of fenbendazole and levamisole treatments in captive Houston Toads (*Bufo [Anaxyrus] houstonensis*). *Journal of Zoo and Wildlife Medicine* **45(3)**, 564–568

Levetiracetam (*S*-Etiracetam, Levetirasetam)
(Desitrend*, Keppra*) POM

Formulations: Oral: 250 mg, 500 mg, 750 mg and 1 g tablets; 100 mg/ml oral 300 ml solution; coated granules 250 mg/sachet. Injectable: 100 mg/ml intravenous solution (5 ml vial); formulated with sodium chloride for injection at 500 mg/100 ml, 1000 mg/100 ml and 1500 mg/100 ml.

Action: The mechanism of anticonvulsant action is unknown but has been shown to bind to the synaptic vesicle protein SV2A within the brain, which may protect against seizures.

Use: As primary or adjunctive maintenance therapy for management of epileptic seizures refractory to conventional therapy. Used at a higher dose, in addition to conventional maintenance therapy, as pulse therapy for cluster seizures. Constant intravenous infusion used for emergency control of status epilepticus. Levetiracetam is rapidly absorbed from the GI tract with peak plasma concentrations reached in <2 hours of oral dosing. Steady state is rapidly achieved within 2 days. Plasma protein binding is minimal. The plasma half-life is short, being around 7 hours in human patients. Withdrawal of levetiracetam therapy or transition to or from another type of antiepileptic therapy should be done gradually. Use with caution and in reduced doses in patients with renal and severe hepatic impairment. Levetiracetam has also been used for the management of neuropathic pain (similar to gabapentin) in human patients.

Safety and handling: Normal precautions should be observed.

Contraindications: No information available.

Adverse reactions: The most commonly reported adverse effects in humans are sedation, weakness and dizziness. Blood dyscrasias such as neutropenia, pancytopenia and thrombocytopenia may also develop.

Drug interactions: Minimal, although there is some evidence to suggest that enzyme-inducing anticonvulsants (including phenobarbital and phenytoin) may modestly reduce levetiracetam levels, but not by clinically relevant amounts.

DOSES
Mammals: Prairie dogs: 20 mg/kg p.o. q8h.
Birds: 50 mg/kg p.o. q8h; 100 mg/kg p.o. q12h; individual variations seen so drug monitoring essential[a].
Reptiles, Amphibians, Fish: No information available.

References
[a] Schnellbacher R, Beaufrère H, Arnold RD, Tully Jr TN, Mayer J and Divers SJ (2014) Pharmacokinetics of levetiracetam in healthy Hispaniolan Amazon parrots (*Amazona ventralis*) after oral administration of a single dose. *Journal of Avian Medicine and Surgery* **28(3)**, 193–200

Levothyroxine (T4, L-Thyroxine)
(Leventa, Soloxine, Thyforon) **POM-V**

Formulations: Oral: 0.1 mg, 0.2 mg, 0.3 mg, 0.5 mg, 0.8 mg tablets; 1 mg/ml solution.

Action: Binds to specific intracellular receptors and alters gene expression.

Use: Treatment of hypothyroidism. No studies have been performed on exotic species and doses are anecdotal. Avian plasma total T4 levels are extremely low and reptile total T4 levels vary widely depending on species and external factors. Currently no European laboratories have tests validated for these levels. Thus, diagnosis of true hypothyroidism in birds and reptiles is controversial and there are few confirmed cases. Levothyroxine has been used to induce moult in birds; however, this is not recommended. Cases of pre-existing cardiac disorders require lower doses initially.

Safety and handling: Normal precautions should be observed.

Contraindications: Uncorrected adrenal insufficiency.

Adverse reactions: Clinical signs of overdosage include tachycardia, excitability, nervousness and excessive panting. May cause feather dystrophy if moult induced too quickly in birds.

Drug interactions: The actions of catecholamines and sympathomimetics are enhanced by thyroxine. Diabetic patients receiving thyroid hormones may have altered insulin requirements; monitor carefully during the initiation of therapy. Oestrogens may increase thyroid requirements by increasing thyroxine-binding globulin. The therapeutic effect of ciclosporin, digoxin and digitoxin may be reduced by thyroid hormones. Tachycardia and hypertension may develop when ketamine is given to patients receiving thyroid hormones. In addition many drugs may affect thyroid function tests and therefore monitoring of therapy.

DOSES
Mammals: Rodents: 5 μg (micrograms)/kg p.o. q12h.
Birds: 0.02 mg/kg p.o. q12–24h. Dissolve 1 mg in 28.4 ml water and give 0.4–0.5 ml/kg q12–24h.

Reptiles: Tortoises: 0.02 mg/kg p.o. q24–48h has been reported for the management of hypothyroidism in a Galapagos tortoise and an African spurred tortoise [1,2].

Amphibians, Fish: No information available.

References

1 Franco KH and Hoover JP (2009) Leveothyroxine as a treatment for presumed hypothyroidism in an adult male African spurred tortoise. *Journal of Herpetological Medicine and Surgery* **19(2)**, 47–49

2 Norton TM, Jacobson ER, Caligiuru R and Kollias GV (1989) Medical management of a Galapagos tortoise (*Geochelone elephantopus*) with hypothyroidism. *Journal of Zoo and Wildlife Medicine* **20**, 212–216

Lidocaine (Lignocaine)
(EMLA, Intubeaze, Lignadrin, Lignol, Locaine, Locovetic, Lidoderm*) **POM-V**

Formulations: Injectable: 1%, 2% solutions (some contain adrenaline). **Topical:** 2% solution (Intubeaze), 4% solution (Xylocaine); 2.5% cream with prilocaine (EMLA); 5% transdermal patches (Lidoderm).

Action: Local anaesthetic action is dependent on reversible blockade of the sodium channel, preventing propagation of an action potential along the nerve fibre. Sensory nerve fibres are blocked before motor nerve fibres, allowing a selective sensory blockade at low doses. Lidocaine also has class 1b antiarrhythmic actions, decreasing the rate of ventricular firing, action potential duration and absolute refractory period, and increasing the relative refractory period. Lidocaine has a rapid onset of action and intermediate duration of action. Addition of adrenaline to lidocaine increases the duration of action by reducing the rate of systemic absorption.

Use: Provision of local or regional analgesia using perineural, infiltration, local i.v. or epidural techniques. It is generally recommended that adrenaline-free solutions be used for epidural administration. Also used to provide systemic analgesia when given i.v. by continuous rate infusion. First-line therapy for rapid or haemodynamically significant ventricular arrhythmias. May also be effective for some supraventricular arrhythmias, such as bypass-mediated supraventricular tachycardia, and for cardioversion of acute-onset or vagally-mediated atrial fibrillation. Widely used topically to desensitize mucous membranes (such as the larynx prior to intubation). EMLA cream is used to anaesthetize the skin before vascular cannulation. It must be placed on the skin for approximately 45–60 min to ensure adequate anaesthesia; covering the skin with an occlusive dressing promotes absorption. EMLA is very useful to facilitate venous catheter placement in the ears of conscious rabbits. Infusions of lidocaine reduce the inhaled concentrations of anaesthetic required to produce anaesthesia and prevent central sensitization to surgical noxious stimuli. Systemic lidocaine is best used in combination with other analgesic drugs to achieve balanced analgesia. Lidocaine will accumulate after prolonged administration, leading to a delayed recovery.

Safety and handling: Normal precautions should be observed.

Contraindications: Do not give lidocaine solutions containing adrenaline i.v. Do not use solutions containing adrenaline for complete ring block of an extremity because of the danger of ischaemic necrosis. Do not use preparations with adrenaline in birds. Use cautiously in small fish: do not overdose small fish or exceed 1–2 mg/kg total dose.

Adverse reactions: Depression, seizures, muscle fasciculations, vomiting, bradycardia and hypotension. Pronounced systemic effects including respiratory depression and sedative effects have been observed in amphibians at high dosages. If reactions are severe, decrease or discontinue administration. Seizures may be controlled with i.v. diazepam or pentobarbital. Monitor the ECG carefully during therapy.

Drug interactions: Cimetidine and propranolol may prolong serum lidocaine clearance if administered concurrently. Other antiarrhythmics may cause increased myocardial depression.

DOSES
Note: 1 mg/kg is 0.05 ml/kg of a 2% solution.
Mammals: Local anaesthesia: apply to the affected area with a small gauge needle to an appropriate volume. Total dose that should be injected should not exceed 4 mg/kg (ideally 1–3 mg/kg). **Rabbits:** 0.3 ml/kg for epidural anaesthesia using 2% solution or 1–2 mg/kg i.v. bolus for cardiac arrhythmias or 2–4 mg/kg intratracheal for cardiac arrhythmias. Intraoperative analgesia given by continuous rate infusion: 1–2 mg/kg loading dose (given slowly over 10–15 min) followed by 50–100 μg (micrograms)/kg/min. Postoperatively, similar dose rates can be used but should be adjusted according to pain assessment and be aware of the likelihood of accumulation, allowing an empirical reduction in dose rate over time [a,b]; Topical: apply thick layer of cream to the skin and cover with a bandage for 45–60 min prior to venepuncture.
Birds: <4 mg/kg as local infusion/nerve block. Do not use preparations with adrenaline [c].
Reptiles, Amphibians: 1–2 mg/kg as local infusion/nerve block; Neuraxial anaesthesia: 2 mg/kg in bearded dragons [d]; 4 mg/kg in turtles [e]. Do not exceed 5 mg/kg total dose per animal due to risk of side effects including cardiotoxicity, respiratory depression and sedation [f].
Fish: 1–2 mg/kg as local infusion/nerve block [1]; Do not exceed 1–2 mg/kg total dose in small fish.

References
[a] Schnellbacher RW, Carpenter JW, Mason DE, KuKanich B, Beaufrère H and Boysen C (2013) Effects of lidocaine administration via continuous rate infusion on the minimum alveolar concentration of isoflurane in New Zealand White rabbits (*Oryctolagus cuniculus*). *American journal of veterinary research* **74(11)**, 1377–1384

b Schnellbacher RW, Divers SJ, Comolli JR et al. (2017) Effects of intravenous administration of lidocaine and buprenorphine on gastrointestinal tract motility and signs of pain in New Zealand White rabbits after ovariohysterectomy. *American journal of veterinary research* **78(12)**, 1359–1371

c da Cunha AF, Strain GM, Rademacher N, Schellbacher R and Tully TM (2013) Palpation and ultrasound-guided brachial plexus blockade in Hispaniolan Amazon parrots (*Amazona ventralis*). *Veterinary Anaesthesia and Analgesia* **40(1)**, 96–102

d Ferreira TH and Mans C (2019) Evaluation of neuraxial anesthesia in bearded dragons (*Pogona vitticeps*). *Veterinary anaesthesia and analgesia* **46(1)**, 126–134

e Mans C (2014) Clinical technique: Intrathecal drug administration in turtles and tortoises. *Journal of Exotic Pet Medicine* **23(1)**, 67–70

f Williams CJ, Alstrup AK, Bertelsen MF, Jensen HM, Leite CA and Wang T (2017) When local anesthesia becomes universal: pronounced systemic effects of subcutaneous lidocaine in bullfrogs (*Lithobates catesbeianus*). *Comparative Biochemistry and Physiology Part A: Molecular & Integrative Physiology* **209**, 41–46

1 Chatigny F, Kamunde C, Creighton CM and Stevens ED (2017) Uses and doses of local anesthetics in fish, amphibians, and reptiles. *Journal of the American Association for Laboratory Animal Science* **56(3)**, 244–253

Lignocaine see Lidocaine

Lincomycin
(Lincocin, Lincoject, Linco-Spectin) POM-V

Formulations: Injectable: 100 mg/ml solution for i.v. or i.m. use. Oral: powder for solution, some formulations combined with other drugs such as spectinomycin (Linco-Spectin).

Action: Lincosamide antibiotic that inhibits bacterial protein synthesis. It is bacteriostatic or bactericidal, depending on the organism and drug concentration. Being a weak base, it is ion-trapped in fluid that is more acidic than plasma and therefore concentrates in prostatic fluid, milk and intracellular fluid.

Use: Active against Gram-positive cocci (including penicillin-resistant staphylococci) and many obligate anaerobes. The lincosamides (lincomycin and clindamycin) are particularly indicated for staphylococcal bone and joint infections. Clindamycin is more active than lincomycin, particularly against obligate anaerobes, and is better absorbed from the gut. Administer slowly if using i.v. route.

Safety and handling: Normal precautions should be observed.

Contraindications: Rapid i.v. administration should be avoided since this can result in collapse due to cardiac depression and peripheral neuromuscular blockade. Do not use lincosamides in rabbits, other small herbivores or hamsters.

Adverse reactions: Human patients on lincomycin may develop colitis. Although not a major veterinary problem, patients developing diarrhoea (particularly if it is haemorrhagic) whilst taking the medication should be monitored carefully. Toxicity is a possibility in patients with liver disease; weigh the risk *versus* the potential benefits before use of this drug in such patients. Lincosamides can cause fatal enterotoxaemia in small herbivores and hamsters. May be nephrotoxic in reptiles.

Drug interactions: The action of neuromuscular blocking agents may be enhanced if given with lincomycin. The absorption of lincomycin may be reduced by kaolin. Lincosamide antimicrobials should not be used in combination with chloramphenicols or macrolides as these combinations are antagonistic.

DOSES
See Appendix for guidelines on responsible antibacterial use.
Mammals: Ferrets: 11 mg/kg p.o. q8h; **Primates:** 5–10 mg/kg i.m. q12h; **Sugar gliders:** 30 mg/kg p.o., s.c., i.m. q24h.
Birds: 50–75 mg/kg p.o., i.m. q12h; **Pigeons:** lincomycin/spectinomycin preparation: 500–750 mg combined activity/l water.
Reptiles: 5 mg/kg i.m. q12–24h.
Amphibians, Fish: No information available.

Liquid paraffin see **Paraffin**

Lomustine (CCNU)
(Lomustine*) **POM**

Formulations: Oral: 40 mg capsule.

Action: Interferes with the synthesis and function of DNA, RNA and proteins. Antitumour activity correlates best with formation of interstrand crosslinking of DNA. Lomustine is highly lipid-soluble, allowing rapid transport across the blood–brain barrier.

Use: Treatment of primary and metastatic brain tumours in humans. Its use in animals is less well defined but has been reported to have some efficacy in the treatment of brain tumours, mast cell tumours, refractory lymphoma, histiocytic sarcoma and epitheliotrophic lymphoma. S-Adenosylmethionine and silybin may be used to prevent or treat lomustine hepatotoxicity.

Safety and handling: Cytotoxic drug: see specialist texts for further advice on chemotherapeutic agents.

Contraindications: Bone marrow suppression. Pre-existing liver disease.

Adverse reactions: Myelosuppression is the dose-limiting toxicity, with neutropenia developing 7 days after administration. Thrombocytopenia can also be seen, often with no other concurrent cytopenias. GI and cumulative dose-related and potentially irreversible hepatic toxicity have been reported in the dog, but not in the ferret.

Drug interactions: Do not use with other myelosuppressive agents. Lomustine requires hepatic microsomal enzyme hydroxylation for the production of antineoplastic metabolites. In humans cimetidine enhances the toxicity of lomustine.

DOSES
See Appendix for chemotherapy protocols in ferrets.

Mammals: Ferrets: anecdotally used in lymphoma at doses extrapolated from cats (cat dose: 40–60 mg/m^2 p.o. q21d, but dosing intervals may need to be increased to 6 weeks).

Birds, Reptiles, Amphibians, Fish: No information available.

Loperamide
(Diareze*, Imodium*, Norimode*) **POM, P, GSL**

Formulations: Oral: 2 mg capsule (Diareze, Imodium, Norimode); 0.2 mg/ml syrup (Imodium).

Action: Opioid agonist that alters GI motility by acting on receptors in the myenteric plexus. It normally has no central action.

Use: Management of non-specific acute and chronic diarrhoea, and irritable bowel syndrome. May be used for symptomatic treatment of severe GI motility problems in rabbits, but for as short a period as possible to avoid GI stasis. Used in birds for cerebral oedema and anuric renal failure.

Safety and handling: Normal precautions should be observed.

Contraindications: Intestinal obstruction.

Adverse reactions: Constipation will occur in some cases.

Drug interactions: No information available.

DOSES
Mammals: Ferrets: 0.2 mg/kg p.o. q12h; **Rabbits:** 0.04–0.2 mg/kg p.o. q8–12h; **Rodents:** 0.1 mg/kg p.o. q8h; **Primates:** 0.04 mg/kg p.o. q8h.

Birds, Reptiles, Amphibians, Fish: No information available.

Lufenuron
(Program, Program plus) **POM-V**

Formulations: Oral: 67.8 mg, 204.9 mg, 409.8 mg tablets (Program); 46 mg, 115 mg, 230 mg, 460 mg lufeneron with milbemycin (ratio of 20 mg lufeneron: 1 mg milbemycin) tablets (Program plus); 133 mg, 266 mg suspension (Program for cats). Injectable: 40 mg, 80 mg as 100 mg/ml suspension (Program).

Action: Inhibition of chitin synthetase leads to a failure of chitin production which means that flea eggs fail to hatch.

Use: Prevention of flea infestation (*Ctenocephalides felis*, *C. canis*). For treatment of flea infestations the additional use of an approved adulticide is recommended. All animals in the household should be treated. Lufenuron has an additional antifungal action but specific doses for the effective treatment of dermatophytosis are currently unknown. Tablets/suspension should be administered with food. Can be administered during pregnancy and lactation (Program). Used to treat crustacean ectoparasites (*Argulus* spp.) in freshwater fish.

Safety and handling: Normal precautions should be observed.

Contraindications: No information available.

Adverse reactions: No information available.

Drug interactions: No information available.

DOSES
Mammals: Ferrets: 30–45 mg/kg p.o. q1month; **Rabbits:** 30 mg/kg p.o. q1month.
Fish: 0.1 mg/l by immersion as required (use suspension formulation)[a].
Birds, Reptiles, Amphibians: No information available.

References
[a] Mayer J, Hensel P, Mejia-Fava J, Brandão J and Divers S (2013) The use of lufenuron to treat fish lice (*Argulus* spp.) in koi (*Cyprinus carpio*). *Journal of Exotic Pet Medicine* 22, 65–69

Malachite green (Aniline green, Bright green)
(Malachite) **ESPA**

Formulations: Immersion: Proprietary formulations are available; also available in combination with formalin.

Action: A biocide (carbinol is the lipid-soluble form) which passes through biological membranes and acts as a cellular respiratory toxin.

Use: For the treatment of fungal infections (water mould) of fish and fish eggs. Some effect against protozoan ectoparasites and myxozoan parasites of fish. Some activity against Gram-positive bacteria in fish. It is strongly recommended that a proprietary formulation is used initially to avoid problems related to purity and enable accurate dosing. Malachite green is absorbed through the gills and cellular toxicity is irreversible. Toxicity is increased at higher temperatures, low pH and low water hardness. It is toxic to some species of small fish and plants. It is inactivated by light, therefore UV and aquarium lights should be switched off during treatment. Manufactured as a dyeing agent; impurities in some forms of malachite green salts are toxic. Must not be used in fish food due to absorption and long persistence of residues in tissues.

Safety and handling: Normal precautions should be observed. Teratogen and suspected carcinogen. Will stain many objects particularly plastics.

Contraindications: Do not use in tetras, small tropical fish or scaleless species.

Adverse reactions: Overdose, particularly in sensitive species, causes irreversible respiratory toxicity.

Drug interactions: Considered to have a synergistic effect with formalin (formaldehyde solution) against protozoan ectoparasites.

DOSES
Fish: 50–60 mg/l for 10–30 seconds by immersion or 1–2 mg/l for 30–60 min by immersion or 0.1 mg/l by prolonged immersion or 100 mg/l applied topically to skin lesions; follow manufacturer's recommendations for proprietary formulations.
Mammals, Birds, Reptiles, Amphibians: No information available.

Mannitol (Cordycepic acid)
(Mannitol*) **POM**

Formulations: Injectable: 10%, 20% solutions.

Action: Mannitol is an inert sugar alcohol that acts as an osmotic diuretic.

Use: Reduction of intracranial pressure (most effective in acute elevations of intracranial pressure), treatment of acute glaucoma and may also be used in the treatment of oliguric renal failure. Reduction in intracranial and intraocular fluid pressure occurs within 15 minutes of the start of a mannitol infusion and lasts for 3–8 hours after the infusion is discontinued; diuresis occurs after 1–3 hours. A 5.07% solution in water is isosmotic with serum. It is recommended that an in-line filter be used when infusing concentrated mannitol. There is some evidence that bolus administration (over 20–30 minutes) may be more effective for reduction of intracranial pressure than continuous administration. When used as treatment for raised intracranial pressure, hypovolaemia should be avoided to maintain cerebral perfusion pressure.

Safety and handling: Any crystals that have formed during storage should be dissolved by warming prior to use. The formation of crystals is a particular problem with the 20% formulations, which are supersaturated.

Contraindications: Prolonged administration may lead to the accumulation of mannitol in the brain and worsening of the cerebral oedema and raised intracranial pressure. Use with care in intracranial haemorrhage (except during intracranial surgery), take care to avoid volume overload in generalized oedema, severe congestive heart failure, pulmonary oedema or anuric renal failure (before rehydration).

Adverse reactions: The most common adverse reactions seen are fluid and electrolyte imbalances. Infusion of high doses may result in circulatory overload and acidosis. Thrombophlebitis may occur and extravasation of the solution may cause oedema and skin necrosis. Mannitol causes diarrhoea if given orally. Rarely mannitol may cause acute renal failure in human patients.

Drug interactions: Diuretic-induced hypokalaemia may occur when ACE inhibitors are used with potassium-depleting diuretics. Potassium-depleting diuretics should be used with care in conjunction with beta-blockers. Nephrotoxicity has been described with concurrent use of mannitol and ciclosporin in human patients. Mannitol may result in temporary impairment of the blood–brain barrier for up to 30 min after administration of high doses. Mannitol should never be added to whole blood for transfusion or given through the same set by which the blood is being infused. Do not add KCl or NaCl to concentrated mannitol solutions (20% or 25%) as a precipitate may form.

DOSES
Mammals: Ferrets: 0.5–1.0 g/kg i.v. infusion over 20 min; **Primates:** 0.25–1.0 g/kg i.v. infusion over 20 min.
Birds: Acute renal failure and cerebral oedema: 0.2–2 mg/kg slow i.v.
Reptiles, Amphibians, Fish: No information available.

Marbofloxacin

(Aurizon, Efex, Marbocyl, Marboxidin, Marfloquin, Softiflox, Ubiflox) **POM-V**

Formulations: Injectable: 200 mg powder for reconstitution giving 10 mg/ml when reconstituted. **Oral:** 5 mg, 20 mg, 80 mg tablets. **Topical:** Compound preparation containing 3 mg/ml of marbofloxacin along with clotrimazole and dexamethasone (aural use).

Action: Broad-spectrum bactericidal antibiotic inhibiting bacterial DNA gyrase. The bactericidal effect is concentration-dependent particularly against Gram-negative bacteria, meaning that pulse-dosing regimens may be effective. Low urinary pH may reduce the activity.

Use: Ideally fluoroquinolone use should be reserved for infections where culture and sensitivity testing predicts a clinical response and where first- and second-line antimicrobials would not be effective. Active against mycoplasmas and many Gram-positive and particularly Gram-negative organisms, including *Pasteurella*, *Staphylococcus*, *Pseudomonas aeruginosa*, *Klebsiella*, *Escherichia coli*, *Proteus* and *Salmonella*. Fluoroquinolones are effective against beta-lactamase-producing bacteria. Marbofloxacin is relatively ineffective in treating obligate anaerobic infections. Fluoroquinolones are highly lipophilic drugs that attain high concentrations within cells in many tissues and are particularly effective in the management of soft tissue, urogenital (including prostatitis) and skin infections. In rabbits, PU/PD has been noted when using the aural preparation due to uptake of corticosteroids and, ideally, a corticosteroid-free preparation should be compounded when an aural fluroquinolone is required.

Safety and handling: Normal precautions should be observed.

Contraindications: No information available.

Adverse reactions: Some animals show GI signs (nausea, vomiting). Use with caution in epileptics until further information is available, as fluoroquinolones potentiate CNS adverse effects when administered concurrently with NSAIDs in humans. Cartilage abnormalities have been reported following the use of other fluoroquinolones in growing animals. Such abnormalities have not been specifically reported following the use of marbofloxacin, but caution is advised.

Drug interactions: Adsorbents and antacids containing cations (Mg^{2+}, Al^{3+}) may bind to fluoroquinolones, preventing their absorption from the GI tract. The absorption of fluoroquinolones may be inhibited by sucralfate and zinc salts; doses should be at least 2 hours apart. Enrofloxacin increases plasma theophylline concentrations. Preliminary data suggest this may not be clinically significant with marbofloxacin unless used in patients with renal insufficiency. Cimetidine may reduce the clearance of fluoroquinolones and should be used with caution in combination.

DOSES

See Appendix for guidelines on responsible antibacterial use.

Mammals: 2–5 mg/kg p.o., s.c., i.m. q24h.

Birds: 10 mg/kg p.o., i.m., i.v. q24h[a]; **Macaws:** 2.5 mg/kg p.o., i.m. q24h[b].

Reptiles: Ball pythons: 10 mg/kg s.c., i.m., p.o. q48h[c]. **Chinese soft-shelled turtles:** 10 mg/kg p.o., i.m.[d]

Amphibians, Fish: No information available.

References

[a] García-Montijano M, González F, Waxman S et al. (2003) Pharmacokinetics of marbofloxacin after oral administration to Eurasian buzzards (*Buteo buteo*). *Journal of Avian Medicine and Surgery* **17(4)**, 185–190

[b] Carpenter JW, Hunter RP, Olsen JH, Henry H, Isaza R and Koch DE (2006) Pharmacokinetics of marbofloxacin in blue and gold macaws (*Ara ararauna*). *American Journal of Veterinary Research* **67(6)**, 947–950

[c] Coke RL, Isaza R, Koch DE, Pellerin MA and Hunter RP (2006) Preliminary single-dose pharmacokinetics of marbofloxacin in ball pythons (*Python regius*). *Journal of Zoo and Wildlife Medicine* **37(1)**, 6–10

[d] Shan Q, Zheng G, Liu S et al. (2015) Pharmacokinetic/pharmacodynamic relationship of marbofloxacin against Aeromonas hydrophila in Chinese soft-shelled turtles (*Trionyx sinensis*). *Journal of Veterinary Pharmacology and Therapeutics* **38(6)**, 537–542

Maropitant

(Cerenia, Prevomax, Vetemex) **POM-V**

Formulations: Injectable: 10 mg/ml solution. **Oral:** 16 mg, 24 mg, 60 mg, 160 mg tablets.

Action: Selective NK-1 receptor antagonist, developed to block substance P from binding within the chemoreceptor trigger zone. Highly protein bound, with a long duration of activity (24 hours).

Use: Treatment and prevention of vomiting in susceptible species, including that caused by chemotherapy and motion sickness. In cases of frequent vomiting, treatment by injection is recommended. It should be used in combination with investigation into the cause of vomiting and with other supportive measures and specific treatments. Tablets best given with food; avoid prolonged fasting before administration. Has been suggested to affect visceral pain in rabbits, reducing the response to colorectal stimulation[a], in addition to increasing colonic peristalsis[b].

Safety and handling: Normal precautions should be observed. Do not attempt to remove the tablet by pushing through the blister packing as this will damage the tablet.

Contraindications: No specific contraindications but it would be sensible not to use maropitant where GI obstruction or perforation could be present or for longer than 48 hours without a definitive diagnosis. Metabolized by the liver so use with caution in patients with hepatic disease.

Adverse reactions: Transient pain reaction during injection is reported with associated hyperexcitability and tachypnoea, but no significant lasting adverse reactions. Pain on injection can be reduced by injecting the product at refrigerated temperatures.

Drug interactions: No compatibility studies exist, and therefore the injection should not be mixed with any other agent. Should not be used concurrently with calcium-channel antagonists as maropitant has an affinity to calcium-channels. Highly bound to plasma proteins and may compete with other highly bound drugs.

DOSES
Mammals: Ferrets, Rabbits: 1 mg/kg s.c. q24h [c].
Birds, Reptiles, Amphibians, Fish: No information available.

References
[a] Okano S, Ikeura Y and Inatomi N (2002) Effects of tachykinin NK1 receptor antagonists on the viscerosensory response caused by colorectal distention in rabbits. *Journal of Pharmacology and Experimental Therapeutics* **300**, 925—931
[b] Onori L, Agio A, Taddei G *et al.* (2003) Peristalsis regulation by tachykin NK1 receptors in the rabbit isolated distal colon. *American Journal of Physiology: Gastrointestinal and Liver Physiology* **285**, G325—G331
[c] Ozawa SM, Hawkins MG, Drazenovich TL, Kass PH and Knych HK (2019) Pharmacokinetics of maropitant citrate in New Zealand White rabbits (*Oryctolagus cuniculus*). *American Journal of Veterinary Research* **80(10)**, 963—968

Mebendazole/Closantel
(Supaverm) **POM-VPS**

Formulations: Oral: 7.5% mebendazole and 5% closantel suspension.

Action: Binds to a structural protein of the parasite microtubules causing paralysis, death and expulsion of the parasites. Closantel uncouples oxidative phosphorylation in the cell mitochondria, resulting in inhibition of ATP synthesis, leading to alterations in energy metabolism and death of the parasite.

Use: For the treatment of external monogenean trematode infestation in koi carp.

Safety and handling: Normal precautions should be observed.

Contraindications: Do not administer to brood fish due to embryotoxic and teratogenic potential. Toxic to many other species.

Adverse reactions: No information available.

Drug interactions: No information available.

DOSES
Fish: 1 ml/400 l by permanent immersion (equivalent to 0.187 mg/l mebendazole and 0.125 mg/l closantel) [a].
Mammals, Birds, Reptiles, Amphibians: No information available.

References
[a] Marshall CJ (1999) Use of Supaverm for the treatment of monogenean infestation in koi carp (*Cyprinus carpio*). *Fish Veterinary Journal* **4**, 33—39

Medetomidine
(Domitor, Dorbene, Dormilan, Medetor, Sedastart, Sedator, Sededorm) **POM-V**

Formulations: Injectable: 1 mg/ml solution.

Action: Agonist at peripheral and central alpha-2 adrenoreceptors producing dose-dependent sedation, muscle relaxation and analgesia.

Use: Provides sedation and premedication when used alone or in combination with opioid analgesics. Medetomidine combined with ketamine is used to provide a short duration (20–30 min) of surgical anaesthesia. Specificity for the alpha-2 receptor is greater for medetomidine than for xylazine, but is lower than for dexmedetomidine. Medetomidine is a potent drug that causes marked changes in the cardiovascular system including an initial peripheral vasoconstriction that results in an increase in blood pressure and a compensatory bradycardia. After 20–30 min vasoconstriction wanes, while blood pressure returns to normal values. Heart rate remains low due to the central sympatholytic effect of alpha-2 agonists. These cardiovascular changes result in a fall in cardiac output; central organ perfusion is well maintained at the expense of redistribution of blood flow away from the peripheral tissues. Respiratory system function is well maintained; respiration rate may fall but is accompanied by an increased depth of respiration. Oxygen supplementation is advisable in all animals. The duration of analgesia from a 10 µg/kg dose is approximately 1 hour in dogs. Combining medetomidine with an opioid provides improved analgesia and sedation. Lower doses of medetomidine should be used in combination with other drugs. Reversal of sedation or premedication with atipamezole shortens the recovery period, which may be advantageous. Analgesia should be provided with other classes of drugs before atipamezole. Using medetomidine in combination with other drugs in the lower dose range can provide good sedation and analgesia with minimal side effects. Similarly to dexmedetomidine, medetomidine may be used in low doses to manage excitation during recovery from anaesthesia and to provide perioperative analgesia when administered by continuous rate infusion. Intramuscular injection of medetomidine has been used in combination with ketamine in elasmobrachs (sharks and rays) and some bony fish.

Safety and handling: Normal precautions should be observed.

Contraindications: Do not use in animals with cardiovascular or other systemic disease. Use in geriatric patients is not advisable. Do not use in pregnant animals. Do not use when vomiting is contraindicated. Not recommended in diabetic animals.

Adverse reactions: Causes diuresis by suppressing ADH secretion, a transient increase in blood glucose by decreasing endogenous insulin secretion, mydriasis and decreased intraocular pressure. Vomiting after i.m. administration is common, so medetomidine should be avoided when vomiting is contraindicated (e.g. foreign body, raised intraocular pressure). Due to effects on blood glucose, use in diabetic animals is not recommended. Spontaneous arousal from deep sedation following stimulation can occur with all alpha-2 agonists; aggressive animals sedated with medetomidine must still be managed with caution.

Drug interactions: When used for premedication, medetomidine will significantly reduce the dose of all other anaesthetic agents required to maintain anaesthesia. Drugs for induction of anaesthesia should be given slowly and to effect to avoid inadvertent overdose, the dose of volatile agent required to maintain anaesthesia can be reduced by up to 70%. Do not use in patients likely to require or receiving sympathomimetic amines.

DOSES
When used for sedation is generally given as part of a combination. See Appendix for sedation protocols in all species.

Mammals: Ferrets: 80–100 µg (micrograms)/kg i.m., s.c. in combination with an opioid and ketamine; **Rabbits:** 0.05–0.1 mg/kg i.v. or 0.1–0.3 mg/kg i.m., s.c. in combination with an opioid and ketamine; **Rodents, Other small mammals:** Doses from 100–200 µg/kg i.p., i.m., s.c. in combination with ketamine and/or opioids or as premedication prior to induction with a volatile anaesthetic.

Birds: See Appendix [a].

Reptiles: 100–200 µg (micrograms)/kg i.m; may be combined with ketamine and/or opioids or midazolam to provide deep sedation/light anaesthesia; **Desert tortoises:** 150 µg/kg i.m. [b]

Fish: 0.05–0.1 mg/kg combined with 1–2 mg/kg ketamine i.m. [c]; **Bonitos:** 0.4 mg/kg combined with 4 mg/kg ketamine i.m.; **Mackerel:** 0.6–4.2 mg/kg combined with 53–228 mg/kg ketamine i.m. [d]; **Sharks:** 0.06–0.08 mg/kg combined with 5 mg/kg ketamine i.m. [e]. Reverse with atipamezole at five times the dose of medetomidine.

Amphibians: No information available.

References
[a] Sandmeier P (2000) Evaluation of medetomidine for short-term immobilization of domestic pigeons (*Columba livia*) and Amazon parrots (*Amazona* species). *Journal of Avian Medicine and Surgery* **14(1)**, 8–14

[b] Sleeman JM and Gaynor J (2000) Sedative and cardiopulmonary effects of medetomidine and reversal with atipamezole in Desert tortoises (*Gopherus agassizii*). *Journal of Zoo and Wildlife Medicine* **31(1)**, 28–35

[c] Williams TD, Christiansen J and Nygren S (1993) A comparison of intramuscular anesthetics in teleosts and elasmobranchs. *Proceedings of the International Association for Aquatic Animal Medicine annual conference, 1993*

[d] Williams TD, Rollins M and Block BA (2004) Intramuscular anesthesia of bonito and Pacific mackerel with ketamine and medetomidine and reversal of anesthesia with atipamezole. *Journal of the American Veterinary Medical Association* **225(3)**, 417–421

[e] Stetter MD (2001) Fish and amphibian anesthesia. *Veterinary Clinics of North America: Exotic Animal Practice* **4(1)**, 69–82

Medroxyprogesterone
(Depo-Provera*, Provera*) **POM**

Formulations: Injectable: 150 mg/ml suspension. **Oral:** 5 mg tablets.

Action: Alters the transcription of DNA leading to alterations in cellular metabolism which mimic progesterone.

Use: Used in primates as a contraceptive. Used in birds to manage feather plucking, persistent ovulation and sexual behavioural problems, but not recommended due to side effects.

Safety and handling: Normal precautions should be observed.

Contraindications: Do not use in pregnancy or diabetes mellitus.

Adverse reactions: Temperament changes (listlessness and depression), increased thirst or appetite, cystic endometrial hyperplasia/pyometra, diabetes mellitus, adrenocortical suppression, reduced libido (males), mammary enlargement/neoplasia and lactation. Subcutaneous injections may cause a permanent local alopecia, skin atrophy and depigmentation. There are many side effects in birds including liver damage, obesity and diabetes mellitus.

Drug interactions: No information available.

DOSES

Mammals: Primates: 5–10 mg/animal p.o. q24h for 5–10 days; 150 mg/animal i.m q30d[a]; **Lemurs:** 5 mg/kg i.m. q6wk.

Birds: Persistent ovulation, Feather plucking, Sexual behavioural problems: 5–50 mg/kg i.m. Use with great care due to side effects. Repeat in 4–6 weeks if necessary.

Reptiles, Amphibians, Fish: No information available.

References
[a] Cruzen CL, Baum ST and Colman RJ (2011) Glucoregulatory function in adult rhesus macaques (*Macaca mulatta*) undergoing treatment with medroxyprogesterone actate for endometriosis. *Journal of the American Association for Laboratory Animal Science* **50(6)**, 921–925

Melatonin
(Circadin*) **POM**

Formulations: Oral: 2 mg tablets. Melatonin is also available in many over-the-counter formulations of various sizes and often with other drugs added.

Action: Hormone which is involved in the neuroendocrine control of seasonal hair loss.

Use: Palliative treatment of adrenocortical disease in ferrets.

Safety and handling: Normal precautions should be observed.

Contraindications: No information available.

Adverse reactions: No information available.

Drug interactions: No information available.

DOSES

Mammals: Ferrets: 0.5 mg p.o. q24h.

Birds, Reptiles, Amphibians, Fish: No information available.

Meloxicam

(Inflacam, Loxicom, Meloxidyl, Meloxivet, **Metacam**, Rheumocam) **POM-V**

Formulations: Oral: 0.5 mg/ml suspension for cats and guinea pigs, 1.5 mg/ml oral suspension for dogs; 1.0 mg, 2.5 mg tablets for dogs. **Injectable:** 2 mg/ml solution for cats, 5 mg/ml solution.

Action: Preferentially inhibits COX-2 enzyme thereby limiting the production of prostaglandins involved in inflammation.

Use: Alleviation of inflammation and pain in both acute and chronic musculoskeletal disorders and the reduction of postoperative pain and inflammation following orthopaedic and soft tissue surgery. All NSAIDs should be administered cautiously in the perioperative period as they may adversely affect renal perfusion during periods of hypotension. If hypotension during anaesthesia is anticipated, delay meloxicam administration until the animal is fully recovered from anaesthesia and is normotensive. Liver disease will prolong the metabolism of meloxicam leading to the potential for drug accumulation and overdose with repeated dosing. The oral dose (standard liquid preparation) may be administered directly into the mouth or mixed with food. Administration to animals with renal disease must be carefully evaluated. Be careful of species differences in effect in reptiles.

Safety and handling: After first opening a bottle of liquid oral suspension use contents within 6 months. Shake the bottle of the oral suspension well before dosing. The shelf-life of a broached bottle of injectable solution is 28 days.

Contraindications: Do not give to dehydrated, hypovolaemic or hypotensive patients or those with GI disease or blood clotting problems. Administration of meloxicam to animals with renal disease must be carefully evaluated and is not advisable in the perioperative period. Do not give to pregnant animals or animals <6 weeks of age.

Adverse reactions: GI signs may occur in all animals after NSAID administration. Stop therapy if this persists beyond 1–2 days. Some animals develop signs with one NSAID and not another. A 1–2-week wash-out period should be allowed before starting another NSAID after cessation of therapy. Stop therapy immediately if GI bleeding is suspected. There is a small risk that NSAIDs may precipitate cardiac failure in humans and this risk in animals is not known.

Drug interactions: Do not administer concurrently or within 24 hours of other NSAIDs and glucocorticoids. Do not administer with other potentially nephrotoxic agents, e.g. aminoglycosides.

DOSES

Mammals: **Ferrets:** 0.2 mg/kg p.o., s.c., i.m. q24h; **Rabbits:** 0.3–0.6 mg/kg s.c., p.o. q12–24h; studies have shown that rabbits may require a dose exceeding 0.3 mg/kg q24h to achieve optimal plasma levels of meloxicam over a 24-hour interval and doses of 1.5 mg/kg s.c., p.o. are well tolerated for 5 days; **Guinea pigs:** licensed at a dose of 0.2 mg/kg q24h on day 1, and 0.1 mg/kg subsequently, with doses of up to 0.5 mg/kg on an individual patient basis where necessary; **Rats:** 1–2 mg/kg s.c., p.o. q24h; **Mice:** 2 mg/kg s.c. p.o. q24h; **Primates:** 0.1 mg/kg p.o. q24h, 0.2 mg/kg i.m. q24h[a]; **Sugar gliders:** 0.2 mg/kg p.o., s.c. q24h; **Hedgehogs:** 0.2 mg/kg p.o., s.c. q24h.

Birds: 0.5–1.0 mg/kg i.m., p.o. q12–24h[b,c]. NB: doses of up to 20 mg/kg p.o. did not result in nephrotoxicity in American kestrels, but therapeutic and toxicology studies show significant species variation.

Reptiles: 0.1–0.5 mg/kg p.o., s.c., i.m. have been suggested although analgesic effect unproven in reptiles; **Bearded dragons:** 0.4 mg/kg i.m. q24h; **Green iguanas:** 0.2 mg/kg i.v., p.o. q24h[d]; **Red-eared sliders:** 0.2 mg/kg i.m., i.v., intracoelomic[e,f].

Amphibians: 0.4 mg/kg p.o., s.c., intracoelomic q24h.

Fish: No information available.

References

[a] Bauer C, Frost P and Kirschner S (2014) Pharmacokinetics of 3 formulations of meloxicam in cynomolgus macaques (*Macaca fascicularis*). *Journal of the American Association of Laboratory Animal Science* **53**, 502–511

[b] Cole GA, Paul-Murphy J, Krugner-Higby L et al. (2009) Analgesic effects of intramuscular administration of meloxicam in Hispaniolan parrots (*Amazona ventralis*) with experimentally induced arthritis. *American Journal of Veterinary Research* **70(12)**, 1471–1476

[c] Lacasse C, Gamble KC and Boothe DM (2013) Pharmacokinetics of a single dose of intravenous and oral meloxicam in Red-tailed Hawks (*Buteo jamaicensis*) and Great Horned Owls (*Bubo virginianus*). *Journal of Avian Medicine and Surgery* **27(3)**, 204–210

[d] Divers SJ, Papich M, McBride M et al. (2010) Pharmacokinetics of meloxicam following intravenous and oral administration in green iguanas (*Iguana iguana*). *American Journal of Veterinary Research* **71(11)**, 1277–1283

[e] Uney K, Altan F, Aboubakr M, Cetin G and Dik B (2016) Pharmacokinetics of meloxicam in red-eared slider turtles (*Trachemys scripta elegans*) after single intravenous and intramuscular injections. *American Journal of Veterinary Research* **77(5)**, 439–444

[f] Di Salvo A, Giorgi M, Catanzaro A, Deli G and Della Rocca G (2016) Pharmacokinetic profiles of meloxicam in turtles (*Trachemys scripta scripta*) after single oral, intracoelomic and intramuscular administrations. *Journal of Veterinary Pharmacology and Therapeutics* **39(1)**, 102–105

Mepivacaine

(Intra-epicaine) **POM-V**

Formulations: Injectable: 2% solution.

Action: Local anaesthetic action is dependent on reversible blockade of the sodium channel, preventing propagation of an action potential along the nerve fibre. Sensory nerve fibres are blocked before motor nerve fibres, allowing a selective sensory blockade at low doses.

Use: Blockade of sensory nerves to produce analgesia following perineural or local infiltration. Instillation into joints to provide intra-articular analgesia. Mepivacaine has less intrinsic vasodilator activity than lidocaine and is thought to be less irritant to tissues. It is of equivalent potency to lidocaine but has a slightly longer duration of action (100−120 minutes). It does not require addition of adrenaline to prolong its effect.

Safety and handling: Normal precautions should be observed.

Contraindications: Mepivacaine should not be injected i.v.

Adverse reactions: Inadvertent i.v. injection may cause convulsions and/or cardiac arrest.

Drug interactions: No information available.

DOSES
Mammals: Use the minimum volume required to achieve an effect. Toxic doses of mepivacaine have not been established in companion animals.
Birds, Reptiles, Amphibians, Fish: No information available.

Metacaine see **Tricaine mesilate**
Metamizole see **Butylscopolamine**

Methadone
(Comfortan, Synthadon) **POM-V CD SCHEDULE 2**

Formulations: Injectable: 10 mg/ml solution. **Oral:** 10 mg tablets.

Action: Analgesia mediated by the mu opioid receptor.

Use: Management of moderate to severe pain in the perioperative period. Incorporation into sedative and pre-anaesthetic medication protocols to provide improved sedation and analgesia. Methadone has similar pharmacological properties to morphine, and is useful in similar situations. It provides profound analgesia with a duration of action of 3−4 hours. Accumulation is likely to occur after prolonged repeated dosing which may allow the dose to be reduced or the dose interval to be extended. Methadone can be given i.v. without causing histamine release and does not cause vomiting when given to animals preoperatively. Transient excitation may occur when methadone is given i.v. Methadone may be administered epidurally to provide analgesia. Respiratory function should be monitored when given i.v. to anaesthetized patients. The response to all opioids appears to vary between individual patients, therefore assessment of pain after administration is imperative. Methadone is metabolized in the liver, and some prolongation of effect may be seen with impaired liver function.

Safety and handling: Normal precautions should be observed.

Contraindications: No information available.

Adverse reactions: In common with other mu agonists, methadone can cause respiratory depression, although this is unlikely when used at clinical doses in conscious animals. Respiratory depression may occur when given i.v. during general anaesthesia due to increased depth of anaesthesia. Methadone will cause constriction of GI sphincters (such as the pyloric sphincter) and may cause a reduction in GI motility when given over a long period. Methadone crosses the placenta and may exert sedative effects in neonates born to dams treated prior to parturition. Severe adverse effects can be treated with naloxone.

Drug interactions: Other CNS depressants (e.g. anaesthetics, antihistamines, barbiturates, phenothiazines, tranquillizers) may cause increased CNS or respiratory depression when used concurrently with narcotic analgesics.

DOSES
Mammals: Analgesia: **Rabbits:** 0.3–0.7 mg/kg slow i.v., i.m.
Birds, Reptiles, Amphibians, Fish: No information available.

Methanediol see **Formaldehyde**
Methanol see **Formaldehyde**

Methimazole (Thiamazole)
(Felimazole, Thyronorm) **POM-V**

Formulations: Oral: 1.25 mg, 2.5 mg, 5 mg tablets; 5 mg/ml solution. Also available as a transdermal formulation on a named patient basis.

Action: Interferes with the synthesis of thyroid hormones by inhibiting peroxidase-catalysed reactions (blocks oxidation of iodide), the iodination of tyrosyl residues in thyroglobulin, and the coupling of mono- or di-iodotyrosines to form T3 and T4. There is no effect on iodine uptake and it does not inhibit peripheral de-iodination of T4 to T3.

Use: Control of thyroid hormone levels in animals with hyperthyroidism. Monitor therapy on the basis of serum thyroxine concentrations (4–6 hours after dosing) and adjust dose accordingly for long-term medical management. Assess haematology, biochemistry and serum total T4 regularly, adjusting dosage as necessary. Transdermal thiamazole gels can also be used, particularly in those that develop GI side effects from the oral formulations. However, this route is not as reliable as oral medication or as safe for humans who apply the gel.

Safety and handling: Normal precautions should be observed.

Contraindications: Do not use in pregnant or lactating animals.

Adverse reactions: Vomiting (in target species capable of this) and inappetence/anorexia may be seen but are often transient. Jaundice, cytopenias, immune-mediated diseases and dermatological changes (pruritus, alopecia and self-induced trauma) are reported but rarely seen. Treatment of hyperthyroidism can decrease glomerular filtration rate, thereby raising serum urea and creatinine values, and can occasionally unmask occult renal failure. Animals that have an adverse reaction to carbimazole are likely also to have an adverse reaction to methimazole.

Drug interactions: Phenobarbital may reduce clinical efficacy. Benzimidazole drugs reduce hepatic oxidation and may lead to increased circulating drug concentrations. Methimazole should be discontinued before iodine-131 treatment.

DOSES
Mammals: Guinea pigs: 0.5–2.0 mg/kg p.o. q24h.
Reptiles: Snakes: 2 mg/kg p.o. q24h for 30 days.
Birds, Amphibians, Fish: No information available.

Methoprene (S-Methoprene)
(Acclaim spray, Amflee Combo, Bob Martin Clear Plus, **Fiproclear Combo**, Fleanil Duo, **Frontline Combo/Plus**, Fyperix Combo, PestiGon Combo, R.I.P. flea spray) **POM-V, NFA-VPS, AVM-GSL**

Formulations: Available in spot-on pipettes of various sizes always in combination with other agents. Those formulations licensed for ferrets contain 50 mg S-methoprene with 60 mg fipronil (Fiproclear Combo, Frontline Combo/Plus). Environmental: S-methoprene with permethrin (Acclaim) or tetramethrine + permethrin (R.I.P. Fleas) household sprays.

Action: Juvenile hormone analogue that inhibits larval development.

Use: Treatment and prevention of flea infestations (*Ctenocephalides canis* and *C. felis*) and ticks (*Ixodes ricinus*). For treatment of flea infestations the topical products should be applied every 4 weeks to all in-contact animals. Bathing between 48 hours before and 24 hours after topical application is not recommended. Minimum treatment interval 4 weeks. Can be used in pregnant and lactating females. Treat infested household as directed with spray; keep away from birds and fish. Environmental sprays also have some efficacy against house dust mites *Dermatophagoides farinae* and *D. pteronyssinus*.

Safety and handling: Normal precautions should be observed.

Contraindications: Do not use on ferrets less than 6 months old.

Adverse reactions: Local pruritus or alopecia may occur at the site of application. May be harmful to aquatic organisms.

Drug interactions: No information available.

DOSES
Mammals: Ferrets: One pipette of 0.5 ml/animal (50 mg fipronil, 60 mg *S*-methoprene) applied topically to back of neck.
Birds, Reptiles, Amphibians, Fish: No information available.

Methotrexate
(Matrex*, Methotrexate*) **POM**

Formulations: Oral: 2.5 mg, 10 mg tablets.

Action: An S-phase-specific antimetabolite antineoplastic agent; competitively inhibits folic acid reductase which is required for purine synthesis, DNA synthesis and cellular replication. This results in inhibition of DNA synthesis and function.

Use: Treatment of lymphoma, although its use in animals is often limited by toxicity. In humans it is used to treat refractory rheumatoid arthritis; however, data are lacking with regards to its use in immune-mediated polyarthritides. Monitor haematological parameters regularly.

Safety and handling: Cytotoxic drug; see specialist texts for further advice on chemotherapeutic agents.

Contraindications: Pre-existing myelosuppression, severe hepatic or renal insufficiency, or hypersensitivity to the drug.

Adverse reactions: GI ulceration, mucositis, hepatotoxicity, nephrotoxicity and haemopoietic toxicity may be seen, particularly with high doses. Low blood pressure and skin reaction are seen in humans.

Drug interactions: Methotrexate is highly bound to serum albumin and thus may be displaced by phenylbutazone, phenytoin, salicylates, sulphonamides and tetracycline, resulting in increased blood levels and toxicity. Folic acid supplements may inhibit the response to methotrexate. Methotrexate increases the cytotoxicity of cytarabine. Cellular uptake is decreased by hydrocortisone, methylprednisolone and penicillins, and is increased by vincristine. Concurrent use of NSAIDs increases the risk of haematological, renal and hepatic toxicity.

DOSES
See Appendix for chemotherapy protocols in ferrets.
Mammals: Ferrets: 0.5 mg/kg i.v. once as part of a chemotherapy protocol.
Birds, Reptiles, Amphibians, Fish: No information available.

Methylthioninium chloride
(Methylene blue)
(Methylthioninium chloride*) **POM, AVM-GSL**

Formulations: Injectable: 10 mg/ml (1% solution). **Immersion:** Several proprietary preparations are available.

Action: Acts as an electron donor to methaemoglobin reductase.

Use: Methaemoglobinaemia. Use an in-line filter if possible. Used for the treatment of protozoans and some monogenean ectoparasites, and external fungal infections in freshwater fish. It is strongly recommended that propriety formulations are used initially to avoid problems related to purity and to enable accurate dosing.

Safety and handling: Normal precautions should be observed.

Contraindications: Do not use unless adequate renal function is demonstrated.

Adverse reactions: May cause a Heinz body haemolytic anaemia and renal failure. Considered to have poor efficacy, stains many objects (especially plastics) and is toxic to some scaleless fish species, plants and nitrifying bacteria in biological filtration systems.

Drug interactions: No information available.

DOSES
Fish: 1–3 mg/l by immersion; follow the manufacturer's recommendation for proprietary formulations.
Mammals, Birds, Reptiles, Amphibians: No information available.

Metoclopramide
(Emeprid, Metomotyl, Vomend, Maxolon*, Metoclopramide*) **POM-V, POM**

Formulations: Injectable: 5 mg/ml solution in 10 ml multidose vials or clear glass ampoules. Oral: 10 mg tablets; 15 mg capsules; 1 mg/ml solution.

Action: Antiemetic and upper GI prokinetic stimulant; distal intestinal motility is not significantly affected. The antiemetic effect is a result of central dopamine (D2) receptor antagonism, and at higher doses $5HT_3$ antagonism, at the chemoreceptor trigger zone. The gastric prokinetic effect is a result of local D2 antagonism and stimulation of muscarinic acetylcholine and $5HT_4$ receptors leading to increases in oesophageal sphincter pressure, the tone and amplitude of gastric contractions and peristaltic activity in the duodenum and jejunum, and relaxing the pyloric sphincter by sensitizing tissues to acetylcholine. There is no effect on gastric, pancreatic or biliary secretions and nor does metoclopramide depend on an intact vagal innervation to affect motility.

Use: Vomiting of many causes can be reduced by this drug. The prokinetic effect may be beneficial in reflux oesophagitis and in emptying the stomach prior to induction of general anaesthesia. High doses are needed to abolish all reflux during anaesthesia. The prokinetic effect may also help to prevent postoperative ileus in rabbits; however, it is only effective in adult rabbits.

Safety and handling: Injection is light-sensitive. Obscure fluid bag if used in a continuous rate infusion.

Contraindications: Do not use where GI obstruction or perforation is present or highly suspected, or for >72 hours without a definitive diagnosis. Relatively contraindicated in epileptic patients.

Adverse reactions: Unusual, and probably relate to relative overdosing and individual variations in bioavailability. They include changes in mentation (depression, nervousness, restlessness) and behaviour. It may also cause sedation and extrapyramidal effects (movement disorders characterized as slow to rapid twisting movements involving the face, neck, trunk or limbs). Metoclopramide reduces renal blood flow, which may exacerbate pre-existing renal disease. Very rarely, allergic reactions may occur.

Drug interactions: The activity of metoclopramide may be inhibited by antimuscarinic drugs (e.g. atropine) and narcotic analgesics. The effects of metoclopramide may decrease (e.g. cimetidine, digoxin) or increase (e.g. oxytetracycline) drug absorption. The absorption of nutrients may be accelerated, thereby altering insulin requirements and/or timing of its effects in diabetics. Phenothiazines may potentiate the extrapyramidal effects of metoclopramide. The CNS effects of metoclopramide may be enhanced by narcotic analgesics or sedatives.

DOSES
Mammals: Ferrets, Rabbits, Guinea pigs: 0.5–1 mg/kg s.c., p.o. q6–12h; **Primates, Hedgehogs:** 0.2–0.5 mg/kg i.m., p.o. q8–24h; **Sugar gliders:** 0.05–0.1 mg/kg i.m., s.c., p.o. q6–12h.
Birds: 0.3–2.0 mg/kg p.o., i.m. q8–24h [a].
Reptiles: 0.05–1 mg/kg p.o., i.m. q24h. Higher doses may be needed in Desert tortoises.
Amphibians, Fish: No information available.

References
[a] Beaufrere H, Nevarez J, Taylor WM *et al.* (2010) Fluoroscopic study of the normal gastrointestinal motility and measurements in the Hispaniolan Amazon parrot (*Amazona ventralis*). *Veterinary Radiology & Ultrasound* **51(4)**, 441–446

Metronidazole
(Eradia, Metrobactin, Stomorgyl, Flagyl*, Metrolyl*, Metronidazole*) **POM-V, POM**

Formulations: Injectable: 5 mg/ml i.v. infusion. **Oral:** 200 mg, 400 mg, 500 mg tablets; 25 mg metronidazole + 46.9 mg spiramycin tablets, 125 mg metronidazole + 234.4 mg spiramycin tablets, 250 mg metronidazole + 469 mg spiramycin tablets (Stomorgyl 2, 10 and 20, respectively); 40 mg/ml, 125 mg/ml oral solution.

Action: Synthetic nitroimidazole with antibacterial and antiprotozoal activity. Its mechanism of action on protozoans is unknown but in bacteria it appears to be reduced spontaneously under anaerobic conditions to compounds that bind to DNA and cause cell death. Spiramycin is a macrolide antibacterial that inhibits bacterial protein synthesis.

Use: Treatment of anaerobic infections, giardiasis and other protozoal infections, and in the management of hepatic encephalopathy. Metronidazole may have effects on the immune system by modulating cell-mediated immune responses. It is absorbed well from the GI tract and diffuses into many tissues including bone, CSF and abscesses. Spiramycin (a constituent of Stomorgyl) is active against Gram-positive aerobes including *Staphylococcus*, *Streptococcus*, *Bacillus* and *Actinomyces*. Metronidazole has been used as an appetite stimulant in reptiles. In ferrets it is used in combination with amoxicillin, and bismuth subsalicylate, ranitidine or omeprazole (triple therapy) for treatment of *Helicobacter mustelae*. In rabbits it is the treatment of choice for enterotoxaemia due to *Clostridium spiroforme*. Metronidazole is frequently used in combination with penicillin or aminoglycoside antimicrobials to improve anaerobic spectrum. Some texts recommend doses in excess of 25 mg/kg. There is a greater risk of adverse effects with rapid i.v. infusion or high total doses. May have a role in chinchillas with giardiasis (however, use with care in this species). Used for the treatment of some protozoan ectoparasites and internal flagellates (e.g. *Hexamita*, *Spironucleus*) in fish.

Safety and handling: Normal precautions should be observed.

Contraindications: Do not administer to Indigo or King snakes due to toxicity. Do not use in very small birds, such as Zebra finches, due to toxicity.

Adverse reactions: Adverse effects in animals are uncommon and are generally limited to vomiting, CNS toxicity (nystagmus, ataxia, knuckling, head tilt and seizures), hepatotoxicity and haematuria. Prolonged therapy or the presence of pre-existing hepatic disease may predispose to CNS toxicity. Use with caution in the first trimester of pregnancy as it may be teratogenic. Anecdotally, has been associated with liver failure in chinchillas. Has been associated with toxicity in Indigo snakes, King snakes and Rattle snakes at doses >40–100 mg/kg.

Drug interactions: Phenobarbital or phenytoin may enhance metabolism of metronidazole. Cimetidine may decrease the metabolism of metronidazole and increase the likelihood of dose-related adverse effects. Spiramycin should not be used concurrently with other antibiotics of the macrolide group as the combination may be antagonistic. Metronidazole is relatively insoluble in water and requires thorough mixing before adding to fish tanks.

DOSES
See Appendix for guidelines on responsible antibacterial use.
Mammals: Ferrets: 15–20 mg/kg p.o. q12h or 50–75 mg/kg p.o. q24h for 14 days with clarithromycin and omeprazole for *Helicobacter*; **Rabbits, Chinchillas, Guinea pigs:** 10–20 mg/kg p.o. q12h or 40 mg/kg p.o. q24h; 50 mg/kg p.o. q12h for 5 days may be required for giardiasis in chinchillas but use with caution; **Other rodents:** 20–40 mg/kg p.o. q24h; **Primates:** 25 mg/kg p.o. q12h; **Sugar gliders:** 80 mg/kg p.o. q24h; 25 mg/kg p.o. q12–24h for 7–10 days; **Hedgehogs:** 20 mg/kg p.o. q12h.
Birds: Raptors: 50 mg/kg p.o. q24h for 5 days; **Parrots:** 30 mg/kg p.o. q12h; **Pigeons:** 40–50 mg/kg p.o. q24h for 5–7 days or 100 mg/kg p.o. q48h for 3 doses or 200 mg/kg p.o. once; **Passerines:** 50 mg/kg p.o. q12h or 200 mg/l water daily for 7 days.
Reptiles:
* Anaerobic bacterial infections: **Green iguanas, Snakes (*Elaphe* species):** 20 mg/kg p.o. q24–48h [a,b].
* Protozoal infections: **Chelonians:** 100–125 mg/kg p.o., repeat after 14 days (use lower doses of 50 mg/kg p.o. q24h for 3–5 days for severe infections); **Chameleons:** 40–60 mg/kg p.o., repeat after 14 days; **Milksnakes:** 40 mg/kg p.o., repeat after 14 days; **Other snakes:** 100 mg/kg p.o., repeat after 14 days.
Amphibians: 50 mg/kg p.o. q24h for 3–5 days or 50 mg/l as a bath for up to 24 hours.
Fish: 25 mg/l by immersion q48h for 3 doses or 100 mg/kg p.o. q24h for 3 days.

References
[a] Kolmstetter CM, Frazier DL, Cox SK and Ramsay EC (2001) Pharmacokinetics of metronidazole in the green iguana (*Iguana iguana*). *Bulletin of the Association of Reptilian and Amphibian Veterinarians* **8(3)**, 4–7
[b] Kolmstetter CM, Cox SK and Ramsay EC (2001) Pharmacokinetics of metronidazole in the yellow rat snake (*Elaphe obsolete quadrivittatta*). *Journal of Herpetological Medicine and Surgery* **11(2)**, 4–8

Miconazole
(Daktarin, Easotic, Malaseb, **Mycozole**, Surolan)
POM-V, ESPA

Formulations: Topical: 2% cream/powder (Daktarin); 2% shampoo (Malaseb); 23 mg/ml suspension with prednisolone and polymyxin (Surolan), 10 mg/ml spray for topical administration (Mycozole).

Action: Inhibits cytochrome P450-dependent synthesis of ergosterol in fungal cells causing increased cell wall permeability and allowing leakage of cellular contents. Miconazole has activity against *Malassezia*, *Cryptococcus*, *Candida* and *Coccidioides*.

Use: Fungal skin and ear infections, including dermatophytosis and chytridiomycosis (amphibians).

Safety and handling: Normal precautions should be observed.

Contraindications: No information available.

Adverse reactions: No information available.

Drug interactions: No information available.

DOSES
Mammals: Rabbits: fungal otitis: 2–12 drops in affected ear q12–24h; dermatophytosis: apply a thin layer of cream topically to affected area twice daily, continue for 2 weeks after a clinical cure and negative fungal cultures. Bathe affected area daily (miconazole/chlorhexidine preparations). Avoid preparations containing steroids.
Amphibians: 5 mg/kg intracoelomic q24h. Topical cream or 0.01% solution for chytridiomycosis[1].
Birds, Reptiles, Fish: No information available.

References
[1] Nichols DK and Lamirande EW (2001) Successful treatment of chytridiomycosis. *Froglog* **46**, 1

Midazolam
(Hypnovel*) **POM**

Formulations: Injectable: 2 mg/ml, 5 mg/ml solutions. **Oral:** 10 mg/ml solution for buccal administration.

Action: Causes neural inhibition by increasing the effect of GABA on the GABA$_A$ receptor, resulting in sedation, anxiolytic effects, hypnotic effects, amnesia, muscle relaxation and anticonvulsive effects. Compared with diazepam it is more potent, has a shorter onset and duration of action and is less irritant to tissues.

Use: Provides sedation with amnesia; as part of a premedication regime, as part of combined anaesthetic protocols, and in the emergency control of epileptic seizures (including status epilepticus). It provides unreliable sedation on its own, although it will sedate depressed animals. It is often used to offset muscle hypertonicity caused by ketamine. It is used with opioids and/or acepromazine for pre-anaesthetic medication in the critically ill. Midazolam can be diluted with saline, but avoid fluids containing calcium as this may result in precipitation of midazolam. Use with caution in severe hypotension, cardiac disease and respiratory disease.

Safety and handling: Normal precautions should be observed.

Contraindications: Avoid in myasthenia gravis and neonates.

Adverse reactions: In human patients, i.v. administration of midazolam has been associated with respiratory depression and severe hypotension. Excitement may occasionally develop.

Drug interactions: Midazolam potentiates the effect of some anaesthetic agents, including propofol and some inhalation agents, reducing the dose required. Concurrent use of midazolam with NSAIDs (in particular diclofenac), antihistamines, barbiturates, opioid analgesics or CNS depressants may enhance the sedative effect. Opioid analgesics may increase the hypnotic and hypotensive effects of midazolam. Erythromycin inhibits the metabolism of midazolam.

DOSES
When used for sedation is generally given as part of a combination. See Appendix for sedation protocols in all species.

Mammals: Ferrets: 0.25–0.5 mg/kg i.v. or 0.3–1.0 mg/kg s.c., i.m.; Rabbits: 0.2–2 mg/kg i.v., i.m.; general anaesthesia: 0.25–1.0 mg/kg i.v. when used with Fentanyl/Fluanisone; Chinchillas: 1 mg/kg i.v. or 2 mg/kg i.m.; Rodents: 2–5 mg/kg i.v., i.m., i.p.; Primates: 0.05–0.1 mg/kg i.v., i.m.; Sugar gliders: 0.1–0.5 mg/kg s.c., i.m., intranasal [a]; Hedgehogs: 0.5–1 mg/kg i.m. [b]

Birds: 0.1–0.5 mg/kg i.m. or 0.05–0.15 mg/kg i.v. (premedicant) or 2–3 mg/kg intranasal [c,d]. Can be combined with butorphanol for premedication.

Reptiles: 0.1–1 mg/kg i.m. for light sedation in snakes, lizards and chelonians [e]; Red-eared sliders: 1.5 mg/kg i.m. provides variable levels of sedation [f]; Can be combined with ketamine and/or opioids/alpha-2 agonists to provide deep sedation/light anaesthesia.

Amphibians, Fish: No information available.

References
[a] Rivas AE, Oye GW and Papendick R (2014) Dermal hemangiosarcoma in a sugar glider (*Petaurus breviceps*). *Journal of Exotic Pet Medicine* **23**, 384–388

[b] LaRue MK, Flesner BK and Higbie CT (2016) Treatment of a thyroid tumour in an African pygmy hedgehog (*Atelerix albiventris*). *Journal of Exotic Pet Medicine* **25**, 226–230

[c] Mans C, Guzman DSM, Lahner LL, Paul-Murphy J and Sladky KK (2012) Sedation and physiologic response to manual restraint after intranasal administration of midazolam in Hispaniolan Amazon parrots (*Amazona ventralis*). *Journal of Avian Medicine and Surgery* **26(3)**, 130–139

[d] Doss GA, Fink DM and Mans C (2018) Assessment of sedation after intranasal administration of midazolam and midazolam-butorphanol in cockatiels (*Nymphicus hollandicus*). *American Journal of Veterinary Research* **79(12)**, 1246–1252

[e] Arnett-Chinn ER, Hadfield CA and Clayton LA (2016) Review of intramuscular midazolam for sedation in reptiles at the National Aquarium, Baltimore. *Journal of Herpetological Medicine and Surgery* **26(1–2)**, 59–63

[f] Oppenhein YC and Moon PF (1995) Sedative effects of midazolam in red-eared slider turtles (*Trachemys scripta elegans*). *Journal of Zoo and Wildlife Medicine* **26**, 409–413

Milbemycin
(Milbemax, Program plus) **POM-V**

Formulations: Oral: 2.5 mg/25 mg, 12.5 mg/125 mg milbemycin/ praziquantel tablets (Milbemax for dogs); 4 mg/10 mg, 16 mg/40 mg (Milbemax for cats); 2.3 mg, 5.75 mg, 11.5 mg, 23 mg milbemycin with lufenuron (ratio 20 mg lufeneron: 1 mg milbemycin) tablets (Program plus).

Action: Interacts with GABA and glutamate gated channels, leading to flaccid paralysis of parasites.

Use: Treatment of adult nematode infestation; roundworms (*Toxocara canis*, *T. cati*), hookworms (*Ancylostoma caninum*, *A. tubaeforme*) and whipworms (*Trichuris vulpis*). The addition of lufeneron provides flea control. For treatment of flea infestations the additional use of an authorized adulticide is recommended. The addition of praziquantel provides control of cestodes (*Dipylidium caninum*, *Taenia* spp., *Echinococcus*, *Mesocestoides*). It is also used for the prevention of heartworm disease (*Dirofilaria immitis*) in countries where this parasite is endemic. Can be used in pregnant and lactating females.

Safety and handling: Normal precautions should be observed.

Contraindications: Do not use in animals suspected of having heartworm disease. Not for use in any animal <0.5 kg.

Adverse reactions: No information available.

Drug interactions: No information available.

DOSES
Mammals: Ferrets: 1.15–2.33 mg/kg p.o. q30d.
Birds, Reptiles, Amphibians, Fish: No information available.

Mineral oil see **Paraffin**

Mirtazapine
(Zispin) **POM**

Formulations: Oral: 15 mg tablets, 15 mg/ml solution.

Action: Tricyclic antidepressant that acts on central alpha-2 receptors which leads to increased noradrenaline levels within the brain. Also inhibits several serotonin receptors and histamine (H1) receptors.

Use: Appetite stimulation. Can also be used as an antiemetic in conjunction with other drugs, but authorized preparations are preferred. Monitor animal carefully when using mirtazapine, particularly if there is also cardiac, hepatic or renal disease.

Safety and handling: Normal precautions should be observed.

Contraindications: Do not use in patients with pre-existing haematological disease.

Adverse reactions: Sedation is common and can be profound. Can affect behaviour in many different ways. Has been associated with blood dyscrasias in humans.

Drug interactions: Several interactions known in humans, principally involving other behaviour-modifying drugs.

DOSES
Mammals: Rabbits: 1.88 mg p.o. q48h; can double dose if needed or increase frequency to q24h but not both.
Birds, Reptiles, Amphibians, Fish: No information available.

Misoprostol
(Cytotec*) **POM**

Formulations: Oral: 200 μg tablet.

Action: Cytoprotection of the gastric mucosa: it inhibits gastric acid secretion and increases bicarbonate and mucus secretion, epithelial cell turnover and mucosal blood flow. It prevents, and promotes healing of, gastric and duodenal ulcers, particularly those associated with the use of NSAIDs. Some reports suggest it may not prevent gastric ulceration caused by methylprednisolone.

Use: Protection against NSAID-induced gastric ulceration. In humans, doses of up to 20 μg/kg p.o. q6–12h are used to manage pre-existing NSAID-induced gastric ulceration, whilst doses of 2–5 μg/kg p.o. q6–8h are used prophylactically to prevent ulceration. Combinations with diclofenac are available for humans, but are not suitable for small animals because of different NSAID pharmacokinetics.

Safety and handling: Women who are or might be pregnant should avoid handling this drug.

Contraindications: Do not use in pregnant animals.

Adverse reactions: Diarrhoea, abdominal pain, nausea, vomiting and abortion.

Drug interactions: Use of misoprostol with gentamicin may exacerbate renal dysfunction.

DOSES
Mammals: Ferrets: 1–5 μg (micrograms)/kg p.o. q8h.
Birds, Reptiles, Amphibians, Fish: No information available.

Mitotane (o,p'-DDD)
(Lysodren*) **POM**

Formulations: Oral: 500 mg tablet or capsule.

Action: Necrosis of the adrenal cortex reducing the production of adrenal cortical hormones.

Use: Management of pituitary-dependent hyperadrenocorticism (HAC). However, other medications are authorized for this condition in dogs (**see Trilostane**). Has been used in the management of adrenal-dependent HAC, but with variable success. Mitotane is available from Europe for animals that have failed trilostane therapy. It should be given with food to improve its absorption from the intestinal tract. Following the initial 7–10 days therapy, an ACTH stimulation test should be performed to monitor the efficacy of therapy. In diabetic animals, the initial dose should be reduced by 30%. The addition of prednisolone is generally not recommended. If switching from trilostane to mitotane, then post-ACTH cortisol concentrations should be >200 nmol/l before starting mitotane. Not recommended to treat adrenal disease in ferrets due to their species-specific adrenal pathophysiology.

Safety and handling: Drug crosses skin and mucous membrane barriers. Wear gloves when handling this drug and avoid inhalation of dust.

Contraindications: No information available.

Adverse reactions: Anorexia, vomiting, diarrhoea and weakness, generally associated with too rapid a drop in plasma cortisol levels. They usually resolve with steroid supplementation. Acute-onset of neurological signs may be seen 2–3 weeks after initiation of therapy, possibly due to rapid growth of a pituitary tumour. Provide supplemental glucocorticoids during periods of stress.

Drug interactions: Barbiturates and corticosteroids increase the hepatic metabolism of mitotane. There may be enhanced CNS depression with concurrent use of CNS depressants. Spironolactone blocks the action of mitotane. Diabetic animals may have rapidly changing insulin requirements during the early stages of therapy.

DOSES
Mammals: Hamsters: 5 mg/animal p.o. q24h for 4 weeks.
Birds, Reptiles, Amphibians, Fish: No information available.

Morphine
(Morphine*, Oramorph*) **POM CD SCHEDULE 2**

Formulations: Injectable: 10 mg/ml, 15 mg/ml, 20 mg/ml, 30 mg/ml solution. **Oral:** 10 mg, 30 mg, 60 mg, 100 mg tablets. In addition there are suspensions, slow-release capsules, and granules in a wide range of strengths. **Rectal:** Suppositories are available in a wide range of strengths.

Action: Analgesia mediated by the mu opioid receptor.

Use: Management of moderate to severe pain in the perioperative period. Incorporation into sedative and pre-anaesthetic medication protocols to provide improved sedation and analgesia. Morphine is the reference opioid with which all others are compared. It provides profound analgesia and forms the mainstay of postoperative analgesic protocols in humans. In most species it has a short duration of action and continuous rate infusions can be used to overcome this limitation. The greater availability of data describing morphine by continuous rate infusion may justify its use over methadone for this method of administration. Accumulation is likely to occur after prolonged repeated dosing, which may allow the dose to be reduced or the dose interval to be extended. Morphine causes histamine release when given rapidly i.v., so it should be diluted and given slowly i.v. It commonly causes vomiting when given to animals preoperatively that are not in pain, therefore morphine should be avoided when vomiting is contraindicated (e.g. animals with raised intraocular pressure). Transient excitation may occur when morphine is given i.v. Preservative-free morphine can be administered into the epidural space where it will provide analgesia for up to 24 hours. Respiratory function should be monitored when morphine is given to anaesthetized patients. The response to all opioids appears to vary between individual patients, therefore assessment of pain after administration is imperative. Morphine is metabolized in the liver, some prolongation of effect may be seen with impaired liver function. Be careful of species differences in effect in reptiles and fish.

Safety and handling: Normal precautions should be observed.

Contraindications: No information available.

Adverse reactions: In common with other mu agonists, morphine can cause respiratory depression, although this is unlikely when used at clinical doses. Respiratory depression may occur when given i.v. during general anaesthesia due to increased depth of anaesthesia. Vomiting is common after morphine administration and it causes constriction of GI sphincters (such as the pyloric sphincter) and may cause a reduction in GI motility when given over a long period. Morphine crosses the placenta and may exert sedative effects in neonates prior to parturition. Severe adverse effects can be treated with naloxone. A paradoxical increase in activity at lower dose rates has been reported in some fish species.

Drug interactions: Other CNS depressants (e.g. anaesthetics, antihistamines, barbiturates, phenothiazines, tranquillizers) may cause increased CNS or respiratory depression when used concurrently with narcotic analgesics.

DOSES

Mammals: Analgesia: **Primates:** 1 mg/kg p.o., s.c., i.m., i.v. q4h; **Ferrets:** 0.5–5 mg/kg i.m., s.c. q2–6h or 0.1 mg/kg epidural once[a]; **Rabbits:** 0.1–0.4 mg/kg/h by CRI; **Rabbits, Rodents:** 0.5–2 mg/kg i.m., s.c. q2–4h. Whilst higher doses have been used in laboratory settings, these are on extremely healthy animals with no current pathology present, unlike clinical cases. Ceiling effects mean that increasing dose does not necessarily correspond to increasing analgesia; in practice, doses of 0.5–2.0 mg/kg are observed to have good analgesic effects.

Reptiles: Analgesia: 1–5 mg/kg i.m., although may result in significant respiratory depression especially at higher doses in debilitated patients; **Red-eared sliders:** 1.5 mg/kg i.m.[b]; **Green iguanas, Bearded dragons:** 1 mg/kg i.m. **Tegus:** 5 mg/kg i.m.[c]

Amphibians: Analgesia: 38–42 mg/kg s.c.[d] May be used at 5 mg/100 ml combined with alfaxalone for immersion anaesthesia.

Fish: Analgesia: **Koi:** 5 mg/kg i.m.[e]; **Goldfish:** 40 mg/kg intracoelomic[f].

Birds: No information available.

References

[a] Sladky KK, Horne WA, Goodrowe KL *et al.* (2000) Evaluation of epidural morphine for postoperative analgesia in ferrets (*Mustela putorius furo*). *Contemporary Topics in Laboratory Animal Science* **39(6)**, 33–38

[b] Sladky KK, Miletic V, Paul-Murphy J *et al.* (2007) Analgesic efficacy and respiratory effects of butorphanol and morphine in turtles. *Journal of the American Veterinary Medical Association* **230(9)**, 1356–1362

[c] Leal WP, Carregaro AB, Bressan TF *et al.* (2017) Antinociceptive efficacy of intramuscular administration of morphine sulfate and butorphanol tartrate in tegus (*Salvator merianae*). *American Journal of Veterinary Research* **78(9)**, 1019–1024

[d] Coble DJ, Taylor DK and Mook DM (2011) Analgesic effects of meloxicam, morphine sulphate, flunixin meglumine and xylazine hydrochloride in African clawed frogs (*Xenopus laevis*). *Journal of the American Association of Laboratory Animal Science* **50(3)**, 355–360

[e] eBaker TR, Baker BB, Johnson SM and Sladky KK (2013) Comparative analgesic efficacy of morphine sulfate and butorphanol tartrate in koi (*Cyprinus carpio*) undergoing unilateral gonadectomy. *Journal of the American Veterinary Medical Association* **243(6)**, 882–890

[f] Newby NC, Wilkie MP and Stevens ED (2009) Morphine uptake, disposition, and analgesic efficacy in the common goldfish (*Carassius auratus*). *Canadian Journal of Zoology* **87(5)**, 388–399

Moxidectin

(**Advocate**, Cydectin, **Moxiclear**, **Prinovox**)
POM-V

Formulations: Topical: 10 mg/ml and 25 mg/ml moxidectin with imidacloprid in spot-on pipette. **Injectable:** 1% solution.

Action: Interacts with GABA and glutamate gated channels, leading to flaccid paralysis of parasites.

Use: Authorized for use in ferrets for treatment and prevention of flea infestation (*Ctenocephalides felis*) and the prevention of heartworm. Used in rabbits for *Psoroptes cuniculi*. Used in birds for mite infestation. Used in lizards for the treatment of nematode infections and mites.

Safety and handling: Normal precautions should be observed.

Contraindications: Do not use larger pipette sizes in ferrets.

Adverse reactions: Transient pruritus and erythema at the site of application may occur. Highly toxic to aquatic organisms.

Drug interactions: No information available.

DOSES
Mammals: Ferrets: 0.4 ml pipette monthly. If under heavy flea pressure can repeat once after 2 weeks; **Rabbits:** 0.2–0.3 mg/kg p.o., repeat in 10 days [a].
Birds: 0.2 mg/kg topically prn.
Reptiles: Bearded dragons, Frillneck lizards: 0.2 ml/kg topically q14d for 3 treatments.
Amphibians: 200 μg (micrograms)/kg s.c. q4months for nematodes.
Fish: No information available.

References
[a] Wagner R and Wendberger U (2000) Field efficacy of moxidectin in dogs and rabbits naturally infested with *Sarcoptes* spp., *Demodex* spp. and *Psoroptes* spp. mites. *Veterinary parasitology* **93(2)**, 149–158

Moxifloxacin
(Moxivig*) **POM**

Formulations: Topical: 0.5% solution (5 mg/ml; 5 ml bottle).

Action: Bactericidal antimicrobial which works by inhibiting the bacterial DNA gyrase enzyme, causing damage to the bacterial DNA. The fluoroquinolones work in a concentration-dependent manner.

Use: Ideally, fluoroquinolone use should be reserved for infections where culture and sensitivity testing predicts a clinical response and where first- and second-line antimicrobials would not be effective. Fourth generation fluoroquinolone with broad-spectrum activity against a wide range of Gram-negative and some Gram-positive aerobes. Active against many ocular pathogens, including *Staphylococcus* spp. and *Pseudomonas aeruginosa*.

Safety and handling: Normal precautions should be observed.

Contraindications: No information available.

Adverse reactions: May cause local irritation after application.

Drug interactions: No information available.

DOSES
See Appendix for guidelines on responsible antibacterial use.
Mammals, Birds, Reptiles: 1 drop in affected eye q12h.
Amphibians, Fish: No information available.

Naloxone
(Naloxone*, Narcan*) **POM**

Formulations: Injectable: 0.02 mg/ml, 0.4 mg/ml solutions.

Action: Competitive antagonist for opioid receptors, reversing the effects of opioid agonists.

Use: Treatment of opioid overdose to reverse the adverse effects of opioid agonists. Also used to identify persistent activity of opioid drugs. Onset of action i.v. is very rapid, but duration is short (30–40 min). Repeated doses or an infusion may be required to manage overdose of longer acting opioids such as morphine and methadone or high-dose fentanyl. Naloxone will also antagonize the effects of endogenous opioids, therefore it can cause antanalgesic effects in opioid naïve subjects. Administration to animals that could be in pain must therefore be considered carefully. Low dose naloxone i.v. will cause a transient elevation of unconsciousness when persistent opioid activity contributes to an unexpectedly long recovery from anaesthesia.

Safety and handling: Normal precautions should be observed.

Contraindications: No information available.

Adverse reactions: Indiscriminate use in animals that have undergone major surgery or trauma will expose the recipient to acute severe discomfort. In such cases the effects of opioid overdose (respiratory depression) should be managed by endotracheal intubation and artificial ventilation. Naloxone should be reserved for emergency situations when the effects of opioid overdose are severe.

Drug interactions: No information available.

DOSES
Mammals: Ferrets: 0.01–0.04 mg/kg i.v., i.m., s.c.; **Rabbits:** 0.01–0.1 mg/kg i.v., i.m., i.p.; **Rodents:** 0.01–0.1 mg/kg s.c., i.v., i.p.; **Primates:** 0.01–0.1 mg/kg s.c., i.m., i.v.; **Hedgehogs:** 0.1–0.16 mg/kg s.c., i.m. [a] Naloxone can be administered as a CRI at 0.02 mg/kg/h i.v. if a longer duration of opioid antagonism is required.
Birds: 2 mg/animal i.v.
Amphibians: 10 mg/kg s.c.
Reptiles, Fish: No Information available.

References
[a] Europaeus HE (1995) Chemical immobilization of free-ranging european hedgehogs (*erinaceus europaeus*). *Journal of Zoo and Wildlife Medicine* **26(2)**, 246–251

Nandrolone
(Laurabolin, Decadurabolin*) **POM-V, POM**

Formulations: Injectable: 25 mg/ml, 50 mg/ml (in oil).

Action: Binds to testosterone receptors and stimulates protein synthesis.

Use: For use wherever excessive tissue breakdown or extensive repair processes are taking place. Has also been advocated in the management of aplastic anaemia and anaemia associated with renal failure; however, may also have adverse effects on renal failure by increasing protein turnover. Monitor haematology to determine the efficacy of treatment and liver enzymes to monitor for hepatotoxicity.

Safety and handling: Normal precautions should be observed.

Contraindications: Do not use in breeding animals, in pregnant animals or in those with diabetes mellitus.

Adverse reactions: Androgenic effects may develop. Use in immature animals may result in early closure of epiphyseal growth plates.

Drug interactions: The concurrent use of anabolic steroids with adrenal steroids may potentiate the development of oedema.

DOSES
Mammals: Ferrets: 1–5 mg/kg i.m. q7d; **Rabbits:** 2 mg/kg s.c., i.m. q7d.
Reptiles: 1 mg/kg i.m. q7–14d.
Birds, Amphibians, Fish: No information available.

Neomycin
(Neopen, Maxitrol*, Nivemycin*) **POM-V, POM**

Formulations: Oral: 500 mg tablets (Nivemycin). **Parenteral:** 100 mg/ml neomycin combined with 200 mg/ml penicillin G (Neopen). **Topical:** Many dermatological, ophthalmic and otic preparations contain 0.25–0.5% neomycin.

Action: A bactericidal antimicrobial agent that inhibits bacterial protein synthesis once it has gained access to the bacterial cell via an oxygen-dependent carrier mechanism. As other aminoglycosides, neomycin operates a concentration-dependent cell killing mechanism, leading to a marked post-antibiotic effect.

Use: Active primarily against Gram-negative bacteria, although some *Staphylococcus* and *Enterococcus* species are sensitive. All obligate anaerobic bacteria and many haemolytic streptococci are resistant. Since parenteral neomycin is extremely nephrotoxic and ototoxic it is used topically for infections of the skin, ear or mucous membranes. It is also used orally to reduce the intestinal bacterial population in the management of hepatic encephalopathy. As with other aminoglycosides it is not absorbed after oral administration unless GI ulceration is present. This drug has been used (often combined with antimuscarinic agents) in the treatment of non-specific bacterial enteritides. However, other antibacterial drugs, if required at all, are better indicated for such use. Neomycin is more active in an alkaline environment.

Safety and handling: Normal precautions should be observed.

Contraindications: For systemic use, do not use in animals with pre-existing renal disease. Do not use ear preparations if the tympanum is ruptured.

Adverse reactions: Systemic toxicity, ototoxicity and nephrotoxicity may very occasionally occur following prolonged high-dose oral therapy or where there is severe GI ulceration/inflammatory bowel disease, as sufficient neomycin may be absorbed. Nephrotoxicity and ototoxicity are potential side effects associated with parenteral use. Some patients may develop a severe diarrhoea/malabsorption syndrome and bacterial or fungal superinfections. Topical ophthalmic preparation may cause local irritation.

Drug interactions: Absorption of digoxin, methotrexate, potassium and vitamin K may be decreased. Other ototoxic and nephrotoxic drugs, e.g. furosemide, should be used with caution in patients on oral neomycin therapy as the combinations are likely to be synergistic.

DOSES
See Appendix for guidelines on responsible antibacterial use.
Mammals: **Ferrets:** 10–20 mg/kg p.o. q6h; **Rabbits:** 30 mg/kg p.o. q12h; **Chinchillas, Guinea pigs:** 15 mg/kg p.o. q12h; **Rats, Mice:** 25 mg/kg p.o. q12h; In-water medication: **Gerbils, Rats, Mice:** 2.6 mg/ml drinking water; **Hamsters:** 0.5 mg/ml drinking water; Ophthalmic: 1 drop/eye q6–8h; Otic: 2–12 drops/ear or apply liberally to skin q4–12h.
Birds: 10 mg/kg p.o. q8–12h.
Reptiles, Amphibians, Fish: No information available.

Nitenpyram
(Bob Martin Flea Tablets, Capstar, Johnson's 4 Fleas) **AVM-GSL**

Formulations: Oral: 11.4 mg, 57 mg tablets.

Action: Postsynaptic binding to insect nicotinic receptors leads to insect paralysis and death. Kills fleas on animal within 30 minutes.

Use: Treatment of fleas. Should be used as part of a fully integrated flea control programme. All animals in the affected household should be treated. Treatment of flystrike in rabbits and rodents. Safe in pregnancy and lactation.

Safety and handling: Normal precautions should be observed.

Contraindications: No information available.

Adverse reactions: Transient increase in pruritus may be seen after administration due to fleas reacting to the product.

Drug interactions: No information available.

DOSES
Mammals: 1 mg/kg p.o. once (minimum dose) or q24h.
Birds, Reptiles, Amphibians, Fish: No information available.

Nitroglycerin(e) see **Glyceryl trinitrate**

Nitrous oxide
(Entonox*, Nitrous oxide*) **POM**

Formulations: Inhalational: 100% nitrous oxide (N_2O) gas. Entonox is N_2O plus oxygen.

Action: Causes CNS depression.

Use: Used with oxygen to carry volatile anaesthetic agents such as isoflurane for the induction and maintenance of anaesthesia. N_2O reduces the concentration of inhalant agent required to maintain anaesthesia. Administration of N_2O at the beginning of volatile agent anaesthesia increases the speed of uptake of volatile agent from the alveoli (via the 2nd gas effect and concentration effect), hastening attainment of a stable plane of volatile agent anaesthesia. Oxygen must be supplemented for 5–10 min after N_2O is discontinued to prevent diffusion hypoxia. N_2O causes minimal respiratory and cardiovascular effects and is a useful addition to a balanced anaesthesia technique. A minimum oxygen concentration of 30% is required during anaesthesia. The inspired concentration of oxygen may fall to critically low levels when N_2O is used in rebreathing circuits during low flow rates. Do not use in such systems unless the inspired oxygen concentration can be measured on a breath-by-breath basis.

Safety and handling: Prolonged exposure can have serious adverse effects on human health. Scavenging is essential. N_2O is not absorbed by charcoal in passive scavenging systems utilizing activated charcoal.

Contraindications: Do not give to patients with air-filled spaces within the body, e.g. pneumothorax or gastric dilatation. N_2O will cause a rapid expansion of any gas-filled space, increasing volume or pressure. It does not appear to cause problems in the normal caecum of hindgut fermenting species. Do not give to animals with marked respiratory compromise, due to the risks of hypoxia.

Adverse reactions: The cobalt ion present in vitamin B12 is oxidized by N_2O so that it is no longer able to act as the cofactor for methionine synthase. The result is reduced synthesis of methionine, thymidine, tetrahydrofolate and DNA. Exposure lasting only a few hours may lead to megaloblastic changes in bone marrow but more prolonged exposure (a few days) may result in agranulocytosis.

Drug interactions: No information available.

DOSES
Mammals, Birds: Inspired concentrations of 50–70%.
Reptiles, Amphibians, Fish: No information available.

Nystatin
(Canaural, Nystan*, Nystatin*) **POM-V, POM**

Formulations: Oral: 100,000 IU/ml suspension. **Topical:** various products.

Action: Binds to ergosterol, a major component of the fungal cell membrane, and forms pores in the membrane that lead to potassium leakage and death of the fungus.

Use: Antifungal agent with a broad spectrum of activity but noted for its activity against *Candida*, particularly *C. albicans*. Not absorbed from the GI tract.

Safety and handling: Normal precautions should be observed.

Contraindications: No information available.

Adverse reactions: Corticosteroid-free preparations are preferred in pregnant animals, birds and rabbits to avoid the systemic effects of corticosteroids.

Drug interactions: No information available.

DOSES
Mammals: All species: Topical: apply to affected areas q8–12h;
Rabbits: 100,000 IU/kg p.o. q12h for GI tract yeast overgrowth;
Chinchillas: 60,000–90,000 IU/kg p.o. q12h for 7–10 days.
Birds: Pigeons: 100,000 IU/kg p.o. q24h for 10 days; **Passerines:** 5000–300,000 IU/kg p.o. q12h for macrorhabdiasis (although there are doubts about its efficacy); **Other birds:** 300,000 IU/kg p.o. q12h[1].
Reptiles: 100,000 IU/kg p.o. q24h for 10 days.
Amphibians: Topical (1% cream) for cutaneous mycoses.
Fish: No information available.

References
[1] Tantaş A, Ak S and Özgür Y (1990) Aetiology, diagnostic criteria and therapeutic findings in candidiasis in parrots. *Veteriner Fakültesi Dergisi (Istanbul)* **16(1/2)**, 181–184

Octreotide
(Sandostatin*, Sandostatin LAR*) **POM**

Formulations: Injectable: 50 µg/ml, 100 µg/ml, 200 µg/ml, 500 µg/ml solutions; depot preparation: 10 mg, 20 mg, 30 mg vials.

Action: Somatostatin analogue that inhibits the release of several hormones.

Use: May be useful in the management of gastric, enteric and pancreatic endocrine tumours (e.g. insulinoma, gastrinoma) and acromegaly. Variable responses have been reported in veterinary medicine. Most recent research suggests that it is not useful in most insulinomas. Tumours not expressing somatostatin receptors will not respond. There is limited information on the use of this drug in veterinary species. In humans doses up to 200 µg/person q8h are used. Similar doses of the aqueous preparation may be required in animals, but dosages for the depot preparation are not known.

Safety and handling: Normal precautions should be observed.

Contraindications: No information available.

Adverse reactions: GI disturbances (anorexia, vomiting, abdominal pain, bloating, diarrhoea and steatorrhoea), hepatopathy and pain at injection sites have been recorded in humans.

Drug interactions: No information available.

DOSES
Mammals: Ferrets: 1–2 µg (micrograms)/kg s.c. q8–12h.
Birds, Reptiles, Amphibians, Fish: No information available.

Ofloxacin
(Exocin*) **POM**

Formulations: Topical: 0.3% solution.

Action: Bactericidal antimicrobial which works by inhibiting the bacterial DNA gyrase enzyme, causing damage to the bacterial DNA. The fluoroquinolones work in a concentration-dependent manner.

Use: Ideally fluoroquinolone use should be reserved for infections where culture and sensitivity testing predicts a clinical response and where first- and second-line antimicrobials would not be effective. For ophthalmic use when other antibacterial agents are ineffective. Active against many ocular pathogens, including *Staphylococcus* and *Pseudomonas aeruginosa*, although there is increasing resistance amongst some staphylococcal and streptococcal organisms. Better corneal penetration than ciprofloxacin.

Safety and handling: Normal precautions should be observed.

Contraindications: No information available.

Adverse reactions: May cause local irritation after application.

Drug interactions: No information available.

DOSES
Mammals: 1 drop to affected eye q6h; loading dose can be used: 1 drop to affected eye q15min for 4 doses.
Birds: 1 drop in affected eye q12h.
Reptiles: 1 drop in affected eye q8–12h.
Amphibians, Fish: No information available.

Oil of cloves see Eugenol

Omeprazole
(Gastrogard, Losec*, Mepradec*, Zanprol*) **POM-V, POM**

Formulations: Oral: 10 mg, 20 mg, 40 mg capsules, gastro-resistant tablets, MUPS (multiple unit pellet system) tablets. Injectable: 40 mg vial for reconstitution for i.v. injection; discard remainder after use.

Action: Proton pump inhibitor. Ten times more potent than cimetidine in inhibiting gastric acid secretion and has a longer duration of activity (>24 hours).

Use: Management of gastric and duodenal ulcers, oesophagitis, and hypersecretory conditions secondary to gastrinoma (Zollinger–Ellison syndrome) or mast cell neoplasia. Gastrogard is licensed for use in equids, but the formulation (370 mg/g paste) makes accurate dosing of small animals impossible. Lansoprazole, rabeprazole and pantoprazole are similar drugs but have no known clinical advantage over omeprazole. Esomeprazole is a newer preparation containing only the active isomer of omeprazole.

Safety and handling: Normal precautions should be observed.

Contraindications: No information available.

Adverse reactions: Chronic suppression of acid secretion has caused hypergastrinaemia in laboratory animals, leading to mucosal cell hyperplasia, rugal hypertrophy and the development of carcinoids, and so treatment for a maximum of 8 weeks has been recommended. However, such problems have not been reported in companion animals. Adverse effects do include nausea, diarrhoea, constipation and skin rashes.

Drug interactions: Omeprazole may enhance the effects of phenytoin. There is a risk of interaction with tacrolimus, mycophenolate mofetil, clopidogrel, digoxin and itraconazole.

DOSES
Mammals: Ferrets: 0.7–4 mg/kg p.o. q24h for a maximum of 8 weeks; **Primates:** 0.4 mg/kg p.o. q12h[a].
Birds, Reptiles, Amphibians, Fish: No information available.

References
[a] Dubois A, Berg DE, Fiala N *et al.* (1998) Cure of *Helicobacter pylori* infection by omeprazole-clarithromycin-based therapy in non-human primates. *Journal of Gastroenterology* **33(1)**, 18–22

Ondansetron
(Zofran*) **POM**

Formulations: Injectable: 2 mg/ml solution in 2 ml and 4 ml ampoules. **Oral:** 4 mg, 8 mg tablets; 4 mg/5 ml syrup. **Rectal:** 16 mg suppositories.

Action: Potent antiemetic effects through action on the GI tract and the chemoreceptor trigger zone. It was developed for, and is particularly useful in, the control of emesis induced by chemotherapeutic drugs.

Use: Indicated for the management of nausea and vomiting in patients who are unable to tolerate, or whose signs are not controlled by, other drugs (e.g. maropitant, metoclopramide). Dolasetron, granisetron, palanosetron and tropisetron are similar drugs but have yet to be extensively used in companion animals.

Safety and handling: Normal precautions should be observed.

Contraindications: Intestinal obstruction.

Adverse reactions: In humans, constipation, headaches, occasional alterations in liver enzymes and, rarely, hypersensitivity reactions have been reported.

Drug interactions: Ondansetron may reduce the effectiveness of tramadol and so the dose of tramadol may need to be increased.

DOSES
Mammals: Ferrets: 1 mg/kg p.o. q12–24h.
Birds, Reptiles, Amphibians, Fish: No information available.

Oxantel see **Pyrantel**

Oxfendazole
(Bovex, Endoworm, Ovidown, Parafend) **POM-VPS**

Formulations: Oral: 2.265% suspension, 5% suspension in combination with selenium and cobalt.

Action: Benzimidazole. Inhibits fumarate reductase system of parasites, thereby blocking the citric acid cycle, and also reduces glucose absorption by the parasite.

Use: Treatment of gastrointestinal parasites, specifically used for oxyurids in chelonians and iguanas. Also thought to have some efficacy against other endoparasites including ascarids, hookworms, whipworms, some cestodes, trematodes and *Giardia*. Avoid using formulations combined with selenium and cobalt.

Safety and handling: Normal precautions should be observed.

Contraindications: No information available.

Adverse reactions: No information available, although other benzimidazoles have been associated with bone marrow suppression and feather abnormalities so these are potential risks.

Drug interactions: No information available.

DOSES
Birds: 10−40 mg/kg p.o. once.
Reptiles: Tortoises: 66 mg/kg p.o. once[a]; **Iguanas:** 25mg/kg p.o. once[b].
Amphibians: 5 mg/kg p.o. once.
Mammals, Fish: No information available.

References
[a] Giannetto S, Brianti E, Poglayen G et al. (2007) Efficacy of oxfendazole and fenbendazole against tortoise (*Testudo hermanni*) oxyurids. *Parasitology Research* **100(5)**, 1069−1073
[b] Kehoe S, Divers S, Mayer J, Comolli J, Verocai G (2019) Efficacy of Single-Dose Oxfendazole to treat nematodiasis in the green iguana (*Iguana iguana*). *Proceedings of the International Conference of Avian, Herpetological and Exotic Mammal Medicine, London*, p. 220

Oxytetracycline
(**Aquatet** [Pharmaq], Engemycin, Oxycare)
POM-V

Formulations: Injectable: 100 mg/ml solution. **Oral:** 50 mg, 100 mg, 250 mg tablets. Feed supplement and soluble powders also available.

Action: Inhibits bacterial protein synthesis. The effect is bacteriostatic.

Use: Active against many Gram-positive and Gram-negative bacteria, rickettsiae, mycoplasmas, spirochaetes and other microbes. One of the less lipid-soluble tetracyclines, it is excreted unchanged in urine and bile and undergoes enterohepatic recirculation. Has been used in combination with nicotinamide in the management of immune-mediated conditions, including discoid lupus erythematosus and lupoid onychodystrophy. Resistance to tetracyclines is widespread. Use with care in rabbits as narrow therapeutic range. Used for the treatment of bacterial disease in fish. High strength formulations for immersion baths for fish should be used since bulking agents may have adverse effects on water quality.

Safety and handling: Normal precautions should be observed.

Contraindications: The concentrated injectable depot formulations used for cattle and sheep should never be given to small animals or fish. Avoid oral dosing in birds, other than for prophylaxis, as tetracyclines are poorly absorbed from the GI tract, rapidly lose potency in drinking water and put birds off drinking water due to their taste.

Adverse reactions: Include vomiting, diarrhoea, depression, hepatotoxicity (rare), fever, hypotension (following i.v. administration) and anorexia. Prolonged use may lead to development of superinfections. Although not well documented in veterinary medicine, tetracyclines induce dose-related functional changes in renal tubules in several species, which may be exacerbated by dehydration, haemoglobinuria, myoglobinuria or concomitant administration of other nephrotoxic drugs. Severe tubular damage has occurred following the use of outdated or improperly stored products and occurs due to the formation of a degradation product. Tetracyclines stain the teeth of children when used in the last 2–3 weeks of pregnancy or the first month of life. Although this phenomenon has not been well documented in animals, it is prudent to restrict the use of tetracyclines in all young animals. Injectable preparations in birds may cause toxicity or muscle necrosis. In rabbits and other small herbivores, higher doses (30 mg/kg) can be associated with enteritis. Injectable depot formulations may produce a sterile fluid-filled cavity at the site of injection in fish.

Drug interactions: The bactericidal action of penicillins may be inhibited by oxytetracycline. Antacids containing divalent or trivalent cations (Mg^{2+}, Ca^{2+}, Al^{3+}), food or milk products bind tetracycline, reducing its absorption. Tetracyclines may increase the nephrotoxic effects of methoxyflurane. The GI effects of tetracyclines may be increased if administered concurrently with theophylline products. Efficacy may be reduced due to chelation when used as a bath treatment for fish in hard water with high levels of divalent metal cations (Ca^{2+}, Mg^{2+}). The drug has a very low bioavailability in some species of fish, including carp and goldfish. If the drug turns the water dark brown when decomposing in fish tanks, 50% of the water should be changed immediately.

DOSES
See Appendix for guidelines on responsible antibacterial use.
Mammals: Ferrets, Hamsters, Gerbils: 20–25 mg/kg i.m. q8–12h; Rabbits: 15 mg/kg i.m. q12h or 30 mg/kg of the 5–10% non-depot preparation s.c. q72h; **Guinea pigs:** 5 mg/kg i.m. q12h; **Chinchillas:** 15 mg/kg i.m. q12h or 50 mg/kg p.o. q12h; **Rats:** 20 mg/kg i.m. q8–12h or 10–20 mg/kg p.o. q8h; **Mice:** 100 mg/kg s.c. q12h or 10–20 mg/kg p.o. q8h; **Primates:** 10 mg/kg s.c., i.m. q24h, 25–50 mg/kg p.o.; **Hedgehogs:** 25–50 mg/kg p.o. q24h.

Birds: Raptors: 25–50 mg/kg p.o. q8h; **Parrots:** 50–100 mg/kg s.c. q2–3d (long-acting preparation); **Pigeons:** 50 mg/kg p.o. q6h or 80 mg/kg i.m. q48h (long-acting preparation) or 130–400 mg/l water [a,b,c]; **Passerines:** 100 mg/kg p.o. q24h or 4–12 mg/l water for 7 days.

Reptiles: 6–10 mg/kg p.o., i.m., i.v. q24h.

Amphibians: 25–50 mg/kg p.o., s.c., i.m. q24h or 100 mg/l for a 1 hour bath.

Fish: 10–100 mg/l (freshwater fish) by prolonged immersion for 1–3 days, if poor response then change 50% of the water and repeat, or 55–83 mg/kg p.o. q24h for 10 days or 10–50 mg/kg i.m., intracoelomic q24h for 5–10 days.

References

[a] Flammer K, Aucoin DP, Whitt DA and Styles DK (1990) Potential use of long-acting injectable oxytetracycline for treatment of chlamydiosis in Goffin's cockatoos. *Avian Diseases* **34(1)**, 228–234

[b] Osofsky A, Tell LA, Kass PH *et al.* (2005) Investigation of Japanese quail (*Coturnix japonica*) as a pharmacokinetic model of cockatiels (*Nymphicus hollandicus*) and Poicephalus parrots via comparison of the pharmacokinetics of a single intravenous injection of oxytetracycline hydrochloride. *Journal of Veterinary Pharmacology and Therapeutics* **28(6)**, 505–513

[c] Teare JA, Schwark WS, Shin SJ and Graham DL (1985) Pharmacokinetics of a long-acting oxytetracycline preparation in ring-necked pheasants, great horned owls and Amazon parrots. *American Journal of Veterinary Research* **46(12)**, 2639

Oxytocin
(Oxytocin S) **POM-V**

Formulations: Injectable: 10 IU/ml solution.

Action: Synthetic oxytocin.

Use: Induces parturition/egg laying when uterine inertia is present (as long as there is no uterine obstruction); evacuates uterine contents; decreases haemorrhage following parturition; and promotes milk 'let-down'. Before oxytocin is used in any species it is important to ensure that there is no evidence of obstructive dystocia and that blood calcium levels are adequate. Calcium supplementation should be administered 1 hour prior to oxytocin if ionized or total blood calcium levels are low. Can also be used i.v. (dose at 25% of i.m. dose, diluted in water for injection). Useful in chelonians, less effective in lizards and snakes. Ineffective in birds.

Safety and handling: Store in refrigerator.

Contraindications: Not recommended for use in egg retention in birds.

Adverse reactions: Overstimulation of the uterus can be hazardous to both mother and fetuses. In birds it can cause painful side effects due to stimulation of smooth muscle.

Drug interactions: Severe hypertension may develop if used with sympathomimetic pressor amines.

DOSES

Mammals: Ferrets: 0.2–3.0 IU/kg s.c., i.m.; **Rabbits:** 0.1–3.0 IU/kg s.c., i.m.; **Rodents:** 0.2–3.0 IU/kg s.c., i.m., i.v.; **Mice:** (milk let-down) 6.25 IU/kg s.c.; **Primates (Common marmosets):** 1–2 IU/animal i.v., i.m.

Birds: Do not use.

Reptiles: Egg retention: 2–10 IU/kg i.m. q90min for a maximum of 3 doses. Start at low end of dose range and better effect if calcium therapy used first. **Red-eared sliders:** 2 IU/kg i.m., i.v. [a]

Amphibians, Fish: No information available.

References

[a] Di Ianni F, Parmigiani E, Pelizzone I et al. (2014) Comparison between intramuscular and intravenous administration of oxytocin in captive-bred red-eared sliders (*Trachemys scripta elegans*) and non-obstructive egg retention. *Journal of Exotic Pet Medicine* **23**, 79–84

Pancreatic enzyme supplements
(Lypex, Pancreatic Enzyme Supplement for Dogs and Cats, Panzym, Tryplase)
AVM-GSL, POM, P

Formulations: Oral: The formulations vary in the amount and type of enzyme present. Readers are referred to individual products for further details. Many other formulations on human market.

Action: Exogenous replacement enzymes.

Use: Pancreatic enzymes (lipase, protease, amylase) are used to control signs of exocrine pancreatic insufficiency (EPI). Fresh raw, or fresh-frozen, pig pancreas (approximately 100 g per meal) is also an effective treatment (and is not a Specified Risk Material) but availability is limited and there is a risk of pathogen ingestion by this method. Non-enteric coated powders and enteric coated granules and tablets are available. Use the manufacturer's recommendations as the minimum required initially; the dose may be reduced empirically once a satisfactory response is achieved. Efficacy may be augmented by antibiotic control of secondary bacterial overgrowth and vitamin B12 therapy for any associated hypocobalaminaemia. Concomitant administration of acid blockers is not cost-effective and there is no requirement for pre-incubation with food. Follow dosing with food or water.

Safety and handling: Powder spilled on hands should be washed off or skin irritation may develop. Avoid inhaling powder as it causes mucous membrane irritation and may trigger asthma attacks in susceptible individuals. These risks are not associated with enteric coated pancreatic granules.

Contraindications: No information available.

Adverse reactions: Contact dermatitis of the lips is occasionally seen with powdered non-coated enzyme. Non-coated pancreatic enzymes may cause oral or oesophageal ulcers, and so dosing should be followed with food or water. High doses may cause diarrhoea and signs of gastrointestinal cramping.

Drug interactions: The effectiveness may be diminished by antacids (magnesium hydroxide, calcium carbonate).

DOSES
Birds: Tryplase: 1 capsule/kg body weight q24h mixed in food.
Mammals, Reptiles, Amphibians, Fish: No information available.

Paracetamol (Acetaminophen)
(Pardale V (paracetamol and codeine phosphate), Paracetamol*, Perfalgan*) **P, POM, POM-V**

Formulations: Oral: 500 mg tablet; 120 mg/5 ml, 250 mg/5 ml suspensions; 400 mg paracetamol and 9 mg codeine phosphate tablet (Pardale V). **Injectable:** 10 mg/ml solution.

Action: It has been proposed that its antipyretic actions are due to prostaglandin synthesis within the CNS; however its exact mechanism of action is unclear.

Use: Control of mild to moderate pain and as an antipyretic. Paracetamol has poor anti-inflammatory effects. It is believed to produce few GI side effects and therefore is commonly administered to patients with gastric ulceration, particularly if traditional NSAIDs are contraindicated; however, there are limited clinical data to support this practice. The licensed oral preparation of paracetamol contains codeine; however, due to a high first pass metabolism of opioids, this codeine is not bioavailable and therefore does not contribute to the analgesia.

Safety and handling: Normal precautions should be observed.

Contraindications: Do not use in snakes[a].

Adverse reactions: Overdose of paracetamol causes liver damage through the production of N-acetyl-p-aminobenzoquinonimine during metabolism, which causes hepatocyte cell death and centrilobular hepatic necrosis. Treatment of overdose with oral methionine or i.v. acetylcysteine is directed at replenishing hepatic glutathione.

Drug interactions: Metoclopramide enhances absorption of paracetamol, thereby enhancing its effects.

DOSES
Mammals: Rabbits: 200–500 mg/kg p.o. is often quoted, but clinical analgesic effects are noted at 10–15 mg/kg, and higher doses are not recommended; **Rodents:** 1–2 mg/ml of drinking water (use flavoured products); **Primates:** 5–10 mg/kg p.o. q6h.
Reptiles: Do not use in snakes[a].
Birds, Amphibians, Fish: No information available.

References
[a] van den Hurk P and Kerkkamp HM (2019) Phylogenetic origins for severe acetaminophen toxicity in snake species compared to other vertebrate taxa. *Comparative Biochemistry and Physiology Part C: Toxicology & Pharmacology* **215**, 18–24

Paraffin (Liquid paraffin, Mineral oil)
(Katalax, Lacri-Lube*, Liquid paraffin oral emulsion*, Simple Eye Ointment*) **AVM-GSL, P**

Formulations: Oral: White soft paraffin paste (Katalax); liquid paraffin (50/50 oil/water mix). **Topical:** 3.5 g, 4 g or 5 g ophthalmic ointment.

Action: Paraffin is a laxative; it softens stool by interfering with intestinal water resorption. It is also a lipid-based tear substitute that mimics the lipid portion of the tear film and helps prevent evaporation of tears.

Use: Paraffin is used to manage constipation. It is beneficial in the management of keratoconjunctivitis sicca, during general anaesthesia and for eyelid paresis. It is a long-acting ocular lubricant and is used when frequency of treatment is not easy. The use of liquid paraffin as an aid to treating reduced GI motility in rabbits has been historically due to the concern that fur accumulation in the GI tract was a contributory factor. This is rarely the case and such products may impair hydration of GI contents, as well as increase the risk of inhalation. Its use is therefore not recommended in this species.

Safety and handling: Normal precautions should be observed.

Contraindications: Do not give orally in patients with a reduced gag reflex.

Adverse reactions: As paraffin is tasteless, normal swallowing may not be elicited if syringing orally; thus inhalation and subsequent lipoid pneumonia are a significant risk. Paraffin ointment may blur vision, although not often a problem in animals.

Drug interactions: Reduced absorption of fat-soluble vitamins may follow prolonged use.

DOSES
Mammals: Ocular: Apply to eye at night or q6–12h prn.
- Ferrets: 10 mm Katalax paste p.o. q12–24h for constipation.

Birds, Reptiles, Amphibians, Fish: No information available.

Paroxetine
(Paxil*, Seroxat*) **POM**

Formulations: Oral: 20 mg, 30 mg tablets; 2 mg/ml liquid suspension.

Action: Blocks serotonin re-uptake in the brain, resulting in antidepressive activity and a raising in motor activity thresholds.

Use: Treatment of behavioural disorders in pet birds, such as feather plucking and self-mutilation.

Safety and handling: Normal precautions should be observed.

Contraindications: Known sensitivity to paroxetine or other SSRIs, history of seizures.

Adverse reactions: Possible reactions include lethargy, decreased appetite and vomiting. Trembling, restlessness, GI disturbances and an apparent paradoxical increase in anxiety may occur in some cases. Owners should be warned of a potential increase in aggression in response to medication.

Drug interactions: Paroxetine should not be used within 2 weeks of treatment with an MAOI (e.g. selegiline) and an MAOI should not be used within 6 weeks of treatment with paroxetine. Paroxetine, like other SSRIs, antagonizes the effects of anticonvulsants and so is not recommended for use with epileptic patients or in association with other agents which lower seizure threshold, e.g. phenothiazines. Caution is warranted if paroxetine is used concomitantly with aspirin or other anticoagulants, since the risk of increased bleeding in the case of tissue trauma may be increased.

DOSES
Birds: 1–2 mg/kg p.o. q12–24h [a].
Mammals, Reptiles, Amphibians, Fish: No information available.

References
[a] van Zeeland YRA, Schoemaker NJ, Haritova A *et al.* (2013) Pharmacokinetics of paroxetine, a selective serotonin reuptake inhibitor in grey parrots (Psittacus erithacus erithacus): influence of pharmaceutical formulation and length of dosing. *Journal of Veterinary Pharmacology and Therapeutics* **36(1)**, 51–58

Penicillamine
(Distamine*, Penicillamine*) **POM**

Formulations: Oral: 125 mg, 250 mg tablets.

Action: Penicillamine is an orally administered chelating agent that binds copper, mercury and lead. It also binds to cystine.

Use: Oral treatment of lead poisoning. May be used in the management of lead toxicity, especially in birds, when injecting EDTA is too difficult or long-term chelation is required. It has a low therapeutic index in birds.

Safety and handling: Normal precautions should be observed.

Contraindications: Moderate to marked renal impairment and a history of penicillamine-related blood dyscrasias. Penicillamine can reduce gastrointestinal absorption of dietary minerals, including zinc, iron, copper and calcium and, therefore, cause deficiencies with long-term use.

Adverse reactions: Serious adverse effects that have been described in humans given penicillamine include leucopenia, thrombocytopenia, fever, lymphadenopathy, skin hypersensitivity reactions and lupus-like reactions. May cause vomiting, hypoglycaemia and death in birds.

Drug interactions: The absorption of penicillamine is decreased if administered with antacids, food, or iron or zinc salts. An increase in the renal and haematological effects of penicillamine have been recorded in humans receiving it with cytotoxic drugs.

DOSES
Mammals: Ferrets: 10 mg/kg p.o. q24h; **Rabbits:** 30 mg/kg p.o. q12h.
Birds: Lead and zinc poisoning: 30–55 mg/kg p.o. q12h.
Reptiles, Amphibians, Fish: No information available.

Penicillin G (Benzyl penicillin)
(Crystapen, Depocillin, Duphapen, Neopen)
POM-V

Formulations: Injectable: comes in a variety of salts (sodium, procaine and benzathine) which affect solubility. Penicillin G sodium (highly soluble): 3 g powder for reconstitution for i.v. use; procaine penicillin (less soluble): 300 mg/ml suspension for s.c. use, slower release.

Action: Binds to penicillin-binding proteins involved in cell wall synthesis, decreasing bacterial cell wall strength and rigidity, and affecting cell division, growth and septum formation. As animal cells lack a cell wall the beta-lactam antibiotics are safe in most species. Kills bacteria in a time-dependent fashion.

Use: A beta-lactamase-susceptible antimicrobial. Narrow spectrum of activity and susceptible to acid degradation in the stomach. Used parenterally to treat infections caused by sensitive organisms (e.g. *Streptococcus*, *Clostridium*, *Borrelia borgderferi*, fusospirochaetes). The sodium salt is absorbed well from s.c. or i.m. sites. Procaine penicillin is sparingly soluble, providing a 'depot' from which it is slowly released. When used for 'blind' therapy of undiagnosed infections, penicillins may be given in conjunction with an aminoglycoside such as gentamicin with or without metronidazole. As penicillin kills in a time-dependent fashion, it is important to maintain tissue concentrations above the MIC for the organism throughout the interdosing interval. Patients with significant renal or hepatic dysfunction may need dosage adjustment.

Safety and handling: After reconstitution penicillin G sodium is stable for 7 days if refrigerated, 24 hours if not.

Contraindications: Use with caution in rabbits, and never orally, though it has been used in injectable forms long term for abscesses and osteomyelitis. Do not use in animals sensitive to beta-lactam antimicrobials. Do not administer penicillins to hamsters, gerbils, guinea pigs, chinchillas or degus. Do not give procaine penicillin to rats and mice.

Adverse reactions: 600 mg of penicillin G sodium contains 1.7 mEq of Na$^+$. This may be clinically important for patients on restricted sodium intakes. The i.m. administration of >600 mg/ml may cause discomfort. Oral doses of penicillins can cause fatal enterotoxaemia in rabbits and other small herbivores.

Drug interactions: Avoid the concomitant use of bacteriostatic antibiotics. The aminoglycosides may inactivate penicillins when mixed in parenteral solutions *in vitro*, but they act synergistically when administered at the same time *in vivo*. Procaine can antagonize the action of sulphonamides and so procaine penicillin G should not be used with them.

DOSES

See Appendix for guidelines on responsible antibacterial use.

Mammals: Ferrets: 20 mg/kg s.c., i.m. q12–24h; Rabbits: 40 mg/kg s.c. once every 7 days for 3 doses for *Treponema cuniculi*; other infections 40 mg/kg s.c. q12–24h[a]; Rats (not procaine): 22 mg/kg s.c., i.m. q24h; Primates: 20–40 mg/kg s.c., i.m. q12h; Sugar gliders: 22–25 mg/kg s.c., i.m. q12–24h; Hedgehogs: 40 mg/kg s.c., i.m. q24h; Chinchillas, Guinea pigs, Hamsters, Gerbils, Degus: Do not use.
Birds, Reptiles, Amphibians, Fish: No information available.

References
[a] Jekl V, Hauptman K, Minarikova A *et al.* (2016) Pharmacokinetic study of benzylpenicillin potassium after intramuscular administration in rabbits. *Veterinary Record* **179(1)**, 18.

Pentamidine isethionate
(Pentacarinat*) **POM**

Formulations: Injectable: 300 mg vials of powder for reconstitution.

Action: Kills protozoans by interacting with DNA. It is rapidly taken up by the parasites by a high-affinity energy-dependent carrier.

Use: Used for treatment of *Pneumocystis* infection. Pentamidine is a toxic drug and the potential to cause toxic damage to the kidney and liver in particular should be carefully considered prior to use.

Safety and handling: Care should be taken by staff handling this drug as it is a highly toxic agent. Similar precautions to those recommended when handling cytotoxic agents used in cancer chemotherapy should be taken.

Contraindications: Impaired liver or kidney function. Never give by rapid i.v. injection due to cardiovascular effects.

Adverse reactions: Pain and necrosis at the injection site, hypotension, nausea, salivation, vomiting and diarrhoea. Hypoglycaemia and blood dyscrasias are also reported in humans.

Drug interactions: No information available.

DOSES

Mammals: Ferrets: 3–4 mg/kg s.c. q48h for *Pneumocystis* pneumonia.

Birds, Reptiles, Amphibians, Fish: No information available.

Pentobarbital (Pentobarbitone)
(Dolethal, Euthasal, Euthatal, **Euthoxin**, Lethobarb, Pentobarbital for euthanasia, Pentoject) **POM-V CD SCHEDULE 3**

Formulations: Injectable: 200 mg/ml, 400 mg/ml, as either a blue, yellow or pink non-sterile aqueous solution.

Action: CNS depressant.

Use: For euthanasia of mammals, birds, reptiles, amphibians and fish. When it is predicted that euthanasia may be problematical (e.g. aggressive patients) it is recommended that premedication with an appropriate sedative is given. The animal should be restrained in order to forestall narcotic excitement until anaesthesia supervenes. The route of choice is i.v. if possible, but alternatives such as intraperitoneal, intracoelomic, intrarenal and intracardiac are possible when venepuncture is difficult to achieve. Intracardiac injection of pentobarbital should be performed under anaesthesia. There is no authorized pentobarbital product in the UK that is suitable for the emergency control of seizures. Fish may need to be immobilized, using an anaesthetic agent immersed in water, to enable accurate intravenous injection of pentobarbital.

Safety and handling: Normal precautions should be observed.

Contraindications: Should not be given i.m. as it is painful and slow to act. Do not use solutions intended for euthanasia to try to control seizures.

Adverse reactions: Narcotic excitement may be seen with agitated animals. Agonal gasping is sometimes seen. In fish, the heart can continue to contract even after brain death and removal from the body.

Drug interactions: Antihistamines and opioids increase the effect of pentobarbital.

DOSES

Mammals: Euthanasia: 150 mg/kg i.v., i.p. as rapidly as possible or to effect.

Birds: Euthanasia: 150 mg/kg i.v.

Reptiles: Euthanasia: 60–100 mg/kg i.v., intracoelomic or intracardiac.

Amphibians: Euthanasia: 60 mg/kg i.v., intracoelomic or via lypmh sacs (e.g. frogs and toads).

Fish: Euthanasia: 60–100 mg/kg i.v., intracoelomic, intracardiac[1].

References
[1] Leary S, Underwood W, Anthony R *et al.* (2013) *AVMA Guidelines for the Euthanasia of Animals: 2013 edition.* American Veterinary Medical Association, Illinois

Pentobarbitone see Pentobarbital

Pentosan polysulphate
(Cartrophen) **POM-V**

Formulations: Injectable: 100 mg/ml solution.

Action: Semi-synthetic polymer of pentose carbohydrates with heparin-like properties that binds to damaged cartilage matrix comprising aggregated proteoglycans and stimulates the synthesis of new aggregated glycosaminoglycan molecules. Ability to inhibit a range of proteolytic enzymes may be of particular importance. Modulates cytokine action, stimulates hyaluronic acid secretion, preserves proteoglycan content and stimulates articular cartilage blood flow, resulting in analgesic and regenerative effects.

Use: Used as a disease modifying agent to reduce the pain and inflammation associated with osteoarthritis in mammals; however, there is no evidence to support its use in exotic species. Administered by aseptic s.c. injection, using an insulin syringe for accurate dosing. The manufacturer recommends monitoring haematocrit and total solids. Based on its use in cats with idiopathic cystitis (because cats suffering from this condition have been shown to have reduced concentrations of GAGs within the protective mucosal layer of the bladder), it has been suggested that pentosan polysulphate may be of benefit in the management of guinea pigs suffering from chronic idiopathic, non-obstructive, lower urinary tract disease. However, there is currently no evidence to support this contention. There is good evidence to suggest that this drug is of minimal value in acute cases.

Safety and handling: Normal precautions should be observed.

Contraindications: Do not use if septic arthritis is present or if renal or hepatic impairment exists. As it may induce spontaneous bleeding, do not use in animals with bleeding disorders.

Adverse reactions: Pain at the injection site has been reported. Because of its fibrinolytic action the possibility of bleeding from undiagnosed tumours or vascular abnormalities exists.

Drug interactions: The manufacturers state that pentosan polysulphate should not be used concurrently with steroids or non-steroidal anti-inflammatory drugs, including aspirin, or used concomitantly with coumarin-based anticoagulants or heparin. However, many animals suffering from osteoarthritis that might benefit from pentosan polysulphate treatment are concurrently receiving NSAID therapy. The risk of bleeding associated with concurrent administration of pentosan polysulphate and COX-2 preferential and COX-2 selective NSAIDs is probably low in animals with no history of blood clotting disorders.

DOSES
Mammals: Rabbits: 3 mg/kg s.c. q5–7d for 4 doses for osteoarthritis; **Guinea pigs:** 3 mg/kg s.c. q5–7d for 4 doses for osteoarthritis and idiopathic cystitis.
Birds, Reptiles, Amphibians, Fish: No information available.

Permanganate of potash see Potassium permanganate
Permethrin see Imidacloprid

Pethidine (Meperidine)
(Pethidine, Demerol*, Meperidine*) **POM-V, POM CD SCHEDULE 2**

Formulations: Injectable: 10–50 mg/ml solutions. 50 mg/ml solution is usually used in veterinary practice.

Action: Analgesia mediated by the mu opioid receptor.

Use: Management of mild to moderate pain. Incorporation into sedative and pre-anaesthetic medication protocols to provide improved sedation and analgesia. Pethidine has a fast onset (10–15 min) and short duration (45–60 min) of action. Frequent redosing is used for analgesia. The short duration of action may be desirable in some circumstances (e.g. when a rapid recovery is required or in animals with compromised liver function). It shares common opioid effects with morphine but also has anticholinergic effects, producing a dry mouth and sometimes an increase in heart rate. Be careful of species differences in effect in reptiles.

Safety and handling: Normal precautions should be observed.

Contraindications: Do not give i.v. Not advisable to use in animals at risk from histamine release (e.g. some skin allergies, asthma, mast cell tumours).

Adverse reactions: Histamine released during i.v. injection causes hypotension, tachycardia and bronchoconstriction. Histamine-mediated reactions may also occur after i.m. injection, resulting in local urticaria. Pethidine crosses the placenta and may exert sedative effects in animals born to dams treated prior to parturition. Severe adverse effects can be treated with naloxone.

Drug interactions: Other CNS depressants (e.g. anaesthetics, antihistamines, barbiturates, phenothiazines, tranquillizers) may cause increased CNS or respiratory depression when used concurrently with narcotic analgesics. Pethidine may produce a serious interaction if administered with monoamine oxidase inhibitors (MAOIs). The mechanism of this interaction is not clear but effects include coma, convulsions and hyperpyrexia.

DOSES
Mammals: Analgesia: **Ferrets:** 5–10 mg/kg i.m., s.c. q2–3h; **Rabbits:** 10 mg/kg i.m., s.c. q2–3h; **Rodents:** 10–20 mg/kg i.m. q2–3h; **Primates:** 2–4 mg/kg i.v., i.m. q2–4h.
Reptiles: Analgesia: **Tortoises:** 20 mg/kg i.m. q12–24h [a].
Birds, Amphibians, Fish: No information available.

References
[a] Wambugu SN, Towett PK, Kiama SG, Abelson KS and Kanui TI (2010) Effects of opioids in the formalin test in the Speke's hinged tortoise (*Kinixy's spekii*). *Journal of Veterinary Pharmacology and Therapeutics* **33(4)**, 347–351

Phenobarbital (Phenobarbitone)
(Epiphen, Epityl, Phenobarbital (non-proprietary), Phenoleptil, Gardenal*) **POM-V, POM CD SCHEDULE 3**

Formulations: Oral: 12.5 mg, 15 mg, 25 mg, 30 mg, 50 mg, 60 mg, 100 mg tablets; 4% (40 mg/ml) solution. **Injectable:** 15 mg/ml, 30 mg/ml, 60 mg/ml, 200 mg/ml solutions (phenobarbital sodium BP).

Action: Thought to mediate its antiepileptic effect through affinity for the GABA$_A$ receptor, resulting in a GABA-ergic effect; GABA being the major inhibitory mammalian neurotransmitter with prolonged opening of the chloride channel. Phenobarbital also blocks the AMPA receptor, inhibiting release of the excitatory neurotransmitter glutamate. This combined potentiation of GABA and inhibition of glutamate leads to reduced neuronal excitability.

Use: Phenobarbital and imepitoin are the initial medications of choice for the management of epileptic seizures due to idiopathic epilepsy. The choice of initial medication is guided by patient requirements: phenobarbital is less expensive and more efficacious, whilst imepitoin has a more rapid onset of action than phenobarbital (does not need to achieve a steady state), does not require the determination of serum concentrations and has a less severe adverse effect profile. Doses are mainly anecdotal in exotic species and information is based on that for dogs. One pharmacokinetic study has been performed in birds. Phenobarbital is rapidly absorbed after oral administration in dogs; maximal plasma concentrations reached within 4–8 hours. Wide range of elimination half-life (40–90 hours) in different dogs. Steady state serum concentrations are not reached until 7–10 days after treatment is initiated and the full clinical effect of a dose cannot be ascertained until this point. Serum concentrations should be determined after starting treatment or dose alterations, once a steady state has been reached.

If <15 µg/ml the dose should be increased accordingly. If seizures are not adequately controlled dose may be increased up to a maximum serum concentration of 45 µg/ml. Plasma concentrations above this level are associated with increased hepatotoxicity. With chronic therapy, induction of the hepatic microsomal enzyme system results in a decreased half-life, particularly during the first 6 months of therapy. As a result, the dose may need to be increased. Phenobarbital levels should be assessed every 6–12 months. Any termination of phenobarbital therapy should be performed gradually with a recommended protocol of: reduce the dose by 25% of the original dose each month (month 1: 75% of the original phenobarbital dose; month 2: 50% of the original phenobarbital dose; month 3: 25% of the original phenobarbital dose).

Safety and handling: Normal precautions should be observed.

Contraindications: Do not administer to animals with impaired hepatic function. Not for use in pregnant and nursing animals, although the risk associated with uncontrolled seizures may be greater than the risk associated with phenobarbital. Do not use to control seizures resulting from hepatic disease (e.g. portosystemic shunt), hypoglycaemia or toxic causes where the clinical signs are mediated through the GABA channels (ivermectin and moxidectin toxicity) as this may exacerbate the seizures. Do not administer high doses by i.v. or i.m. injection in animals with marked respiratory depression.

Adverse reactions: Sedation, ataxia, polyphagia and PU/PD. Polyphagia and PU/PD are likely to persist throughout therapy. Ataxia and sedation occur commonly following initiation of therapy but usually resolve within 1 week, although they may continue if high doses are used. Hepatic toxicity is rare, but may occur at high serum concentrations (or as a rare idiosyncratic reaction within 2 weeks of starting treatment). Hyperexcitability has been reported in dogs on subtherapeutic dose levels. Haematological abnormalities, including neutropenia, anaemia and thrombocytopenia, may occur. Long-term administration in the absence of hepatotoxicity is associated with: moderate increase in liver size on abdominal radiographs; no change in liver echogenicity or architecture on ultrasonography; no evidence of morphological liver damage on histology; significant increase in ALP and, to a lesser extent, ALT activity; transiently decreased albumin (up to 6 months after starting therapy) and increased GGT; and no changes in AST, bilirubin or fasting bile acids. Therefore, liver function should be assessed by other parameters, in particular a bile acid assay, persistent decrease in albumin levels, serum AST, bilirubin and ultrasonographic examination of the liver. Phenobarbital treatment does not affect adrenal function tests (ACTH stimulation test and low dose dexamethasone test) despite acceleration of dexamethasone metabolism. Phenobarbital significantly decreases total T4 and free T4, and cholesterol levels tend to increase towards the upper limits of the normal range.

Drug interactions: The effect of phenobarbital may be increased by other CNS depressants (antihistamines, narcotics, phenothiazines). Phenobarbital may enhance the metabolism of, and therefore decrease the effect of, corticosteroids, beta-blockers, metronidazole and theophylline. Barbiturates may enhance the effects of other antiepileptics. Cimetidine, itraconazole and chloramphenicol increase serum phenobarbital concentration through inhibition of the hepatic microsomal enzyme system.

DOSES
Mammals: Ferrets: 1–2 mg/kg p.o. q12–24h or 2–10 mg/kg/h i.v. CRI; **Guinea pigs, Gerbils:** 10–25 mg/kg i.v., i.p. q12–24h; **Primates:** 1–6 mg/kg p.o. q24h, 2 mg/kg i.v.
Birds: 3.5–7 mg/kg p.o. q12h [a].
Reptiles, Amphibians, Fish: No information available.

References
[a] Powers LV and Papich MG (2011) Pharmacokinetics of orally administered phenobarbital in African grey parrots (*Psittacus erithacus erithacus*). *Journal of Veterinary Pharmacology and Therapeutics* **34(6)**, 615–617

Phenobarbitone see Phenobarbital
Phenoxetol see Phenoxyethanol

Phenoxybenzamine
(Dibenyline*) **POM**

Formulations: Oral: 10 mg capsule. **Injectable:** 50 mg/ml solution.

Action: An alpha-adrenergic blocker that irreversibly blocks presynaptic and postsynaptic receptors, producing a so-called chemical sympathectomy.

Use: Reflex dyssynergia/urethral spasm. If concurrent beta-blockers are also used (for severe tachycardia/arrhythmias), only start these once alpha blockade is in place (to avoid a hypertensive crisis). Use with extreme caution in animals with pre-existing cardiovascular disease.

Safety and handling: Normal precautions should be observed.

Contraindications: No information available.

Adverse reactions: Adverse effects associated with alpha-adrenergic blockade include hypotension, miosis, tachycardia and nasal congestion.

Drug interactions: There is an increased risk of a first dose hypotensive effect if administered with beta-blockers or diuretics. Phenoxybenzamine will antagonize effects of alpha-adrenergic sympathomimetic agents (e.g. phenylephrine).

DOSES
Mammals: Ferrets: 0.5–1 mg/kg p.o. q12h.
Birds, Reptiles, Amphibians, Fish: No information available.

Phenoxyethanol (Ethylene glycol monophenyl ether, Phenoxetol)
(**Aqua-sed**, Masuizai Koi Sedate) **ESPA**

Formulations: Immersion: 100% liquid.

Action: Precise mechanism of action is unknown but may involve an effect on nerve cell membranes and suppress activity in the CNS.

Use: For the sedation, immobilization, anaesthesia and euthanasia of fish. The drug is fairly soluble but requires vigorous whisking into water to improve solubility. It does not accumulate in the fish tissues after induction of anaesthesia and therefore can be used for prolonged periods. It is considered safer and more potent at lower temperatures. It has some antibacterial properties and has been included at low concentrations in some proprietary formulations.

Safety and handling: Irritant. Normal precautions should be observed.

Contraindications: No information available.

Adverse reactions: There can be a long induction time, and hyperactivity during induction and recovery. There is a narrow safety margin in some species and there may be involuntary muscle activity during anaesthesia.

Drug interactions: No information available.

DOSES
Fish: Anaesthesia: 0.1–0.5 ml/l by immersion; Euthanasia: 2.0 ml/l by immersion [1,2].
Mammals, Birds, Reptiles, Amphibians: No information available.

References
[1] Ross LG and Ross B (1999) *Anaesthesia and Sedative Techniques for Aquatic Animals.* Blackwell Science, Oxford
[2] Sneddon LU (2012) Clinical anaesthesia and analgesia in fish. *Journal of Exotic Pet Medicine* **21**, 32–43
[3] Underwood W, Anthony R, Cartner S *et al.* (2013) *AVMA Guidelines for the Euthanasia of Animals: 2013 edition.* American Veterinary Medical Association, Illinois

Phenylephrine
(Phenylephrine hydrochloride*) **POM**

Formulations: Injectable: 1% (10 mg/ml) solution. Ophthalmic: 2.5%, 10% solution (single-dose vials).

Action: Directly stimulates the alpha-adrenergic receptors in the iris dilator musculature.

Use: When applied topically to the eye causes vasoconstriction and mydriasis (pupil dilation). Ophthalmic uses include mydriasis prior to intraocular surgery (often in conjunction with atropine) and differentiation of involvement of superficial conjunctival vasculature from deep episcleral vasculature (by vasoconstriction). It is also used in the diagnosis of Horner's syndrome (HS) (denervation hypersensitivity) by determining the time to pupillary dilation, following administration of 1% phenylephrine topically to both eyes. Essentially, the shorter the time to pupillary dilation, the closer the lesion to the iris: <20 minutes suggests third-order HS; 20–45 min suggests second-order HS; 60–90 min suggests first-order HS or no sympathetic denervation of the eye. If 10% phenylephrine is used, mydriasis occurs in 5–8 minutes in post-ganglionic (third-order neuron) lesions. Vasoconstrictors should be used with care. Although they raise blood pressure, they do so at the expense of perfusion of vital organs (e.g. kidney). In many patients with shock, peripheral resistance is already high and to raise it further is unhelpful.

Safety and handling: Normal precautions should be observed.

Contraindications: No information available.

Adverse reactions: These include hypertension, tachycardia and reflex bradycardia.

Drug interactions: There is a risk of arrhythmias if phenylephrine is used in patients receiving digoxin or with volatile anaesthetic agents. When used concurrently with oxytocic agents the pressor effects may be enhanced, leading to severe hypertension.

DOSES
Mammals: Ophthalmic use: 1 drop approximately 2 hours before intraocular surgery. 1 drop as a single dose for vasoconstriction. 1 drop to both eyes for diagnosis of Horner's syndrome.
* **Primates:** 1–2 µg (micrograms)/kg i.v. as a bolus followed by 0.5–1 µg/kg/min CRI.

Birds, Reptiles, Amphibians, Fish: No information available.

Phenylpropanolamine
(Diphenylpyraline)
(Propalin, Urilin) **POM-V**

Formulations: Oral: 40 mg/ml syrup.

Action: Increases urethral outflow resistance and has some peripheral vasoconstrictive effects.

Use: Treatment of incontinence secondary to urinary sphincter incompetence. May also be useful in the management of nasal congestion. Incontinence may recur if doses are delayed or missed. The onset of action may take several days.

Safety and handling: Normal precautions should be observed.

Contraindications: No information available.

Adverse reactions: May include restlessness, aggressiveness, irritability and hypertension. Cardiotoxicity has been reported.

Drug interactions: No information available.

DOSES
Mammals: Rabbits: 5–10 mg/animal p.o. q12h, reducing to lowest effective dose gradually.
Birds, Reptiles, Amphibians, Fish: No information available.

Phenytoin (Diphenylhydantoin)
(Epanutin*) POM

Formulations: Oral: 25 mg, 50 mg, 100 mg, 300 mg capsules; 50 mg chewable tablets; 30 mg/5 ml suspension.

Action: Diminishes the spread of focal neural discharges. Its action appears to be a stabilizing effect on synaptic junctions and it depresses motor areas of the cortex without depressing sensory areas.

Use: Used for control of epilepsy in primates. Hepatic function should be monitored every 6–12 months in patients on chronic therapy.

Safety and handling: Normal precautions should be observed.

Contraindications: No information available.

Adverse reactions: Adverse effects include ataxia, vomiting, hepatic toxicity, peripheral neuropathy, toxic epidermal necrolysis and pyrexia.

Drug interactions: A large number of potential drug interactions are reported in human patients, in particular complex interactions with other antiepileptics. The plasma concentration of phenytoin may be increased by cimetidine, diazepam, metronidazole, phenylbutazone, sulphonamides and trimethoprim. The absorption, effects or plasma concentration of phenytoin may be decreased by antacids, barbiturates and calcium. The metabolism of corticosteroids, doxycycline, theophylline and thyroxine may be increased by phenytoin. The analgesic properties of pethidine may be reduced by phenytoin, whereas the toxic effects may be enhanced. Concomitant administration of two or more antiepileptics may enhance toxicity without a corresponding increase in antiepileptic effect.

DOSES
Mammals: Primates: 2.5 mg/kg p.o. q12h.
Birds, Reptiles, Amphibians, Fish: No information available.

Phytomenadione see Vitamin K1

Pimobendan
(Cardisure, Fortekor-Plus, Pimocard, Vetmedin)
POM-V

Formulations: Injectable: 0.75 mg/ml solution (5 ml vial, Vetmedin). Oral: 5 mg hard capsules or 1.25 mg, 5 mg or 10 mg chewable tablets (Vetmedin); 1.25 mg, 2.5 mg, 5 mg, 10 mg flavoured tablets (Cardisure, Pimocard). Available in compound preparations with benazepril (1.25 mg pimobendan/2.5 mg benazepril; 5 mg pimobendan/10 mg benazepril) (Fortekor-Plus).

Action: Inodilator producing both positive inotropic and vasodilatory effects. Inotropic effects are mediated via sensitization of the myocardial contractile apparatus to intracellular calcium and by phosphodiesterase (PDE) III inhibition. Calcium sensitization allows for a positive inotropic effect without an increase in myocardial oxygen demand. Vasodilation is mediated by PDE III and V inhibition, resulting in arterio- and venodilation.

Use: Use in exotic species is anecdotal and extrapolated from use in dogs. Indicated for use with concurrent congestive heart failure therapy (e.g. furosemide, ACE inhibitors). The presence of food may reduce bioavailability.

Safety and handling: Normal precautions should be observed.

Contraindications: Do not use in hypertrophic cardiomyopathy and in cases where augmentation of cardiac output via increased contractility is not possible (e.g. aortic stenosis).

Adverse reactions: A moderate positive chronotropic effect and vomiting may occur in some cases, which may be avoided by dose reduction.

Drug interactions: The positive inotropic effects are attenuated by drugs such as beta-blockers and calcium-channel blockers (especially verapamil). No interaction with digitalis glycosides has been noted.

DOSES
Mammals: Ferrets: 0.5 mg/kg p.o. q12h; **Rabbits:** 0.1–0.3 mg/kg p.o. q12–24h; **Rodents:** 0.2–0.4 mg/kg p.o. q12h; **Primates:** 0.2 mg/kg p.o. q24h; **Sugar gliders:** 0.3–0.5 mg/kg p.o. q12h; **Hedgehogs:** 0.3 mg/kg p.o. q12h.

Birds: 0.25 mg/kg p.o. q12h [a] has been used for clinical cases, although pharmacokinetic studies in Amazon parrots indicate that doses up to 10 mg/kg p.o. q12h may be required for optimal effect [b,1].

Reptiles, Amphibians, Fish: No information available.

References
[a] Sedacca CD, Campbell TW, Bright JM, Webb BT and Aboellail TA (2009) Chronic cor pulmonale secondary to pulmonary atherosclerosis in an African grey parrot. *Journal of the American Veterinary Medical Association* **234(8)**, 1055–1059

[b] Guzman DS, Beaufrere H, KuKanich B *et al.* (2014) Pharmacokinetics of single oral dose of pimobendan in Hispaniolan Amazon parrots (*Amazona ventralis*). *Journal of Avian Medicine and Surgery* **28(2)**, 95–101

[1] Fitzgerald BC, Dias S and Martorell J (2018) Cardiovascular Drugs in Avian, Small Mammal, and Reptile Medicine. *Veterinary Clinics: Exotic Animal Practice* **21(2)**, 399–442

Piperacillin
(Tazocin*) **POM**

Formulations: Injectable: 2.25 g, 4.5 g powder (2 g or 4 g piperacillin sodium + 0.25 g or 0.5 g tazobactam (Tazocin)).

Action: Beta-lactam antibiotics bind penicillin-binding proteins involved in cell wall synthesis, decreasing bacterial cell wall strength and rigidity, and affecting cell division, growth and septum formation. As animal cells lack a cell wall the beta-lactam antibiotics are extremely safe in most species. The effect is bactericidal and killing occurs in a time-dependent fashion.

Use: Piperacillin is a ureidopenicillin, classified with ticarcillin as an antipseudomonal penicillin. It is reserved for life-threatening infections (e.g. endocarditis or septicaemia) where culture and sensitivity testing predict a clinical response. These include infections caused by *Pseudomonas aeruginosa* and *Bacteroides fragilis* in neutropenic patients, although it has activity against other Gram-negative bacilli including *Proteus*. For pseudomonal septicaemias, antipseudomonal penicillins should be given with an aminoglycoside (e.g. gentamicin) as there is a synergistic effect. Piperacillin should usually be combined with a beta-lactamase inhibitor and therefore is co-formulated with tazobactam. Experience in veterinary species is limited, and doses are largely empirical.

Safety and handling: Normal precautions should be observed.

Contraindications: Avoid use in animals with reported sensitivity to penicillins. Do not administer to rabbits, guinea pigs, chinchillas, hamsters, gerbils or degus.

Adverse reactions: Nausea, diarrhoea and skin rashes are the commonest adverse effects in humans. Painful if given by i.m. injection. The sodium content of each formulation may be clinically important for patients on restricted sodium intakes. Avoid use in animals with reported sensitivity to penicillins. Avoid administration in small herbivores (e.g. rabbits), hamsters and gerbils as penicillins can cause fatal enterotoxaemia.

Drug interactions: Piperacillin enhances the effects of non-depolarizing muscle relaxants. Gentamicin inactivates piperacillin if mixed in the same syringe. Clinical experience with this drug is limited. There is synergism between the beta-lactams and the aminoglycosides.

DOSES
See Appendix for guidelines on responsible antibacterial use.
Mammals: Primates: 80–100 mg/kg i.m., i.v. q8h;
Hedgehogs: 10 mg/kg s.c. q8–12h; **Rabbits, Chinchillas, Guinea pigs, Hamsters, Gerbils, Degus:** Do not use.
Birds: 100 mg/kg i.m., i.v. q12h[a].

Reptiles:
- **Chelonians, Lizards:** 50–100 mg/kg i.m. q24h for 7–14 days; may be nebulized diluted 100 mg piperacillin/10 ml saline for 15–20 min q8–12h for lower respiratory tract infections.
- **Blood pythons:** <100 mg/kg i.m. q48h[b].

Amphibians: 100 mg/kg s.c., i.m. q24h.

Fish: No information available.

References
[a] Robbins PK, Tell LA, Needham ML and Craigmaill AL (2000) Pharmacokinetics of piperacillin after intramuscular injection in red-tailed hawks (*Buteo jamaicensis*) and great horned owls (*Bubo virginianus*). *Journal of Zoo and Wildlife Medicine* **31(1)**, 47–51

[b] Hilf M, Swanson D, Wagner R and Yu VL (1991) Pharmacokinetics of piperacillin in blood pythons (*Python curtus*) and *in vitro* evaluation of efficacy against aerobic Gram-negative bacteria. *Journal of Zoo and Wildlife Medicine* **22(2)**, 199–203

Piperazine
(Biozine, Easy Round Wormer, Piperazine Citrate Worm Tablets, Puppy Easy Worm Syrup, Roundworm, **Soluverm**) **AVM-GSL**

Formulations: Oral: 100 mg, 105 mg, 416 mg, 500 mg tablets; 500 mg/g (50% w/w), 510 mg/g (51% w/w) powder; 58 mg/ml syrup.

Action: An anti-ascaridial anthelmintic that blocks acetylcholine, thus affecting neurotransmission and paralysing the adult worm; it has no larvicidal activity.

Use: Active against *Ascaris* spp. Ineffective against tapeworms and lung worms. Piperazine may be used in pregnant animals. Used for the treatment of non-encysted gastrointestinal nematodes in fish.

Safety and handling: Normal precautions should be observed.

Contraindications: No information available.

Adverse reactions: Uncommon but occasionally vomiting or muscle tremors and ataxia have been reported.

Drug interactions: Piperazine and pyrantel have antagonistic mechanisms of action; do not use together.

DOSES
Mammals: Ferrets: 50–100 mg/kg p.o., repeat in 2–3 weeks; Rabbits: 200 mg/kg p.o., repeat in 2–3 weeks; **Chinchillas:** 100 mg/kg p.o. q24h for 2 doses; **Primates:** 65 mg/kg p.o. q24h for 10 days; **Sugar gliders:** 50 mg/kg p.o. q24h. In-water medication (7 days on, 7 days off, 7 days on) at the following doses, is also possible: **Guinea pigs, Hamsters:** 10 mg/ml; **Rats, Mice:** 4–5 mg/ml.

Birds: Pigeons: 1.9 g/l water; **Passerines:** 3.7 g/l water for 12h. Repeat in 2–3 weeks.

Amphibians: 50 mg/kg p.o., repeat in 14 days.

Fish: 10 mg/kg in feed q24h for 3 doses or 110 mg/kg in feed once.

Reptiles: No information available.

Piroxicam
(Brexidol*, Feldene*, Piroxicam*) **POM**

Formulations: Oral: 10 mg, 20 mg capsules; 20 mg dissolving tablet. **Injectable:** 20 mg/ml solution.

Action: Inhibition of COX enzymes limits the production of prostaglandins involved in inflammation. Also limits tumour growth but the mechanism is still to be determined.

Use: In veterinary medicine, piroxicam has been used to treat certain tumours expressing COX receptors, e.g. transitional cell carcinoma of the bladder, prostatic carcinoma and colonic-rectal carcinoma and polyps. Piroxicam suppositories are available in the human field and may be useful in the management of colorectal polyps/neoplasia. Other NSAIDs are authorized for veterinary use in various inflammatory conditions but there is no information on the effect of these drugs in neoplastic conditions.

Safety and handling: Normal precautions should be observed.

Contraindications: Gastric ulceration, renal disease, concurrent use of corticosteroids.

Adverse reactions: As a non-specific COX inhibitor it may cause general adverse effects associated with NSAIDs, including GI toxicity, gastric ulceration and renal papillary necrosis (particularly if patient is dehydrated). There is a small risk that NSAIDs may precipitate cardiac failure in humans and this risk in animals is unknown.

Drug interactions: Do not use with corticosteroids or other NSAIDs (increased risk of gastric ulceration). Concurrent use with diuretics or aminoglycosides may increase risk of nephrotoxicity. Piroxicam is highly protein bound and may displace other protein bound drugs. The clinical significance of this is not well established.

DOSES
Mammals: Rabbits: 0.2 mg/kg p.o. q8h; **Mice:** 3.4–20 mg/kg p.o. q24h.
Birds: 0.5–0.8 mg/kg p.o. q12h[1].
Reptiles, Amphibians, Fish: No information available.

References
[1] Hawkins MG and Paul-Murphy J (2011) Avian analgesia. *Veterinary Clinics of North America: Exotic Animal Practice* **14(1)**, 61–80

PMSG see **Serum gonadotrophin**

Polysulphated glycosaminoglycan
(Adequan) **POM-V**

Formulations: Injectable: 100 mg/ml solution for i.m. injection.

Action: Precursor to mucopolysaccharides, enzyme inhibitor, stimulates chondrocytes and synovial cells. Binds to damaged cartilage matrix consisting of aggregated proteoglycans and stimulates the synthesis of new glycosaminoglycan molecules and inhibits proteolytic enzymes.

Use: Acts as a chondroprotective agent in the adjunctive management of non-infectious and non-immune-mediated arthritides. For intra-articular use surgical preparation of the joint is necessary and for both preparations aseptic technique is mandatory. Not a replacement, but rather an adjunct for other therapies.

Safety and handling: Normal precautions should be observed.

Contraindications: Not for use in patients where arthrotomy is anticipated because of a possible increase in bleeding. Not for use when infection is present or suspected.

Adverse reactions: Intra-articular injection may cause pain and inflammation. Although rare, joint sepsis is possible.

Drug interactions: None described to date.

DOSES
Mammals: Rabbits: 2.2 mg/kg s.c., i.m. q3d for 21–28 days, then q14d as needed; **Primates:** 2 mg/kg i.m. q3–5d for 2–3 months.
Birds, Reptiles, Amphibians, Fish: No information available.

Polyvinyl alcohol
(Liquifilm Tears*, Sno Tears*) **P**

Formulations: Ophthalmic: 1.4%, 10 ml, 15 ml.

Action: Polyvinyl alcohol is a synthetic resin tear substitute (lacromimetic).

Use: It is used for lubrication of dry eyes. In cases of keratoconjunctivitis sicca (KCS or dry eye) it will improve ocular surface lubrication, tear retention and patient comfort while lacrostimulation therapy (e.g. topical ciclosporin) is initiated. It is more adherent and less viscous than hypromellose. Patient compliance is poor if administered >q4h; consider using a longer acting tear replacement.

Safety and handling: Normal precautions should be observed.

Contraindications: No information available.

Adverse reactions: No information available.

Drug interactions: No information available.

DOSES
Mammals: 1 drop per eye q1h.
Birds, Reptiles, Amphibians, Fish: No information available.

Polyvinylpyrrolidone–iodine complex see Povidone–iodine

Potassium bromide
(Epilease, Libromide, Potassium bromide solution) **POM-V, AVM-GSL**

Formulations: Oral: 325 mg tablets; 100 mg, 250 mg, 1000 mg capsules; 250 mg/ml solution.

Action: Within the CNS it competes with transmembrane chloride transport and inhibits sodium, resulting in membrane hyperpolarization and elevation of the seizure threshold. Bromide competes with chloride in postsynaptic anion channels following activation by inhibitory neurotransmitters and therefore potentiates the effect of GABA. Acts synergistically with other therapeutic agents that have GABA-ergic effects (such as phenobarbital).

Use: Control of seizures in which the seizures are refractory to treatment with phenobarbital or where the use of phenobarbital or imepitoin is contraindicated. KBr is usually used in conjunction with phenobarbital. Although not authorized for this use, KBr has been used in conjunction with imepitoin. Bromide has a long half-life (>20 days) and steady state plasma concentrations may not be achieved for 3–4 months. Monitoring of serum drug concentrations should be performed and dose levels adjusted accordingly. The serum KBr concentration should reach 0.8–1.5 mg/ml to be therapeutic. The slow rise of plasma bromide levels after enteral administration limits its usefulness in status epilepticus. Bromide is well absorbed from the GI tract and eliminated slowly by the kidney in competition with chloride. High levels of dietary salt increase renal elimination of bromide. Consequently, it is important that the diet be kept constant once bromide therapy has started. Bromide will be measured in assays for chloride and will therefore produce falsely high 'chloride' results. Use with caution in renal disease.

Safety and handling: Normal precautions should be observed.

Contraindications: No information available.

Adverse reactions: Ataxia, sedation and somnolence are seen with overdosage. Skin reactions have been reported in animals with pre-existing skin diseases, e.g. flea bite dermatitis. Vomiting may occur after oral administration, particularly if high concentrations

(>250 mg/ml) are used. Polyphagia, polydipsia and pancreatitis have also been reported. In the case of acute bromide toxicity, 0.9% NaCl i.v. is the treatment of choice. Less commonly behavioural changes, including irritability or restlessness, may be evident.

Drug interactions: Bromide competes with chloride for renal reabsorption. Increased dietary salt, administration of fluids or drugs containing chloride, and use of loop diuretics (e.g. furosemide) may result in increased bromide excretion and decreased serum bromide concentrations.

DOSES
Mammals: Ferrets: 22–30 mg/kg p.o. q24h in combination with phenobarbital; 70–80 mg/kg p.o. q24h if used alone.
Birds, Reptiles, Amphibians, Fish: No information available.

Potassium citrate
(Cystopurin*, Potassium citrate BP*) **AVM-GSL**

Formulations: Oral: 30% solution. Various preparations are available.

Action: Enhances renal tubular resorption of calcium and alkalinizes urine.

Use: Management of calcium oxalate and urate urolithiasis, and fungal urinary tract infections. May be used to treat hypokalaemia, although potassium chloride or gluconate is preferred. Used to treat some forms of metabolic acidosis.

Safety and handling: Normal precautions should be observed.

Contraindications: Renal impairment or cardiac disease.

Adverse reactions: Rare, but may include GI signs and hyperkalaemia.

Drug interactions: No information available.

DOSES
Mammals: Rabbits: 33 mg/kg p.o. q8h; Guinea pigs: 10–30 mg/kg p.o. q12h.
Birds, Reptiles, Amphibians, Fish: No information available.

Potassium permanganate
(Permanganate of potash)
(Permanganate dip) **ESPA**

Formulations: Immersion: crystals for dissolution in water; solution (proprietary formulations are available).

Action: Oxidization of organic matter.

Use: Treatment of external bacterial infections and ectoparasites in freshwater fish. Used to disinfect aquarium plants and kill algae. Best used as a separate 30–60 min bath treatment. Effective treatment in ponds requires 2 mg/l of active chemical to be maintained throughout the treatment period. The permanganate ion (pink colour in solution) reacts with organic matter and is reduced to inactive manganese dioxide (clear or light brown colour). If the colour change takes place within 12 hours, more potassium permanganate should be added in 2 mg/l increments with care until the light pink colour is restored. Toxic at high pH because manganese dioxide may precipitate on to the gills. Stains many materials. Used in birds for cautery of broken bleeding nails/talons.

Safety and handling: Normal precautions may be observed.

Contraindications: Do not use in sea water. Not recommended for use in aquaria since many species are sensitive to this chemical.

Adverse reactions: No information available.

Drug interactions: Do not use with formalin.

DOSES
Fish: External bacteria and parasites: 5 mg/l by immersion for 30–60 min or 2 mg/l by prolonged immersion (follow manufacturer's recommendations for proprietary formulations); Plant disinfection: 10 mg/l by immersion for 5–10 min.
Birds: Effective by direct application for cautery of broken bleeding nails/talons.
Mammals, Reptiles, Amphibians: No information available.

Potentiated sulphonamides see Trimethoprim/Sulphonamide

Povidone–iodine (Iodophor, Polyvinylpyrrolidone–iodine complex, PVP) (Tamodine, Betadine*, Vetasept*) **ESPA**

Formulations: Topical: 7.5% w/w povidone–iodine (0.75% w/w available iodine) solution.

Action: Biocidal effect on a broad range of organisms (bacteria, fungi, viruses, protozoa) by killing cells through iodination of lipids and oxidation of cytoplasmic and membrane compounds.

Use: Clean and dress wounds in fish.

Safety and handling: Normal precautions should be observed.

Contraindications: Care should be taken when using with iodine-sensitive patients since potential for iodine to be absorbed by some animals (e.g. use in axolotls may cause metamorphosis).

Adverse reactions: No information available.

Drug interactions: No information available.

DOSES

Fish: Topical: Apply undiluted with a cotton bud or swab to wet surface and rinse with fresh water.

Mammals, Birds, Reptiles, Amphibians: No information available.

Pralidoxime
(Pralidoxime*) **POM**

Formulations: Powder for reconstitution: 1 g vial which produces 200 mg/ml solution.

Action: Reactivates the cholinesterase enzyme damaged by organophosphate (OP) and allows the destruction of accumulated acetylcholine at the synapse to be resumed. In addition, pralidoxime detoxifies certain OPs by direct chemical inactivation and retards the 'ageing' of phosphorylated cholinesterase to a non-reactive form.

Use: Management of OP toxicity. Most effective if given within 24 hours. Pralidoxime does not appreciably enter the CNS, thus CNS toxicity is not reversed. If given within 24 hours of exposure, treatment is usually only required for 24–36 hours. Respiratory support may be necessary. Treatment of OP toxicity should also include atropine. Use at a reduced dose with renal failure.

Safety and handling: Normal precautions should be observed.

Contraindications: Do not use for poisoning due to carbamate or OP compounds without anticholinesterase activity.

Adverse reactions: Nausea, tachycardia, hyperventilation and muscular weakness are reported in humans.

Drug interactions: Aminophylline, morphine, phenothiazines or theophylline should be avoided in these patients.

DOSES

Birds: 10–100 mg/kg i.m., i.v. q24h prn [1].

Mammals, Reptiles, Amphibians, Fish: No information available.

References
[1] Dell K (2012) Clinical management of seizures in avian patients. *Journal of Exotic Pet Medicine* **21(2)**, 132–139

Praziquantel

(Bob Martin 2 in 1 Dewormer, Bob Martin 3 in 1 Dewormer, Bob Martin Spot-on Dewormer, Cazitel Plus, Cestem Flavoured, Dolpac, Droncit, Droncit Spot-on, Drontal cat, Drontal plus, Endoguard, **Fluke-Solve**, **Fluke-Solve Aquarium**, Milbemax for cats, Milbemax for dogs, Plerion, Prazitel, Profender Spot-on) **POM-V, NFA-VPS, AVM-GSL**

Formulations: Oral: 50 mg and 175 mg praziquantel with pyrantel and febantel tablets (Bob Martin 3 in 1 Dewormer, Cazitel Plus, Cestem Flavoured, Drontal plus, Endoguard, Prazitel); 10 mg, 25 mg, 50 mg and 125 mg praziquantel with oxantel and pyrantel tablets (Dolpac, Plerion); 20 mg and 30 mg praziquantel with pyrantel tablets (Bob Martin 2 in 1 Dewormer, Drontal cat); 25 mg and 125 mg praziquantel with milbemycin tablets (Milbemax for dogs); 10 mg and 40 mg praziquantel with milbemycin tablets (Milbemax for cats). **Topical:** 20 mg, 30 mg, 60 mg, 96 mg in spot-on pipette (Bob Martin Spot-on Dewormer, Droncit Spot-on); 85.8 mg/ml praziquantel with emodepside in spot-on pipettes (Profender Spot-on). Immersion: 10 g, 100 g sachets (Fluke-Solve)

Action: Cestocide that increases cell membrane permeability of susceptible worms, resulting in loss of intracellular calcium and paralysis. This allows the parasites to be phagocytosed or digested.

Use: Used for the treatment of trematodes and cestodes including skin and gill trematode infections and tapeworms in ornamental fish.

Safety and handling: Normal precautions should be observed. Solutions containing emodepside should not be handled by women of child-bearing age.

Contraindications: Do not use at the same time as any other fish or pond treatments. Turn off UV and carbon filters for 24 hours after adding product to water.

Adverse reactions: Oral administration can occasionally result in anorexia, vomiting, lethargy and diarrhoea.

Drug interactions: No information available.

DOSES

Mammals: Ferrets: 5–10 mg/kg p.o., repeat in 10–14 days; Rabbits: 5–10 mg/kg p.o., repeat in 10 days; **Gerbils, Rats, Mice:** 30 mg/kg p.o. q14d (for 3 treatments); **Primates:** 20 mg/kg (cestodes) or 40 mg/kg (trematodes) p.o. once; **Hedgehogs:** 7 mg/kg p.o., repeat in 14 days.
Birds: 10mg/kg i.m.; 10–20 mg/kg p.o., repeat in 10–14 days.

Reptiles: 5–8 mg/kg p.o., repeat in 2 weeks in most species. Profender has been used topically in a variety of reptile species at doses up to 1.12 ml/kg, corresponding to 24 mg emodepside and 96 mg praziquantel/kg, once [a,b].

Amphibians: 8–24 mg/kg p.o. q7–21d or 10 mg/l bath for 3 hours repeat q7–21d.

Fish: 2 mg/l by immersion, repeat every 3 weeks for 3 doses.

References

[a] Schilliger L, Betremieux O, Rochet J, Krebber R and Schaper R (2009) Absorption and efficacy of a spot-on combination containing emodepside plus praziquantel in reptiles. *Revue de Médecine Vétérinaire* **160(12)**, 557–561

[b] Tang PK, Pellett S, Blake D and Hedley J (2017) Efficacy of a Topical Formulation Containing Emodepside and Praziquantel (Profender®, Bayer) against Nematodes in Captive Tortoises. *Journal of Herpetological Medicine and Surgery* **27(3)**, 116–122

Prazosin
(Hypovase*, Prazosin*) **POM**

Formulations: Oral: 0.5 mg, 1 mg, 2 mg, 5 mg tablets.

Action: Prazosin is a postsynaptic alpha-1 blocking agent causing arterial and venous vasodilation. This leads to reduction in blood pressure and systemic vascular resistance.

Use: Adjunctive therapy of congestive heart failure secondary to mitral regurgitation in cases that are refractory to standard therapy. May be useful in promoting urine flow in patients with functional urethral obstruction and in the management of systemic or pulmonary hypertension. Efficacy may decline over time. Not often used.

Safety and handling: Normal precautions should be observed.

Contraindications: Hypotension, renal failure.

Adverse reactions: Hypotension, syncope, drowsiness, weakness, GI upsets.

Drug interactions: Concomitant use of beta-blockers (e.g. propranolol) or diuretics (e.g. furosemide) may increase the risk of a first dose hypotensive effect. Calcium-channel blockers may cause additive hypotension. Prazosin is highly protein-bound and so may be displaced by, or displace, other highly protein-bound drugs (e.g. sulphonamide) from plasma proteins.

DOSES

Mammals: Ferrets: 0.05–0.1 mg/kg p.o. q8h for urethral smooth muscle relaxation.

Birds, Reptiles, Amphibians, Fish: No information available.

Prednisolone
(PLT, Prednicare, Prednidale, Pred-forte*) **POM-V**

Formulations: Ophthalmic: Prednisolone acetate 0.5%, 1% suspensions in 5 ml, 10 ml bottles (Pred-forte). **Topical:** Prednisolone is a component of many topical dermatological, otic and ophthalmic preparations. **Injectable:** Prednisolone sodium succinate 10 mg/ml solution; 7.5 mg/ml suspension plus 2.5 mg/ml dexamethasone. **Oral:** 1 mg, 5 mg, 25 mg tablets. PLT is a compound preparation containing cinchophen.

Action: Binds to specific cytoplasmic receptors which then enter the nucleus and alter the transcription of DNA, leading to alterations in cellular metabolism which result in anti-inflammatory, immunosuppressive and antifibrotic effects. Also has glucocorticoid activity.

Use: Management of chronic allergic/inflammatory conditions (e.g. atopy, inflammatory bowel disease), immune-mediated conditions, hypoadrenocorticism, and lymphoproliferative and other neoplasms. In combination with cinchophen (PLT) it is used in the management of osteoarthritis. Prednisolone has approximately 4 times the anti-inflammatory potency and half the relative mineralocorticoid potency of hydrocortisone. It, like methylprednisolone, is considered to have an intermediate duration of activity and is suitable for alternate-day use. Animals on chronic therapy should be tapered off their steroids when discontinuing the drug. There are no studies comparing protocols for tapering immunosuppressive or anti-inflammatory therapy; it is appropriate to adjust the therapy according to laboratory or clinical parameters. For example, cases with immune-mediated haemolytic anaemia should have their therapy adjusted following monitoring of their haematocrit. There is no evidence that long-term low doses of glucocorticoids do, or do not, prevent relapse of immune-mediated conditions. Impaired wound healing and delayed recovery from infections may be seen. Use glucocorticoids with care in rabbits as they are sensitive to these drugs. If using in birds must make sure bird is genuinely pruritic and underlying infectious disease, e.g. aspergillosis, chlamydiosis, has been excluded before use. The use of steroids in most cases of shock and spinal cord injury is of no benefit and may be detrimental. Has been used as part of the chemotherapy protocol in one green iguana.

Safety and handling: Shake suspension before use.

Contraindications: Do not use in pregnant animals. Systemic corticosteroids are generally contraindicated in patients with renal disease and diabetes mellitus. Topical corticosteroids are contraindicated in ulcerative keratitis.

Adverse reactions: Prolonged use of glucocorticoids suppresses the hypothalamic–pituitary axis (HPA), causing adrenal atrophy, and may cause significant proteinuria and glomerular changes. Catabolic effects of glucocorticoids lead to weight loss and cutaneous atrophy. Iatrogenic hyperadrenocorticism may develop with chronic use. Vomiting, diarrhoea and GI ulceration may develop; the latter may be more severe when corticosteroids are used in animals with neurological injury. Hyperglycaemia and decreased serum T4 values may be seen in patients receiving prednisolone. Corticosteroids should be used with care in birds as there is a high risk of immunosuppression and side effects, such as hepatopathy and a diabetes mellitus-like syndrome. In rabbits, even small single doses can potentially cause severe adverse reactions. Ferrets are particularly susceptible to GI ulceration, and concurrent gastric protectants may be advisable, especially in stressed animals.

Drug interactions: There is an increased risk of GI ulceration if used concurrently with NSAIDs. Hypokalaemia may develop if acetazolamide, amphotericin B or potassium-depleting diuretics (e.g. furosemide, thiazides) are administered concomitantly with corticosteroids. Glucocorticoids may antagonize the effect of insulin. The metabolism of corticosteroids may be enhanced by phenytoin or phenobarbital and decreased by antifungals (e.g. itraconazole).

DOSES

See Appendix for chemotherapy protocols in ferrets.

Mammals: **Ferrets:** lymphoma; anti-inflammatory: 1–2 mg/kg p.o. q24h; postoperative management of adrenalectomy: 0.25–0.5 mg/kg p.o. q12h, taper to q48h; **Rabbits:** anti-inflammatory: 0.25–0.5 mg/kg p.o. q12h for 3 days, then q24h for 3 days, then q48h; **Primates:** anti-inflammatory: 0.5 mg/kg p.o., s.c., i.m. q24h; allergy, autoimmune disease: up to 2 mg/kg p.o., s.c., i.m. q24h; **Sugar gliders:** anti-inflammatory: 0.1–0.2 mg/kg p.o., s.c., i.m. q24h; **Hedgehogs:** allergy: 2.5 mg/kg p.o., s.c., i.m. q12h; **Others:** anti-inflammatory: 1.25–2.5 mg/kg p.o. q24h. Ophthalmic: Dosage frequency and duration of therapy is dependent upon the type of lesion and response to therapy. Usually 1 drop in the affected eye(s) q4–24h, tapering in response to therapy. Care should be exercised in rabbits, as they are highly sensitive to the effects of steroids, even in topical preparations.

Birds: Pruritus: 1 mg/kg p.o. q12h, reduced to minimum effective dose as quickly as possible.

Reptiles: Analgesic, Anti-inflammatory: 2–5 mg/kg p.o. q24–48h; Lymphoma: 2 mg/kg p.o. q24h for 2 weeks, then 1 mg/kg p.o. q24h as part of the chemotherapy protocol in a green iguana[1].

Amphibians, Fish: No information available.

References

[1] Folland DW, Johnston MS, Thamm DH and Reavill D (2011) Diagnosis and management of lymphoma in a green iguana (*Iguana iguana*). *Journal of the American Veterinary Medical Association* **239(7)**, 985–991

Prochlorperazine
(Buccastem*, Prochlorperazine*, Stemetil*) **POM**

Formulations: Injectable: 12.5 mg/ml solution in 1 ml ampoule. Oral: 3 mg, 5 mg tablets; 5 mg/ml syrup.

Action: Blocks dopamine, muscarinic acetylcholine and 5-HT3 receptors in chemoreceptor trigger zone and vomiting centre.

Use: Predominantly to control motion sickness and emesis associated with vestibular disease.

Safety and handling: Normal precautions should be observed.

Contraindications: No information available.

Adverse reactions: Sedation, depression, hypotension and extrapyramidal reactions (rigidity, tremors, weakness, restlessness, etc.).

Drug interactions: CNS depressant agents (e.g. anaesthetics, narcotic analgesics) may cause additive CNS depression if used with prochlorperazine. Antacids or antidiarrhoeal preparations (e.g. bismuth subsalicylate or kaolin/pectin mixtures) may reduce GI absorption of oral phenothiazines. Increased blood levels of both drugs may result if propranolol is administered with phenothiazines. Phenothiazines block alpha-adrenergic receptors, which may lead to unopposed beta activity causing vasodilation and increased cardiac rate if adrenaline is given.

DOSES
Mammals: Rabbits: 0.2–0.5 mg/kg p.o. q8h for torticollis.
Birds, Reptiles, Amphibians, Fish: No information available.

Progesterone
(Progesterone*) **POM**

Formulations: Injectable: 25 mg/ml oily solution.

Action: Binds to specific cytoplasmic receptors, which then enter the nucleus and alter the transcription of DNA leading to alterations in cellular metabolism.

Use: Induction of ovulation in conjunction with hCG or PMSG in amphibians.

Safety and handling: Normal precautions should be observed.

Contraindications: No information available.

Adverse reactions: No information available.

Drug interactions: No information available.

DOSES
Amphibians: 1–5 mg/kg s.c., i.m. once.
Mammals, Birds, Reptiles, Fish: No information available.

Proligestone
(Delvosteron) **POM-V**

Formulations: Injectable: 100 mg/ml suspension.

Action: Alters the transcription of DNA, leading to alterations in cellular metabolism which mimic those caused by progesterone.

Use: Postponement of oestrus in the jill ferret, and treatment and prevention of false pregnancy in the rabbit. As coat colour changes may occasionally occur, injection into the medial side of the flank fold is recommended for thin-skinned or show animals.

Safety and handling: Normal precautions should be observed.

Contraindications: Best avoided in diabetic animals, as insulin requirements are likely to change unpredictably. Do not use in birds.

Adverse reactions: Proligestone does not appear to be associated with as many or as serious adverse effects as other progestogens (e.g. megestrol acetate, medroxyprogesterone acetate). However, adverse effects associated with long-term progestogen use, e.g. temperament changes (listlessness and depression), increased thirst or appetite, cystic endometrial hyperplasia/pyometra, diabetes mellitus, acromegaly, adrenocortical suppression, mammary enlargement/neoplasia and lactation, may be expected. Irritation at the site of injection may occur and calcinosis circumscripta at the injection site has been reported.

Drug interactions: No information available.

DOSES

Mammals: Ferrets: 50 mg/animal s.c., if no response give 25 mg/animal after 7 days, repeat at further 7 days; **Rabbits:** 30 mg/kg for pseudopregnancy.
Birds: Do not use.
Reptiles, Amphibians, Fish: No information available.

Propentofylline
(Vitofyllin, Vivitonin) **POM-V**

Formulations: Oral: 50 mg, 100 mg tablets.

Action: Propentofylline is a xanthine derivative that increases blood flow to the heart, muscle and CNS via inhibition of phosphodiesterase. It also has an antiarrhythmic action, bronchodilator effects, positive inotropic and chronotropic effects on the heart, inhibitory effects on platelet aggregation and reduces peripheral vascular resistance.

Use: Anecdotally used in raptors for wing tip oedema and in parrots for egg yolk peritonitis.

Safety and handling: Normal precautions should be observed.

Contraindications: No information available.

Adverse reactions: May increase myocardial oxygen demand.

Drug interactions: No information available.

DOSES
Birds: 5 mg/kg p.o. q12h.
Mammals, Reptiles, Amphibians, Fish: No information available.

Propofol
(Norofol, Procare, PropoFlo Plus, PropoFol, Rapinovet) **POM-V**

Formulations: Injectable: 10 mg/ml solution: lipid emulsion available both without a preservative or antibacterial or with a preservative (benzyl alcohol), 20 ml, 50 ml and 100 ml glass bottles. The solution containing a preservative can be used for up to 28 days after the vial is first broached.

Action: The mechanism of action is not fully understood but it is thought to involve modulation of the inhibitory activity of GABA at GABA receptors.

Use: Induction of anaesthesia and maintenance of anaesthesia using intermittent boluses or a continuous rate infusion. The solution containing benzyl alcohol preservative should not be used for maintenance of anaesthesia by continuous rate infusion due to the risk of toxicity caused by prolonged administration. Injection i.v. produces a rapid loss of consciousness as the CNS takes up the highly lipophilic drug. Over the next few minutes propofol distributes to peripheral tissues and the concentration in the CNS falls such that, in the absence of further doses, the patient wakes up. Propofol does not have analgesic properties, therefore it is better used in combination with other drugs to maintain anaesthesia; for example, a continuous rate infusion of a potent opioid. Considerable care must be taken with administration in hypovolaemic animals and those with diminished cardiopulmonary, hepatic and renal reserves. Propofol has been used by immersion to induce general anaesthesia in a few species of fish (koi, goldfish and trout).

Safety and handling: Shake the lipid emulsion well before use and do not mix with other therapeutic agents or therapeutic fluids prior to administration. If using a preparation that contains no bacteriostat, opened bottles should be stored in a refrigerator and used within 8 hours or discarded. Once broached, the lipid preparation with a preservative has a shelf-life of 28 days.

Contraindications: No information available.

Adverse reactions: The rapid injection of large doses causes apnoea, cyanosis, bradycardia and severe hypotension. Problems are less likely when injection is made over 30–60 seconds. Propofol is not irritant to tissues but a pain reaction is commonly evident during i.v. injection; the underlying mechanism causing pain is unknown.

Drug interactions: No information available.

DOSES

Mammals: Ferrets: 2–8 mg/kg i.v.; **Rabbits:** unpremedicated 7.5–15 mg/kg i.v.; premedicated 2–6 mg/kg i.v.; **Rats:** 7.5–10 mg/kg i.v.; **Mice:** 12–26 mg/kg i.v.; **Primates:** 2.5–5 mg/kg i.v. followed by 0.3–0.4 mg/kg/min CRI.

Birds: 10 mg/kg i.v. by slow infusion to effect: supplemental doses up to 3 mg/kg [a,b]; 0.5 mg/kg/min i.v. infusion as CRI.

Reptiles: 5–10 mg/kg i.v., intraosseous; **Red-eared sliders:** 10–20 mg/kg i.v. (higher doses required for successful intubation) [c]; **Bearded dragons:** 10mg/kg i.v. [d]; **Green iguanas:** 5–10 mg/kg intraosseous; **Brown tree snakes:** 5 mg/kg i.v.

Amphibians: Leopard frogs: 10 mg/kg injected in the sublingual plexus area (achieves sedative–light anaesthesia). **Tiger salamanders:** 10–35 mg/kg intracoelomic gives induction in 30 minutes and recovery in 24 hours [e]. Euthanasia: 60–100 mg/kg intracoelomic or 100–400 mg/kg topically, remove and rinse after induction.

Fish: Anaesthesia: 2.5–10 mg/l by immersion [f].

References

[a] Langlois I, Harvey RC, Jones MP and Schumacher J (2003) Cardiopulmonary and anesthetic effects of isoflurane and propofol in Hispaniolan Amazon parrots (*Amazona ventralis*). *Journal of Avian Medicine and Surgery* **17(1)**, 4–10

[b] Müller K, Holzapfel J and Brunnberg L (2011) Total intravenous anaesthesia by boluses or by continuous rate infusion of propofol in mute swans (*Cygnus olor*). *Veterinary Anaesthesia and Analgesia* **38(4)**, 286–291

[c] Ziolo MS and Bertelsen MF (2009) Effects of propofol administered via the supravertebral sinus in red-eared sliders. *Journal of the American Veterinary Medical Association* **234(3)**, 390–393

[d] Perrin KL and Bertelsen MF (2017). Intravenous Alfaxalone and Propofol Anesthesia in the Bearded Dragon (*Pogona vitticeps*). *Journal of Herpetological Medicine and Surgery* **27(3)**, 123–126

[e] Mitchell MA, Riggs SM, Singleton CB *et al.* (2009) Evaluating the clinical and cardiopulmonary effects of clove oil and propofol in tiger salamanders (*Ambystoma tigrinum*). *Journal of Exotic Pet Medicine* **18**, 50–56

[f] Oda A, Bailey KM, Lewbart GA, Griffith EH and Posner LP (2014) Physiologic and biochemical assessments of koi (*Cyprinus carpio*) following immersion in propofol. *Journal of the American Veterinary Medical Association* **245(11)**, 1286–1291

Propranolol
(Inderal*, Propranolol*) **POM**

Formulations: Injectable: 1 mg/ml solution. **Oral:** 10 mg, 40 mg, 80 mg, 160 mg tablets.

Action: Non-selective beta-blocker. Blocks the chronotropic and inotropic effects of beta-1 adrenergic stimulation on the heart, thereby reducing myocardial oxygen demand. Blocks the dilatory effects of beta-2 adrenergic stimulation on the vasculature and bronchial smooth muscle. The antihypertensive effects are mediated through reducing cardiac output, altering the baroreceptor reflex sensitivity and blocking peripheral adrenoceptors.

Use: Management of cardiac arrhythmias (sinus tachycardia, atrial fibrillation or flutter, supraventricular tachycardia, ventricular arrhythmias), hypertrophic cardiomyopathy or obstructive heart disease. Potential efficacy as an additional antihypertensive drug and can be used in phaeochromocytoma if combined with an alpha-blocker. Used to reverse some of the clinical features of thyrotoxicosis prior to surgery in patients with hyperthyroidism. May be used in behavioural therapy to reduce somatic signs of anxiety and is therefore useful in the management of situational anxieties and behavioural problems where contextual anxiety is a component. Some authors suggest using propranolol in combination with phenobarbital for the management of fear- and phobia-related behaviour problems. There is a significant difference between i.v. and oral doses. This is a consequence of propranolol's lower bioavailability when administered orally as a result of decreased absorption and a high first pass effect. Wean off slowly when using chronic therapy.

Safety and handling: Normal precautions should be observed.

Contraindications: Do not use in patients with bradyarrhythmias, acute or decompensated congestive heart failure. Relatively contraindicated in animals with medically controlled congestive heart failure as is poorly tolerated. Do not administer concurrently with alpha-adrenergic agonists (e.g. adrenaline).

Adverse reactions: Bradycardia, AV block, myocardial depression, heart failure, syncope, hypotension, hypoglycaemia, bronchospasm, diarrhoea and peripheral vasoconstriction. Depression and lethargy are occasionally seen as a result of CNS penetration. Propranolol may exacerbate any pre-existing renal impairment. Sudden withdrawal of propranolol may result in exacerbation of arrhythmias or the development of hypertension.

Drug interactions: The hypotensive effect of propranolol is enhanced by many agents that depress myocardial activity including anaesthetic agents, phenothiazines, antihypertensive drugs, diuretics and diazepam. There is an increased risk of bradycardia, severe hypotension, heart failure and AV block if propranolol is used concurrently with calcium-channel blockers. Concurrent digoxin administration potentiates bradycardia. The metabolism of propranolol is accelerated by thyroid hormones, thus reducing its effect. The dose of propranolol may need to be decreased when initiating carbimazole therapy. Oral aluminium hydroxide preparations reduce propranolol absorption. Cimetidine may decrease the metabolism of propranolol, thereby increasing its levels in the blood. Propranolol enhances the effects of muscle relaxants (e.g. suxamethonium, tubocurarine). Hepatic enzyme induction by phenobarbital or phenytoin may increase the rate of metabolism of propranolol. There is an increased risk of lidocaine toxicity if administered with propranolol due to a reduction in lidocaine clearance. The bronchodilatory effects of theophylline may be blocked by propranolol. Although the use of propranolol is not contraindicated in patients with diabetes mellitus, insulin requirements should be monitored as propranolol may enhance the hypoglycaemic effect of insulin.

DOSES
Mammals: Ferrets: 0.2–2 mg/kg p.o., s.c. q12–24h for hypertrophic cardiomyopathy.
Birds: Supraventricular tachycardia: 0.04 mg/kg slow i.v.
Reptiles, Amphibians, Fish: No information available.

Prostaglandin E2 see Dinoprostone
Prostaglandin F2 see Dinoprost tromethamine

Proxymetacaine (Proparacaine)
(Proxymetacaine*) POM

Formulations: Ophthalmic: 0.5% ($\pm$ fluorescein 0.25%), 1.0% solution (single-use vials).

Action: Local anaesthetic action is dependent on reversible blockade of the sodium channel, preventing propagation of an action potential along the nerve fibre. Sensory nerve fibres are blocked before motor nerve fibres, allowing a selective sensory blockade at low doses.

Use: Proxymetacaine is used on the ocular surface (cornea and conjunctival sac), the external auditory meatus and the nares. It acts rapidly (within 10 seconds) and provides anaesthesia for 25–55 minutes in the conjunctival sac depending on the species. Serial application increases duration and depth of anaesthesia. Topical anaesthetics block reflex tear production and should not be applied before a Schirmer tear test.

Safety and handling: Store in refrigerator and in the dark; reduced efficacy if stored at room temperature for >2 weeks.

Contraindications: Do not use for therapeutic purposes.

Adverse reactions: Conjunctival hyperaemia is common; local irritation manifested by chemosis may occasionally occur for several hours after administration (less likely than with tetracaine). All topical anaesthetics are toxic to the corneal epithelium and delay healing of ulcers.

Drug interactions: No information available.

DOSES
Mammals: Ophthalmic: 1–2 drops/eye; duration 1 hour in rabbits.
Birds, Reptiles, Amphibians, Fish: No information available.

PVP see **Povidone–iodine**

Pyrantel

(Bob Martin 2 in 1 Dewormer, Bob Martin 3 in 1 Dewormer, Cazitel Plus, Cestem Flavoured, Dolpac, Drontal cat, Drontal plus, Drontal puppy, Endoguard Flavour/Plus, Plerion, Prazitel) **POM-V**

Formulations: Oral: Pyrantel with praziquantel and febantel (50 mg, 50 mg, 150 mg; 175 mg, 175 mg, 525 mg) tablets (Bob Martin 3 in 1 Dewormer, Cazitel Plus, Cestem Flavoured, Drontal plus, Endoguard, Prazitel); pyrantel with praziquantel and oxantel (10 mg, 10 mg, 40 mg; 25 mg, 25 mg, 100 mg; 50 mg, 50 mg, 200 mg; 125 mg, 125 mg, 500 mg) tablets (Dolpac, Plerion); pyrantel embonate with praziquantel (230 mg, 20 mg; 345 mg, 30 mg) tablets (Bob Martin 2 in 1 Dewormer, Drontal cat); 14.4 mg/ml pyrantel embonate with 15 mg/ml febantel suspension (Drontal puppy). **Note:** some formulations and doses give content of pyrantel (febantel, oxantel) in terms of pyrantel embonate/pamonate (50 mg pyrantel is equivalent to 144 mg pyrantel embonate/pamonate).

Action: A cholinergic agonist which interferes with neuronal transmission in parasites and thereby kills them. Febantel and oxantel are derivatives of pyrantel with increased activity against whipworms.

Use: Control of *Toxocara canis*, *Toxascaris leonina*, *Trichuris vulpis*, *Uncinaria stenocephala*, *Ancylostoma caninum* and *A. braziliensis*.

Safety and handling: Normal precautions should be observed.

Contraindications: Safety has not been established in pregnant or lactating animals and therefore its use is not recommended.

Adverse reactions: Vomiting and diarrhoea may be observed.

Drug interactions: The addition of febantel or oxantel has a synergistic effect. Do not use with levamisole, piperazine or cholinesterase inhibitors.

DOSES

Mammals: Ferrets: 4.4 mg/kg (pyrantel embonate) p.o., repeat in 14 days; **Rabbits:** 5–10 mg/kg (pyrantel embonate/pamoate) p.o., repeat in 10–21 days; **Rodents:** 50 mg/kg (pyrantel embonate/pamoate) p.o., repeat as required; **Primates:** 11 mg/kg p.o., repeat in 14 days[a].
Reptiles: 5 mg/kg p.o., repeat in 14 days.
Amphibians: 5 mg/kg p.o. q14d.
Birds, Fish: No information available.

References
[a] Bentzel DE and Bacon DJ (2007) Comparison of various anthelmintic therapies for the treatment of *Trypanoxyuris microon* infection in owl monkeys (*Aotus nancymae*). *Comparative Medicine* **2**, 206–209

Pyrimethamine
(Daraprim*, Fansidar*) **P**

Formulations: Oral: 25 mg tablet. Fansidar also contains sulfadoxine.

Action: Interference with folate metabolism of the parasite and thereby prevents purine synthesis (and therefore DNA synthesis).

Use: Infections caused by *Toxoplasma gondii*, *Neospora caninum* and *Plasmodium* spp. Should not be used in pregnant or lactating animals without adequate folate supplementation. Used in birds to treat atoxoplasmosis, sarcocystosis and leucocytozoonosis.

Safety and handling: Normal precautions should be observed.

Contraindications: No information available.

Adverse reactions: Depression, anorexia and reversible bone marrow suppression (within 6 days of the start of therapy). Folate supplementation (5 mg/day) may prevent bone marrow suppression.

Drug interactions: Increased antifolate effect if given with phenytoin or sulphonamides. Folate supplementation for the host will reduce the efficacy of the drug if given concomitantly and should thus be given a few hours before pyrimethamine.

DOSES
Mammals: Ferrets: 0.5 mg/kg p.o. q12h; **Primates:** Toxoplasmosis: 2 mg/kg p.o. q24h for 3 days, then 1 mg/kg p.o. q24h for 28 days; *Plasmodium:* 10 mg/kg p.o. q24h; *Encephalitozoon cuniculi:* 0.5 mg/kg p.o. q12h. Monitor for folate deficiency and supplement with folate.
Birds: 0.5–1 mg/kg p.o. q12h for 28 days[1].
Reptiles, Amphibians, Fish: No information available.

References
[1] Doneley RJ (2009) Bacterial and parasitic diseases of parrots. *Veterinary Clinics of North America: Exotic Animal Practice* **12(3)**, 417–432

Pyriproxyfen
(Indorex household spray) **AVM-GSL**

Formulations: Environmental spray.

Action: Juvenile hormone analogue. Arrests the development of flea larvae in the environment.

Use: Use as part of a comprehensive flea control programme in ferrets and rabbits (anecdotal) in conjunction with on-animal adulticide products. Anecdotally has been used in aviaries to control tick infestations.

Safety and handling: Normal precautions should be observed.

The product should not enter watercourses as this may be dangerous for fish and other organisms.

Contraindications: Do not use directly on animals.

Adverse reactions: None reported.

Drug interactions: None reported.

DOSES
Use in the environment as directed.

Ranitidine
(Ranitidine*, Zantac*) **POM**

Formulations: Injectable: 25 mg/ml solution. **Oral:** 75 mg, 150 mg, 300 mg tablets; 15 mg/ml syrup.

Action: Ranitidine is a histamine (H2) receptor antagonist blocking histamine-induced gastric acid secretion. It is more potent than cimetidine but has lower bioavailability (50%) and undergoes hepatic metabolism. It also has a prokinetic effect through stimulation of local muscarinic acetylcholine receptors, which may be of benefit when gastrointestinal motility is impaired.

Use: Management of gastric and duodenal ulcers, idiopathic, uraemic or drug-related erosive gastritis, oesophagitis, and hypersecretory conditions secondary to gastrinoma or mast cell neoplasia. Often used prophylactically in ferrets to prevent stress-associated gastric ulceration. If used for the treatment of ulceration, then treatment should continue for 2 weeks after remission of clinical signs which means typically a 1 month course. Absorption is not clinically significantly affected by food intake, anticholinergic agents or antacids. Used for its prokinetic effect in rabbits, chinchillas and guinea pigs. Currently cimetidine is the only antiulcer drug with a veterinary market authorization. However, the use of ranitidine is justified under the cascade when predominantly used for its prokinetic effect.

Safety and handling: Normal precautions should be observed.

Contraindications: No information available.

Adverse reactions: Rarely reported but include cardiac arrhythmias and hypotension, particularly if administered rapidly i.v.

Drug interactions: It is advisable, though not essential, that sucralfate is administered 2 hours before H2 blockers. Stagger oral doses of ranitidine when used with other antacids, digoxin or metoclopramide by 2 hours as it may reduce their absorption or effect.

DOSES
Mammals: Ferrets: 3.5 mg/kg p.o. q12h; **Rabbits:** 4–6 mg/kg p.o., s.c. q8–24h; **Guinea pigs, Chinchillas:** 5 mg/kg p.o. q12h as a prokinetic; **Primates:** 0.5 mg/kg p.o. q12h (anti-ulcer).
Birds, Reptiles, Amphibians, Fish: No information available.

Retinol see **Vitamin A**

Rifampin (Rifampicin)
(Rifadin*, Rifampicin*, Rimactane*) POM

Formulations: Oral: 150 mg, 300 mg capsules; 20 mg/ml syrup.

Action: Bactericidal drug binding to the beta subunit of RNA polymerase and causing abortive initiation of RNA synthesis.

Use: Wide spectrum of antimicrobial activity including bacteria (particularly Gram-positives), *Chlamydia*, *Rickettsia*, some protozoans and poxviruses. Very active against *Staphylococcus aureus* and *Mycobacterium tuberculosis*. Gram-negative aerobic bacteria are usually innately resistant. Obligate anaerobes (Gram-positive or -negative) are usually susceptible. Exact indications for small animal veterinary practice remain to be fully established. It has been suggested as part of the combination of treatments for mycobacterial infections in primates in combination with ethambutol and isoniazid. It may also have a place in the management of chlamydiosis, erhlichiosis and bartonellosis. Chromosomal mutations readily lead to resistance, therefore rifampin should be used in combination with other antimicrobial drugs to prevent the emergence of resistant organisms. Various combinations of clarithromycin, enrofloxacin, clofaxamine and doxycycline have been used with rifampin in the management of mycobacteriosis, including in birds. Until controlled studies are conducted to investigate the value of rifampin in these infections, recommendations remain empirical.

Safety and handling: Women of child-bearing age should not handle crushed or broken tablets or the syrup without the use of gloves.

Contraindications: Rifampin may be teratogenic at high doses and should not be administered to pregnant animals. It should not be administered to animals with liver disease.

Adverse reactions: Rifampin metabolites may colour urine, saliva and faeces orange–red.

Drug interactions: Rifampin is a potent hepatic enzyme inducer and increases the rate of metabolism of other drugs in humans, including barbiturates, theophylline and itraconazole. Increased dosages of these drugs may be required if used in combination with rifampin.

DOSES
See Appendix for guidelines on responsible antibacterial use.
Mammals: Rabbits: 40 mg/kg p.o. q12h rifampin in conjunction with 50 mg/kg p.o. q24h azithromycin or 80 mg/kg p.o. q12h clarithromycin for *Staphylococcus* osteomyelitis; Primates: 22.5 mg/kg p.o. q24h for 6 weeks, then reduce to 15 mg/kg p.o. q24h for 1 year[a].
Birds: 10–20 mg/kg p.o. q12–24h.
Reptiles, Amphibians, Fish: No information available.

References
[a] Wolf RH, Gibson SV, Watson EA *et al.* (1988) Multidrug chemotherapy of tuberculosis in rhesus monkeys. *Laboratory Animal Science* **38**, 25–33

Rocuronium
(Esmeron*) **POM**

Formulations: Injectable: 10 mg/ml solution.

Action: Inhibits the actions of acetylcholine at the neuromuscular junction by binding competitively to the nicotinic acetylcholine receptor on the post-junctional membrane.

Use: Provision of neuromuscular blockade during anaesthesia. This may be to improve surgical access through muscle relaxation, facilitate positive pressure ventilation or intraocular surgery. Rocuronium is very similar to vecuronium but it has a more rapid onset of action and shorter duration to spontaneous recovery. Its availability in aqueous solution and longer shelf-life increase convenience. Monitoring (using a nerve stimulator) and reversal of the neuromuscular blockade is recommended to ensure complete recovery before the end of anaesthesia. The neuromuscular blockade caused by rocuronium can be rapidly reversed using sugammadex (a cyclodextrin developed to reverse aminosteroidal neuromuscular blocking agents) at a dose of 8 mg/kg i.v. in dogs. Hypothermia, acidosis and hypokalaemia will prolong the duration of action of neuromuscular blockade. Hepatic disease may prolong duration of action of rocuronium; atracurium is preferred in this group of patients. The effects of renal disease on duration of action of rocuronium require further investigation.

Safety and handling: Normal precautions should be observed.

Contraindications: Do not administer unless the animal is adequately anaesthetized and facilities to provide positive pressure ventilation are available.

Adverse reactions: Causes an increase in heart rate and a mild hypertension when used at high doses.

Drug interactions: Neuromuscular blockade is more prolonged when rocuronium is given in combination with volatile anaesthetics, aminoglycosides, clindamycin and lincomycin.

DOSES
Birds: Kestrels: 0.12 mg/eye topically [a,b].
Reptiles: 0.25–0.5 mg/kg i.m. Not recommended as a substitute for analgesia or general anaesthesia.
Mammals, Amphibians, Fish: No information available.

References
[a] Barsotti G, Briganti A, Spratte JR, Ceccherelli R and Breghi G (2010) Mydriatic effect of topically applied rocuronium bromide in tawny owls (*Strix aluco*): comparison between two protocols. *Veterinary Ophthalmology* **13(S1)**, 9–13
[b] Barsotti G, Briganti A, Spratte JR, Ceccherelli R and Breghi G (2012) Safety and efficacy of bilateral topical application of rocuronium bromide for mydriasis in European kestrels (*Falco tinnunculus*). *Journal of Avian Medicine and Surgery* **26(1)**, 1–5

S-Adenosylmethionine (SAMe)
(Denamarin, Denosyl, Doxion, Hepatosyl Plus, Samylin, Zentonil Advanced, Zentonil Plus) **GSL**

Formulations: Oral: 90 mg, 100 mg, 200 mg, 225 mg, 400 mg, 425 mg tablets; 50 mg, 100 mg, 200 mg capsules; 75 mg, 300 mg, 400 mg powder.

Action: *S*-Adenosylmethionine (SAMe) is an endogenous molecule synthesized by cells throughout the body and is a component of several biochemical pathways. SAMe is especially important in hepatocytes because of their central role in metabolism. In humans, antidepressant effects of SAMe are also documented.

Use: Adjunctive treatment for liver disease, especially for acute hepatotoxin-induced liver disease. SAMe has been shown to increase hepatic glutathione levels; a potent antioxidant which protects hepatocytes from toxins and death. Can also be used in patients on long-term therapy with potentially hepatotoxic drugs. The use as an antidepressant therapy in animals has yet to be established. The safety of exogenous SAMe has not been proven in pregnancy; therefore, it should be used with caution.

Safety and handling: Normal precautions should be observed.

Contraindications: No information available.

Adverse reactions: None reported. GI signs (nausea, vomiting, diarrhoea), dry mouth, headache, sweating and dizziness are occasionally reported in humans.

Drug interactions: Concurrent use of SAMe with tramadol, meperidine, pentazocine, MAOIs including selegiline, SSRIs such as fluoxetine, or other antidepressants (e.g. amitriptyline) could cause additive serotonergic effects. SAMe may increase the clearance of drugs that undergo hepatic glucuronidation, including paracetamol, diazepam and morphine.

DOSES
Mammals: Ferrets, Rodents: 20–100 mg/kg p.o. daily for liver support.
Reptiles: 30 mg/kg p.o. daily for liver support.
Birds, Amphibians, Fish: No information available.

Salbutamol
(Ventolin*) **POM**

Formulations: Inhalational: 100 µg per metered inhalation (Evohaler). Injectable: 0.5 mg/ml.

Action: Selective beta-2 stimulation causes smooth muscle relaxation and bronchodilation.

Use: Treatment of bronchospasm in inflammatory airway disease and irritation. Used in rats for mycoplasmosis-related chronic obstructive pulmonary disease (COPD).

Safety and handling: Normal precautions should be observed.

Contraindications: No information available.

Adverse reactions: In humans side effects of the beta-2 agonists include headache, muscle cramps and palpitation. Other side effects include tachycardia, arrhythmias, peripheral vasodilation, and disturbances of sleep and behaviour.

Drug interactions: In humans there is an increased risk of side effects if salbutamol is used by patients also taking diuretics, digoxin, theophylline or corticosteroids.

DOSES
Mammals: Rats: 100 μg (micrograms)/animal q4–6h (use a small chamber) or as needed for relief of bronchospasm.
Birds: 0.05 mg/kg s.c., i.m., i.v. q8h.
Reptiles, Amphibians, Fish: No information available.

Selamectin
(Stronghold) **POM-V**

Formulations: Topical: Spot-on pipettes of various sizes containing 6% or 12% selamectin.

Action: Interacts with GABA and glutamate-gated channels leading to flaccid paralysis of the parasite.

Use: Treatment and prevention of flea and ear mite infestations, *Trixascaris*, *Cheyletiella*, sarcoptic acariasis, biting lice, hookworms (*Ancylostoma tubaeforme*), adult roundworms (*Toxocara canis*, *T. cati*) and prevention of heartworm disease (*Dirofilaria immitis*). Frequent shampooing may reduce the efficacy of the product. Can be used in lactation and pregnancy.

Safety and handling: Highly toxic to aquatic organisms; therefore, take care with disposal.

Contraindications: None.

Adverse reactions: Transient pruritus and erythema at the site of application may occur. Do not use in chelonians as could potentially cause neurotoxicity and death similar to ivermectin.

Drug interactions: No information available.

DOSES
Mammals: Ferrets, Rabbits, Rodents: 6–15 mg/kg monthly; Sugar gliders, Hedgehogs: 6–18 mg/kg monthly.
Birds: 20 mg/kg single dose[1].

Reptiles: Do not use in chelonians.
Amphibians: Bullfrogs: 6 mg/kg single-dose[a].
Fish: No information available.

References

[a] D'Agostino JJ, West G, Boothe DM, Jayanna PK, Snider T and Hoover JP (2007) Plasma pharmacokinetics of selamectin after a single topical administration in the American bullfrog (*Rana catesbeiana*). *Journal of Zoo and Wildlife Medicine* **38(1)**, 51–55

[1] DiGeronimo PM (2016) Therapeutic Review: Selamectin. *Journal of Exotic Pet Medicine* **25**, 80–83

Serum gonadotrophin (PMSG, Equine chorionic gonadotrophin)
(PMSG-Intervet) **POM-V**

Formulations: Injectable: 5000 IU freeze-dried plug.

Action: Mimics action of FSH.

Use: Induction of oestrus by stimulation of ovarian follicle development. Increases spermatogenesis, though with low efficiency. Induction of ovulation in amphibians.

Safety and handling: Normal precautions should be observed.

Contraindications: No information available.

Adverse reactions: Anaphylactoid reactions may occur rarely.

Drug interactions: No information available.

DOSES
Mammals: Guinea pigs: 1000 IU/animal i.m., repeat in 7–10 days.
Amphibians: Induction of ovulation: 50–200 IU s.c., i.m. followed by 600 IU hCG after 72 h; **Barred frogs:** 2 doses of PMSG (50 IU and 25 IU at 6 and 4 days, respectively), prior to 2 doses of 100 IU hCG 24 h apart[a].
Birds, Reptiles, Fish: No information available.

References

[a] Clulow J, Clulow S, Guo J, French AJ, Mahony MJ and Archer M (2012) Optimisation of an oviposition protocol employing human chorionic and pregnant mare serum gonadotropins in the barred frog (*Mixophyes fasciolatus*) (*Myobatrachidae*). *Reproductive Biology and Endocrinology* **10**, 60

Sevoflurane
(SevoFlo) **POM-V**

Formulations: Inhalational: 250 ml bottle.

Action: The mechanism of action of volatile anaesthetic agents is not fully understood.

Use: Induction and maintenance of anaesthesia. Sevoflurane is potent and highly volatile so should only be delivered from a suitable calibrated vaporizer. It is less soluble in blood than isoflurane; therefore, induction and recovery from anaesthesia is quicker. Sevoflurane has a less pungent smell than isoflurane and induction of anaesthesia using chambers or masks is usually well tolerated in small animals. The concentration of sevoflurane required to maintain anaesthesia depends on the other drugs used in the anaesthesia protocol; the concentration should be adjusted according to clinical assessment of anaesthetic depth. The cessation of administration results in rapid recovery, which may occasionally be associated with signs of agitation. Sevoflurane does not sensitize the myocardium to catecholamines to the extent that halothane does.

Safety and handling: Measures should be adopted to prevent contamination of the environment.

Contraindications: No information available.

Adverse reactions: Causes a dose-dependent hypotension that does not wane with time. The effects of sevoflurane on respiration are dose-dependent and comparable with isoflurane. Sevoflurane crosses the placental barrier and will affect neonates delivered by caesarean section. Sevoflurane is degraded by soda lime to compounds that are nephrotoxic in rats (principally Compound A). Conditions accelerating degradation (i.e. low gas flows, high absorbent temperatures and high sevoflurane concentrations) should be avoided in long operations.

Drug interactions: Opioid agonists, benzodiazepines and nitrous oxide reduce the concentration of sevoflurane required to achieve surgical anaesthesia. The effects of sevoflurane on the duration of action of non-depolarizing neuromuscular blocking agents are similar to those of isoflurane, i.e. greater potentiation compared with halothane.

DOSES

Mammals, Birds: The expired concentration required to maintain surgical anaesthesia in 50% of recipients is about 2.5% in most animals (minimum alveolar concentration)[a,b]. The MAC in rabbits is 3.7%. Administration of other anaesthetic agents and opioid analgesics reduces the dose requirement of sevoflurane; therefore, the dose should be adjusted according to individual requirement. 6–8% sevoflurane concentration is required to induce anaesthesia in unpremedicated patients.

Reptiles: Induction: 6–8% in 100% oxygen; Maintenance: 3–5% in 100% oxygen[c,d].

Amphibians: Induction: 37.5 µl/g of a topical mixture (3 parts liquid sevoflurane, 3.5 parts KY jelly, 1.5 parts distilled water) in a closed chamber[e]; Gaseous chamber induction: In cane toads, 1.75% sevoflurane resulted in loss of righting reflex within 15 minutes in 50% of toads (*Rhinella marina*)[f].

Fish: No information available.

References

[a] Joyner PH, Jones MP, Ward D, Gompf RE, Zagaya N and Sleeman JM (2008) Induction and recovery characteristics and cardiopulmonary effects of sevoflurane and isoflurane in bald eagles. *American Journal of Veterinary Research* **69(1)**, 13–22

[b] Phair KA, Larsen RS, Wack RF, Shilo-Benjamini Y and Pypendop BH (2012) Determination of the minimum anesthetic concentration of sevoflurane in thick-billed parrots (*Rhynchopsitta pachyrhyncha*). *American Journal of Veterinary Research* **73(9)**, 1350–1355

[c] Barter LS, Hawkins MG, Brosnan RJ, Antognini JF and Pypendop BH (2006) Median effective dose of isoflurane, sevoflurane, and desflurane in green iguanas. *American Journal of Veterinary Research* **67(3)**, 392–397

[d] Bertelsen MF, Mosley C, Crawshaw GJ, Dyson D and Smith DA (2005) Inhalation anesthesia in Dumeril's monitor (*Varanus dumerili*) with isoflurane, sevoflurane, and nitrous oxide: effects of inspired gases on induction and recovery. *Journal of Zoo and Wildlife Medicine* **36(1)**, 62–69

[e] Zec S, Clark-Price SC, Coleman DA and Mitchell MA (2014) Loss and Return of Righting Reflex in American Green Tree Frogs (*Hyla cinerea*) after Topical Application of Compounded Sevoflurane or Isoflurane Jelly: A Pilot Study. *Journal of Herpetological Medicine and Surgery* **24(3)**, 72–76

[f] Morrison KE, Strahl-Heldreth D and Clark-Price SC (2016) Isoflurane, sevoflurane and desflurane use in cane toads (*Rhinella marina*). *Veterinary Record Open* **3(1)**, 185

Silver sulfadiazine
(Flamazine*) **POM**

Formulations: Topical: 1% cream (water-soluble).

Action: Slowly releases silver in concentrations that are toxic to bacteria and yeasts. The sulfadiazine component also has anti-infective qualities.

Use: Topical antibacterial and antifungal drug particularly active against Gram-negative organisms such as *Pseudomonas aeruginosa*. Used in the management of second- and third-degree burns, and flystrike. Up to 10% may be absorbed, depending on the size of area treated. Used for the postoperative treatment of skin wounds and localized external bacterial infections in fish.

Safety and handling: Use gloves.

Contraindications: Do not use in neonates or pregnant animals.

Adverse reactions: Patients hypersensitive to sulphonamides may react to silver sulfadiazine. It may accumulate in patients with impaired hepatic or renal function.

Drug interactions: No information available.

DOSES
See Appendix for guidelines on responsible antibacterial use.
Mammals: Apply sparingly to wounds q12–24h. Otitis (resistant *Pseudomonas*/refractory *Malassezia*): Dilute 1:1 with sterile water and apply topically.
Birds:
- Burns/skin infection: Apply antiseptically to the affected area to a thickness of approximately 1.5 mm. Initially, apply as often as necessary to keep wound covered, then reduce as healing occurs to once a day applications. Dressings may be applied if necessary. Keep the affected area clean.

- Otitis (resistant *Pseudomonas*/refractory *Malassezia*): Dilute 1:1 with sterile water and apply topically.

Reptiles, Amphibians: Apply topically to wounds q24–72h.

Fish: Apply topically to wounds keeping site out of water for 30–60 seconds.

Silybin (Milk thistle, Silibinin, Silymarin)
(Denamarin, Doxion, Hepatosyl Plus, Marin, Samylin, Zentonil Advanced) **AVM-GSL**

Formulations: Oral: 9 mg, 24 mg, 25 mg, 35 mg, 40 mg, 50 mg, 70 mg, 100 mg tablets; 10 mg, 40 mg, 53 mg powder.

Action: Silybin is the active component of milk thistle or silymarin. It acts as an antioxidant and free radical scavenger, promotes hepatocyte protein synthesis, increases the level of glutathione, and stimulates biliary flow and the production of hepatoprotective bile acids. It also inhibits leucotriene production so reducing the inflammatory response.

Use: Adjunctive treatment for liver disease, especially for acute hepatotoxin-induced liver disease. Silybin has been shown to increase hepatic glutathione levels; a potent antioxidant which protects hepatocytes from toxic damage. Can also be used in patients on long-term therapy with potentially hepatotoxic drugs.

Safety and handling: Normal precautions should be observed.

Contraindications: No information available.

Adverse reactions: GI signs, pruritus and headaches have been recognized in primates.

Drug interactions: Silybin may inhibit microsomal cytochrome P450 isoenzyme 2C9 (CYP2C9). May increase plasma levels of beta-blockers (e.g. propranolol), calcium-channel blockers (e.g. verapamil), diazepam, lidocaine, metronidazole, pethidine and theophylline. Silymarin may increase the clearance of drugs that undergo hepatic glucuronidation, including paracetamol, diazepam and morphine. Clinical significance has not been determined for this interaction and the usefulness of silymarin for treating paracetamol toxicity has not been determined.

DOSES
Mammals: Ferrets: 50–250 mg/kg p.o. q24h. (Note: rabbits and herbivorous rodents may denature active principles in the stomach.)
Birds: 50–75 mg/kg p.o. q12h.
Reptiles, Amphibians, Fish: No information available.

Sodium bicarbonate
(Sodium bicarbonate*) **POM**

Formulations: Injectable: 1.26%, 4.2%, 8.4% solutions for i.v. infusion (8.4% solution = 1 mmol/ml). **Oral:** 300 mg, 500 mg, 600 mg tablets; 100% BP powder.

Action: Provision of bicarbonate ions.

Use: Management of severe metabolic acidosis, to alkalinize urine, and as an adjunctive therapy in the treatment of hypercalcaemic or hyperkalaemic crisis. Active correction of acid–base imbalance requires blood gas analysis. Do not attempt specific therapy unless this facility is immediately available. 1 g of sodium bicarbonate provides 11.9 mEq of Na^+ and 11.9 mEq of bicarbonate. In hypocalcaemic patients use sodium bicarbonate cautiously and administer slowly. As oral sodium bicarbonate (especially at higher doses) may contribute significant amounts of sodium, use with caution in patients on salt-restricted intakes, e.g. those with congestive heart failure. Used for buffering water in fish tanks (i.e. increasing alkalinity) and for raising pH during the use of some acidic anaesthetic agents by immersion (e.g. tricaine).

Safety and handling: Normal precautions should be observed.

Contraindications: Should not be used in animals that are unable to effectively expel carbon dioxide (e.g. hypoventilating, hypercapnoeic patients).

Adverse reactions: Excessive use of sodium bicarbonate i.v. can lead to metabolic alkalosis, hypernatraemia, congestive heart failure, a shift in the oxygen dissociation curve causing decreased tissue oxygenation, and paradoxical CNS acidosis leading to respiratory arrest.

Drug interactions: Sodium bicarbonate is incompatible with many drugs and calcium salts: do not mix unless checked beforehand. Alkalinization of the urine by sodium bicarbonate decreases the excretion of quinidine and sympathomimetic drugs, and increases the excretion of aspirin, phenobarbital and tetracyclines (especially doxycycline).

DOSES
Mammals:
- Severe metabolic acidosis: mmol $NaHCO_3$ required = base deficit $\times$ 0.5 $\times$ body weight (kg) (0.3 is recommended instead of 0.5 in some references). Give half the dose slowly i.v. over 3–4 hours, recheck blood gases and clinically re-evaluate the patient. Avoid over-alkalinization.
- Acutely critical situations (e.g. cardiac arrest): 1 mmol/kg i.v. over 1–2 min followed by 0.5 mmol/kg at intervals of 10 min during the arrest.
- Adjunctive therapy of hypercalcaemia: 0.5–1 mmol/kg i.v. over 30 min.

- Adjunctive therapy of hyperkalaemia: 2–3 mmol/kg i.v. over 30 min.
- Metabolic acidosis secondary to renal failure or to alkalinize the urine: Initial dose 8–12 mg/kg p.o q8h and then adjust dose to maintain total CO_2 concentrations at 18–24 mEq/l. The dose may be increased to 50 mg/kg to adjust urine pH in patients with normal renal, hepatic and cardiac function.

Fish: Add powder as required to the aquarium water and monitor pH using a digital pH meter [1].

Birds, Reptiles, Amphibians: No information available.

References
[1] Noga EJ (2010) *Fish Disease – Diagnosis and Treatment, 2nd edn.* Wiley-Blackwell, Oxford

Sodium chloride
(Aqupharm, Hypertonic saline, Sodium chloride, Vetivex) **POM-V**

Formulations: Injectable: 0.45% to 7% NaCl solutions; 0.18% NaCl with 4% glucose and 0.9% NaCl with 5% glucose solutions. **Oral:** 300 mg, 600 mg tablets. **Ophthalmic:** 5% ointment (compounded by an ocular pharmacy). **Immersion:** crystals for dissolution in water.

Action: Expands plasma volume and replaces lost extracellular fluid. In freshwater aquaria and ponds, nitrite toxicity resulting from poor water quality causes oxidation of haemoglobin to methaemoglobin. Chloride ions inhibit nitrite absorption through the gill epithelium and reduce the toxic effect in fish. It also reduces the osmotic pressure between the freshwater environment and the fish tissues.

Use: When used for fluid replacement NaCl (0.45% and 0.9%) will expand the plasma volume compartment. Compared with colloids, 2.5 to 3.0 times as much fluid must be given because the crystalloid is distributed to other sites. Normal saline is also the treatment of choice for patients with hypercalcaemia or hyperchloraemic alkalosis. Sodium chloride solutions are often used as a drug diluent. Hypertonic saline is used to expand the circulating blood volume rapidly in animals with shock, particularly during the preoperative period. The hypertonic ophthalmic ointment is used in the management of corneal oedema. Hypertonic saline solutions have very high sodium concentrations and it is important to monitor serum sodium concentrations before and after their administration; maintenance with an isotonic crystalloid is usually required after administration to correct electrolyte and fluid disturbances created by the administration of the hypertonic solution. Oral sodium supplementation is recommended by some authors in the long-term management of hypoadrenocorticism. Used for the treatment of external protozoans in amphibians and fish. Used as a short-term bath to control external bacterial and parasitic infections and help remove excess mucus from gills. Reduces stress associated with transportation in fish. Used for the reduction of toxicity due to poor water quality and to aid the healing of wounds in freshwater fish. Inadequate biological filtration or water changes results in increased nitrite levels in the environment, which adversely affects fish health and causes methaemoglobinaemia. Although salt will reduce the toxic effects of poor water quality, it is essential that the underlying causes are addressed. Do not use salt with yellow prussate of soda (YPS, sodium ferrocyanide) added as an anti-caking agent or iodized salt. Use lower dose rates initially for prolonged immersion, since small fish and some species (e.g. catfish) are sensitive to salt. Fish must be observed during high salt concentration baths and should be removed if exhibiting signs of distress (i.e. loss of activity and balance). Remove plants that may not tolerate salt before prolonged immersion treatments.

Safety and handling: Hypertonic saline solutions should be regarded as drugs and not as intravenous fluids and should be stored separately to prevent confusion.

Contraindications: Do not use if zeolite is used in the filtration system as this will cause the release of absorbed ammonia into the environment.

Adverse reactions: Peripheral oedema is more likely to occur after crystalloids because muscle and subcutaneous capillaries are less permeable to protein. Normal saline contains higher amounts of chloride than plasma, which will increase the risk of acidosis. The degree of acidosis is not likely to be a problem in a healthy patient but acidosis may be exacerbated in a compromised patient. Hypertonic saline administered at fluid rates >1 ml/kg/min can cause a vagally mediated bradycardia, therefore the rate of fluid administration must be carefully controlled. The ophthalmic ointment may cause a stinging sensation.

Drug interactions: No information available.

DOSES
Fluid therapy: fluid requirements depend on the degree of dehydration and ongoing losses.
Mammals:
- Corneal oedema: apply a small amount of ointment q4–24h.
- Hypotension/shock: 5 ml/kg of 7.5% solution over 5–10 minutes. Solutions of this concentration are hypertonic, therefore they should be used with caution and with other appropriate fluid replacement strategies. Hypertonic NaCl may be combined with colloid solutions to stabilize the increase in vascular volume provided by the hypertonic solution.

Amphibians: External protozoans: 6 g/l as a 24 h bath for 3–5 days.
Fish:
- External protozoans: 6 g/l as a 24 h bath for 3–5 days.
- Ectoparasite control: 30 g/l as a bath for 5–10 min weekly or as needed.
- Osmoregulation: 1–5 g/l by prolonged immersion.

Birds, Reptiles: No information available.

Spiramycin see **Metronidazole**

Streptomycin
(Devomycin) **POM-V**

Formulations: Injectable: Streptomycin (250 mg/ml); Streptomycin (150 mg/ml) with dihydrostreptomycin (150 mg/ml) (Devomycin D).

Action: Inhibits bacterial protein synthesis, resulting in a bactericidal effect that is concentration-dependent.

Use: Active against a range of Gram-negative and some Gram-positive pathogens although resistance is quite widespread and it is less active than other aminoglycosides. It is specifically indicated in the treatment of infections caused by *Leptospira* and *Mycobacterium tuberculosis* (in combination with other drugs). Aminoglycosides require an oxygen-rich environment to be effective, thus they are ineffective in sites of low oxygen tension (abscesses, exudates) and all obligate anaerobes are resistant. Use of streptomycin is limited and if an aminoglycoside is indicated other members of the family are more commonly employed (e.g. gentamicin). There is a marked post-antibiotic effect, allowing the use of pulse-dosing regimens which may limit toxicity. Dosing 2–3 times a week is used to treat mycobacteriosis in humans.

Safety and handling: Normal precautions should be observed.

Contraindications: Do not use in guinea pigs, hamsters, gerbils, rats and mice. Do not use in raptors and use with caution in other bird breeds.

Adverse reactions: Streptomycin is one of the more ototoxic aminoglycosides, interfering with balance and hearing, which can be permanent. Nephrotoxicosis may be a problem but is less likely than with other aminoglycosides. Toxic to certain rodents and birds, especially raptors (neurotoxic). Fatal reaction to streptomycin and penicillin reported in parrots. Oral doses can cause fatal enterotoxaemia in rabbits and potentially other small herbivores.

Drug interactions: Increased risk of nephrotoxicity when used with cephalosporins (notably cefalotin) and cytotoxic drugs. Ototoxicity is increased with loop diuretics. The effects of neostigmine and pyridostigmine may be antagonized by aminoglycosides. The effect of non-depolarizing muscle relaxants (e.g. pancuronium) may be enhanced. Penicillin and streptomycin act synergistically. Aminoglycosides may be chemically inactivated by beta-lactam antibiotics (e.g. penicillins, cephalosporins) or heparin when mixed *in vitro*.

DOSES

See Appendix for guidelines on responsible antibacterial use.

Mammals: Rabbits: 50 mg/kg streptomycin in combination with 40 mg/kg penicillin s.c. q24h. Do not use in guinea pigs, hamsters, gerbils, rats and mice.

Birds: Not recommended[a].

Reptiles, Amphibians, Fish: No information available.

References
[a] Hauser H (1960) Fatal reaction to streptomycin and penicillin in parrots with pulmonary mycosis. *Monatshefte fur Veterinarmedizin* **15**, 632–634

Sucralfate
(Antepsin*, Antepsin suspension*, Carafate*) **POM**

Formulations: Oral: 1 g tablet; 0.2 g/ml suspension.

Action: In an acidic medium an aluminium ion detaches from the compound, leaving a very polar, relatively non-absorbable ion. This ion then binds to proteinaceous exudates in the upper GI tract, forming a chemical diffusion barrier over ulcer sites, preventing further erosion from acid, pepsin and bile salts. However, its major action appears to relate to stimulation of mucosal defences and repair mechanisms (stimulation of bicarbonate and PGE production and binding of epidermal growth factor). These effects are seen at neutral pH.

Use: Treatment of oesophageal, gastric and duodenal ulceration, used with an H2 receptor antagonist or proton pump inhibitor but given separately. The efficacy of sucralfate as a phosphate binder in renal failure is uncertain.

Safety and handling: Normal precautions should be observed.

Contraindications: Perforated ulcer.

Adverse reactions: Minimal; constipation is the main problem in humans. Bezoar formation and hypophosphataemia are also reported in humans.

Drug interactions: Sucralfate may decrease the bioavailability of H2 antagonists, phenytoin and tetracycline. Although there is little evidence to suggest that this is of clinical importance, it may be a wise precaution to administer sucralfate at least 2 hours before these drugs. Sucralfate interferes significantly with the absorption of fluoroquinolones and digoxin.

DOSES

Mammals: Ferrets: 25–125 mg/kg p.o. q6–12h; **Rabbits:** 25 mg/kg p.o. q8–12h; **Rodents:** 25–50 mg/kg p.o. q6–8h; **Primates:** 500 mg/animal p.o. q6–12h; **Hedgehogs:** 10 mg/kg p.o. q8–12h.

Birds: 25 mg/kg p.o. q8h.

Reptiles: 500–1000 mg/kg p.o. q6–8h.

Amphibians, Fish: No information available.

Sulfadimethoxine
(Coxi Plus, Coxidin) **POM-V**

Formulations: Oral: 1000 mg/4 g sachet.

Action: Competitively inhibits bacterial and protozoal synthesis of folic acid.

Use: Coccidiosis in ferrets, hedgehogs, primates, rabbits, birds and reptiles; atoxoplasmosis in passerine birds. Use with care in reptiles with reduced renal function, renal failure or dehydration.

Safety and handling: Normal precautions should be observed.

Contraindications: No information available.

Adverse reactions: No information available.

Drug interactions: No information available.

DOSES
Mammals: Ferrets: 50 mg/kg p.o. once, then 25 mg/kg p.o. q24h for 5–10 days; **Rabbits, Rodents:** 50 mg/kg p.o. once, then 25 mg/kg p.o. q24h for 10–20 days; **Primates:** 50 mg/kg p.o. once, then 25 mg/kg p.o. q24h; **Hedgehogs:** 2–20 mg/kg p.o. q24h for 2–5 days, repeat in 5 days or 10 mg/kg p.o. q24h for 5–7 days; **Other small mammals:** 10–15 mg/kg p.o. q12h.
Birds: 1 g/l of drinking water daily for 2 days, then 3 days off and 2 days on.
Reptiles: 90 mg/kg p.o. once, then 45 mg/kg p.o. q24h for 5–7 days.
Amphibians, Fish: No information available.

Sulfasalazine
(Salazopyrin*, Sulphasalazine*) **POM**

Formulations: Oral: 500 mg tablet; 250 mg/ml suspension.

Action: Sulfasalazine is a pro-drug: a diazo bond binding sulfapyridine to 5-ASA is cleaved by colonic bacteria to release free 5-ASA, which acts locally in high concentrations in the colon as an anti-inflammatory.

Use: Used in the management of colitis. There is a significant risk of keratoconjunctivitis sicca and periodic Schirmer tear tests should be performed.

Safety and handling: Normal precautions should be observed.

Contraindications: No information available.

Adverse reactions: Uncommon but include keratoconjunctivitis sicca (KCS), vomiting, allergic dermatitis and cholestatic jaundice. Owners should be made aware of the seriousness of KCS and what signs to monitor. The cause of the KCS is not clear. Historically sulfapyridine has been blamed. Olsalazine has been recommended as the incidence of KCS is less with its use, though not completely abolished. It is possible that 5-ASA may sometimes be responsible.

Drug interactions: The absorption of digoxin may be inhibited by sulfasalazine, and the measurement of serum folate concentration may be interfered with. Sulfasalazine may cause a reduction in serum thyroxine concentrations.

DOSES
Mammals: Ferrets: 62.5–125 mg/animal p.o. q8–24h.
Birds, Reptiles, Amphibians, Fish: No information available.

Sulphonamide see Trimethoprim/sulphonamide

T4 see **Levothyroxine**

Telmisartan
(Semintra) **POM-V**

Formulations: Oral: 4 mg/ml solution, 10 mg/ml solution.

Action: Angiotensin II receptor (type AT1) antagonist which acts to inhibit the effects of angiotensin (i.e. vasoconstriction; increased aldosterone synthesis; sodium and water retention; and renal, vascular and cardiac remodelling). In the kidney, angiotensin II may result in glomerular capillary hypertension and increased protein in the glomerular filtrate, which could trigger or potentiate interstitial fibrosis.

Use: Suggested for the reduction of proteinuria associated with chronic kidney disease in rats and rabbits. Telmisartan is authorized for use in cats, in which it has been shown to delay deterioration in proteinuria over 6 months in cats with chronic kidney disease (IRIS stages IIa to IV, urine specific gravity <1.035 and no co-morbidities). It is used, off licence, to treat protein-losing nephropathy in rats, and chronic kidney disease in rabbits. Monitoring of blood pressure is recommended in animals that develop clinical signs referable to hypotension or those undergoing general anaesthesia. There is some evidence of efficacy in reducing hypertension in rabbits [a,b]. Rats and rabbits have been shown to be the most sensitive species to telmisartan-related gastrointestinal damage, and so if any signs of GI disturbance are noted treatment should be discontinued [c].

Safety and handling: Normal precautions should be observed.

Contraindications: The safety of telmisartan has not been established in breeding, pregnant, lactating or skeletally immature animals.

Adverse reactions: Mild and transient GI signs (inappetance, diarrhoea, and regurgitation and vomiting in those species in which this is possible). Rats and rabbits are considered most sensitive to gastrointestinal inflammation and ulceration. Healthy cats administered 5 times the recommended dose for 6 months experienced decreases in blood pressure and RBC count and increases in blood urea nitrogen, this may be a consideration in other species.

Drug interactions: Avoid concurrent use of ACE inhibitors.

DOSES
Mammals: Rats, Rabbits: 1 mg/kg p.o. q24h.
Birds, Reptiles, Amphibians, Fish: No information available.

References
[a] Maeda S, Nishizaki M, Yamawake N et al. (2010) Effect of High-dose Telmisartan on the Prevention of Recurrent Atrial Fibrillation in Hypertensive Patients. *Journal of Atrial Fibrillation* **3(3)**, 289
[b] Hu ZP, Fang XL, Qian HY, Fang N, Wang BN and Wang Y (2014) Telmisartan prevents angiotensin II-induced endothelial dysfunction in rabbit aorta via activating HGF/Met system and PPARγ pathway. *Fundamental & Clinical Pharmacology* **28(5)**, 501–511
[c] European Medicines Agency (2005) Micardis: EPAR–Scientific Discussion. Available from: https://www.ema.europa.eu/en/medicines/human/EPAR/micardis

Terbinafine
(Lamisil*) POM

Formulations: Oral: 250 mg tablets. **Topical:** 1% cream.

Action: Inhibits ergosterol synthesis by inhibiting squalene epoxidase, an enzyme that is part of the fungal cell wall synthesis pathway.

Use: Management of dermatophytosis, subcutaneous and systemic fungal infections in mammals, and aspergillosis in birds. Optimal therapeutic regimes are still under investigation. Pre-treatment and monitoring CBC, renal and liver function tests are advised.

Safety and handling: Normal precautions should be observed.

Contraindications: No information available.

Adverse reactions: Vomiting, diarrhoea, increased liver enzymes and pruritus.

Drug interactions: No information available.

DOSES
Mammals: Rodents: 10–30 mg/kg p.o. q24h for 4–6 weeks; Hedgehogs: Doses of 100 mg/kg p.o. q12h are reported [a], although 20–30 mg/kg appears clinically effective in resolving dermatophytosis.
Birds: 10–15 mg/kg p.o. q12h or nebulization of 1 mg/ml for 20 min q8h [b,c,d].
Reptiles, Amphibians, Fish: No information available.

References
[a] Bexton S and Nelson H (2016) Comparsion of two systemic antifungal agents, itraconazole and terbinafine, for the treatment of dermatophytosis in Europaean hedgehogs (*Erinaceus europaeus*). *Veterinary Dermatology* **27**, 500–e133
[b] Bechert U, Christensen JM, Poppenga R, Fahmy SA and Redig P (2010) Pharmacokinetics of terbinafine after single oral dose administration in red-tailed hawks (*Buteo jamaicensis*). *Journal of Avian Medicine and Surgery* **24(2)**, 122–130
[c] Emery LC, Cox SK and Souza MJ (2012) Pharmacokinetics of nebulized terbinafine in Hispaniolan Amazon parrots (*Amazona ventralis*). *Journal of Avian Medicine and Surgery* **26(3)**, 161–166
[d] Evans EE, Emery LC, Cox SK and Souza MJ (2013) Pharmacokinetics of terbinafine after oral administration of a single dose to Hispaniolan Amazon parrots (*Amazona ventralis*). *American Journal of Veterinary Research* **74(6)**, 835–838

Terbutaline
(Bricanyl*, Monovent*) POM

Formulations: Injectable: 0.5 mg/ml solution. **Oral:** 5 mg tablets; 1.5 mg/5 ml syrup.

Action: Selective beta-2 adrenergic agonist that directly stimulates bronchodilation.

Use: Bronchodilation. Use with caution in patients with diabetes mellitus, hyperthyroidism, hypertension or seizure disorders.

Safety and handling: Normal precautions should be observed.

Contraindications: No information available.

Adverse reactions: Fine tremor, tachycardia, hypokalaemia, hypotension and hypersensitivity reactions. Administration i.m. may be painful.

Drug interactions: There is an increased risk of hypokalaemia if theophylline or high doses of corticosteroids are given with high doses of terbutaline. Use with digitalis glycosides or inhalational anaesthetics may increase the risk of cardiac arrhythmias. Beta-blockers may antagonize its effects. Other sympathomimetic amines may increase the risk of adverse cardiovascular effects.

DOSES
Mammals: Rabbits: 0.312–1.25 mg/animal p.o. q8h; **Rats:** 5 mg/kg p.o. q12h.
Birds: 0.1 mg/kg i.m. in an emergency.
Reptiles, Amphibians, Fish: No information available.

Tetracaine (Amethocaine)
(Amethocaine hydrochloride*) POM

Formulations: Ophthalmic: 0.5%, 1% solution (single-use vials).

Action: Local anaesthetic action is dependent on reversible blockade of the sodium channel, preventing propagation of an action potential along the nerve fibre. Sensory nerve fibres are blocked before motor nerve fibres, allowing a selective sensory blockade at low doses.

Use: Local anaesthesia of the ocular surface (cornea and conjunctival sac). Although effective, it is rarely used in veterinary practice. An alternative topical ophthalmic anaesthetic such as proxymetacaine is advised. Duration of action has not been reported in companion animal species. Topical anaesthetics block reflex tear production and should not be applied before a Schirmer tear test.

Safety and handling: Store in refrigerator.

Contraindications: Do not use for therapeutic purposes.

Adverse reactions: Tetracaine often causes marked conjunctival irritation, chemosis and pain on application. All topical anaesthetics are toxic to the corneal epithelium and delay healing of ulcers.

Drug interactions: No information available.

DOSES
Mammals, Birds: Ophthalmic: 1 drop per eye, single application.
Reptiles, Amphibians, Fish: No information available.

Tetracosactide (Tetracosactrin, ACTH) (Synacthen*) **POM**

Formulations: Injectable: 0.25 mg/ml solution for intravenous use. In the event of availability problems, an alternative lyophilized formulation (0.25 mg/ml) for intramuscular use may be imported on a named patient basis.

Action: ACTH analogue that binds to specific receptors on the cell membrane of adrenocortical cells and induces the production of steroids from cholesterol.

Use: To stimulate cortisol production in the diagnosis of hypo- (but not hyper-) adrenocorticism (Addison's disease) in ferrets. Availability problems at time of writing. It is recommended to use lower doses than previously published and reserve for diagnosis of hypoadrenocorticism.

Safety and handling: Normal precautions should be observed. Small aliquots of the intravenous and intramuscular preparations may be frozen and thawed once without undue loss of activity.

Contraindications: No information available.

Adverse reactions: None reported.

Drug interactions: None reported.
Mammals: Ferrets: 1 µg (micrograms)/kg i.m. for diagnosis of hypoadrenocorticism.
Birds, Reptiles, Amphibians, Fish: No information available.

Theophylline (Corvental-D) **POM-V**

Formulations: Oral: 100 mg, 200 mg, 500 mg sustained-release capsules.

Action: Causes inhibition of phosphodiesterase, alteration of intracellular calcium, release of catecholamine, and antagonism of adenosine and prostaglandin, leading to bronchodilation and other effects.

Use: Spasmolytic agent and has a mild diuretic action. It has been used in the treatment of small airway disease. Beneficial effects include bronchodilation, enhanced mucociliary clearance stimulation of the respiratory centre, increased sensitivity to $PaCO_2$, increased diaphragmatic contractility, stabilization of mast cells and a mild inotropic effect. Theophylline has a low therapeutic index and should be dosed on a lean body weight basis. Administer with caution in patients with severe cardiac disease, gastric ulcers, hyperthyroidism, renal or hepatic disease, severe hypoxia or severe hypertension. Therapeutic plasma theophylline values are 5–20 µg/ml.

Safety and handling: Normal precautions should be observed.

Contraindications: Patients with a known history of arrhythmias or seizures.

Adverse reactions: Vomiting, diarrhoea, polydipsia, polyuria, reduced appetite, tachycardia, arrhythmias, nausea, twitching, restlessness, agitation, excitement and convulsions. Most adverse effects are related to the serum level and may be symptomatic of toxic serum concentrations. The severity of these effects may be decreased by the use of modified-release preparations. They are more likely to be seen with more frequent administration.

Drug interactions: Agents that may increase the serum levels of theophylline include cimetidine, diltiazem, erythromycin, fluoroquinolones and allopurinol. Phenobarbital may decrease the serum concentration of theophylline. Theophylline may decrease the effects of pancuronium. Theophylline and beta-adrenergic blockers (e.g. propranolol) may antagonize each other's effects. Theophylline administration with halothane may cause an increased incidence of cardiac dysrhythmias and with ketamine an increased incidence of seizures.

DOSES
Mammals: Ferrets: 4.25–10 mg/kg p.o. q8–12h; **Guinea pigs, Rats:** 10–20 mg/kg p.o. q8–12h.
Birds: 10mg/kg p.o. q12h.
Reptiles, Amphibians, Fish: No information available.

Thiamazole see **Methimazole**
Thiamine see **Vitamin B1**
ʟ-Thyroxine see **Levothyroxine**

Ticarcillin
(Timentin*) **POM**

Formulations: Injectable: 3 g ticarcillin and 200 mg clavulanic acid powder for reconstitution.

Action: Beta-lactam antibiotics bind penicillin-binding proteins involved in cell wall synthesis, decreasing bacterial cell wall strength and rigidity, and affecting cell division, growth and septum formation. The effect is bactericidal and killing occurs in a time-dependent fashion. Clavulanic acid acts as a non-competitive 'suicide' inhibitor for beta-lactamase enzymes.

Use: A carboxypenicillin that, like piperacillin, is indicated for the treatment of serious (usually but not exclusively life-threatening) infections caused by *Pseudomonas aeruginosa*, although it also has activity against certain other Gram-negative bacilli including *Proteus* spp. and *Bacteroides fragilis*. For *Pseudomonas* septicaemias antipseudomonal penicillins are often given with an aminoglycoside (e.g. gentamicin) as there is a synergistic effect. As ticarcillin kills bacteria by a time-dependent mechanism, dosing regimens should be designed to maintain tissue concentration above the MIC throughout the interdosing interval. Pharmacokinetic information on the ticarcillin/clavulanic acid combination is limited in veterinary species. After reconstitution it is stable for 48–72 hours.

Safety and handling: Normal precautions should be observed.

Contraindications: Avoid use in animals with reported sensitivity to penicillins. Do not administer to rabbits, guinea pigs, chinchillas, hamsters, gerbils or degus.

Adverse reactions: Nausea, diarrhoea and skin rashes may be seen. Can cause fatal enterotoxaemia in small herbivores (e.g. rabbits), hamsters and gerbils.

Drug interactions: Do not mix with aminoglycosides in the same syringe because there is mutual inactivation. There is synergism *in vivo* between the beta-lactams and the aminoglycosides.

DOSES
See Appendix for guidelines on responsible antibacterial use.
Mammals: Rabbits, Guinea pigs, Chinchillas, Hamsters, Gerbils: Do not use.
Birds: 150–200 mg/kg i.v., i.m. q8–12h [a].
Reptiles: 50–100 mg/kg i.m. q24–48h [b].
Amphibians, Fish: No Information available.

References
[a] Schroeder EC, Frazier DL, Morris PJ et al. (1997) Pharmacokinetics of ticarcillin and amikacin in blue-fronted Amazon parrots (*Amazona aestiva aestiva*). *Journal of Avian Medicine and Surgery* **11(4)**, 260–267

[b] Manire CA, Hunter RP, Koch DE, Byrd L and Rhinehart HL (2005) Pharmacokinetics of ticarcillin in the Loggerhead sea turtle (*Caretta caretta*) after single intravenous and intramuscular injections. *Journal of Zoological Wildlife Medicine* **36(1)**, 44–53

Timolol maleate
(Azarga*, CoSopt*, Timolol*, Timoptol*) **POM**

Formulations: Ophthalmic: 0.25%, 0.5% solutions (5 ml bottle, single-use vials; 0.5% solution most commonly used); 1% brinzolamide with 0.5% timolol (Azarga); 2% dorzolamide with 0.5% timolol (CoSopt) (5 ml bottle, single-use vials).

Action: A topical non-selective beta-blocker that decreases aqueous humour production via beta-adrenoreceptor blockade in the ciliary body. **See also Dorzolamide.**

Use: Management of glaucoma. It can be used alone or in combination with other topical glaucoma drugs, such as a topical carbonic anhydrase inhibitor. Dorzolamide/timolol or brinzolamide/timolol may be more effective than either drug alone. The combination causes miosis and is therefore not the drug of choice in uveitis or anterior lens luxation. Although no specific guidelines are available, it may be appropriate to use 0.25% solution in smaller patients.

Safety and handling: Normal precautions should be observed.

Contraindications: Avoid in uncontrolled heart failure and asthma.

Adverse reactions: Ocular adverse effects include miosis, conjunctival hyperaemia and local irritation. Systemic absorption may occur following topical application causing bradycardia and reduced blood pressure.

Drug interactions: Additive adverse effects may develop if given concurrently with oral beta-blockers. Concomitant administration of timolol with verapamil may cause a bradycardia and asystole. Prolonged AV conduction times may result if used with calcium antagonists or digoxin.

DOSES
Mammals: Rabbits: 1 drop per eye q12h.
Birds, Reptiles, Amphibians, Fish: No information available.

TMS see **Tricaine mesilate**

Tobramycin
(Nebcin*, Tobramycin*) **POM**

Formulations: Injectable: 40 mg/ml solution.

Action: Aminoglycosides inhibit bacterial protein synthesis. They are bactericidal and their mechanism of killing is concentration-dependent, leading to a marked post-antibiotic effect, allowing pulse-dosing regimens which may limit toxicity.

Use: Treatment of Gram-negative infections. It is less active against most Gram-negative organisms than gentamicin, but appears to be more active against *Pseudomonas aeruginosa*. Aminoglycosides are ineffective at sites of low oxygen tension (e.g. abscesses) and all obligate anaerobic bacteria are resistant. The doses below are for general guidance only, and should be assessed according to the clinical response. Cellular casts found in the urine sediment are an early sign of nephrotoxicity. Monitor renal function during use. If giving i.v., administer slowly. Geriatric animals or those with decreased renal function should only be given this drug systemically when absolutely necessary and then q12h or less frequently.

Safety and handling: Normal precautions should be observed.

Contraindications: Do not use ophthalmic product where corneal ulceration is present. Aminoglycosides may be contraindicated in small herbivores.

Adverse reactions: Tobramycin is considered to be less nephrotoxic than gentamicin.

Drug interactions: Avoid concurrent use of other nephrotoxic, ototoxic or neurotoxic agents (e.g. amphotericin B, furosemide). Increase monitoring and adjust dosages when these drugs must be used together. Aminoglycosides may be chemically inactivated by beta-lactam antibiotics (e.g. penicillins, cephalosporins) or heparin when mixed *in vitro*. The effect of non-depolarizing muscle relaxants (e.g. pancuronium) may be enhanced by aminoglycosides. Synergism may occur when aminoglycosides are used with penicillins or cephalosporins.

DOSES
See Appendix for guidelines on responsible antibacterial use.
Birds: 2.5–5 mg/kg i.m. q8–12h.
Reptiles: 2.5 mg/kg i.m. q24–72h. Concurrent fluid therapy advised, especially if hydration status poor or uncertain.
Mammals, Amphibians, Fish: No Information available.

Tolfenamic acid
(Tolfedine) **POM-V**

Formulations: Injectable: 40 mg/ml solution. Oral: 6 mg, 20 mg, 60 mg tablets.

Action: Inhibition of cyclo-oxygenase but uncertain if preferentially inhibits COX-2 over COX-1. COX inhibition limits the production of prostaglandins involved in inflammation. Also reported to have a direct antagonistic action on prostaglandin receptors.

Use: Alleviation of acute and chronic inflammation and pain. Liver disease will prolong the metabolism of tolfenamic acid leading to the potential for drug accumulation and overdose with repeated dosing. Use with caution in renal diseases and in the perioperative period, as may adversely affect renal perfusion during periods of hypotension. There is emerging evidence, using *in vitro* models and dog tumour cell lines, that tolfenamic acid may have anticancer activity against some tumour types.

Safety and handling: Normal precautions should be observed.

Contraindications: Do not give to dehydrated, hypovolaemic or hypotensive patients or those with GI disease or blood clotting problems. Do not give to pregnant animals or animals <6 weeks old.

Adverse reactions: GI signs may occur in all animals after NSAID administration. Stop therapy if this persists beyond 1–2 days. Some animals develop signs with one NSAID drug and not another. A 1–2-week wash-out period should be allowed before starting another NSAID after cessation of therapy. Stop therapy immediately if GI bleeding is suspected. There is a small risk that NSAIDs may precipitate cardiac failure in humans and this risk in animals is unknown.

Drug interactions: Do not administer concurrently with, or within 24 hours of, other NSAIDs and glucocorticoids. Do not administer with other potentially nephrotoxic agents, e.g. aminoglycosides.

DOSES

Mammals: Guinea pigs: 2 mg/kg s.c. q24h.
Birds, Reptiles, Amphibians, Fish: No information available.

Toltrazuril (Triazinone)
(Baycox, Zorabel) POM-V

Formulations: Oral: 25 mg/ml, 50 mg/ml solution.

Action: Damages all intracellular development stages of *Eimeria* spp. Interferes with the division of the nucleus and with the activity of the mitochondria, which are responsible for the respiratory metabolism of coccidia. In the magrometes, toltrazuril damages the so-called wall-forming bodies. In all intracellular developmental stages, severe vacuolization occurs due to inflation of the endoplasmic reticulum.

Use: For the treatment of coccidiosis in rabbits and microsporidiosis (e.g. *Glugae*) in fish. The highly alkaline solution is unpalatable and irritant and should be diluted with at least an equal volume of water immediately prior to oral administration in rabbits. It has been used experimentally and effectively against a number of parasites in fish.

Safety and handling: Normal precautions should be observed.

Contraindications: No information available.

Adverse reactions: In rabbits, oral irritation when concentrated solutions are used; higher doses have resulted in transient inappetence.

Drug interactions: No information available.

DOSES

Mammals: Rabbits: 2.5–10 mg/kg p.o. q24h for 2–3 days, repeat in 7–14 days[a].
Birds: Raptors: Coccidiosis 10 mg/kg p.o. q24h for 2 doses; repeat weekly for 3 weeks; **Blue-crowned laughing thrush:** 10 mg/kg p.o. q24h for 2 doses; repeat weekly as needed[b].
Fish: 5–20 mg/l by immersion for 1–4 hours q48h, repeated 3 times.
Reptiles, Amphibians: No information available.

References

[a] Redrobe SP, Gakos G, Elliot SC, Saunders R, Martin S and Morgan ER (2010) Comparison of toltazuril and sulphadimethoxine in the treatment of intestinal coccidiosis in pet rabbits. *Veterinary Record* **167(8)**, 287–290

[b] Jamriška J, Lavilla LA, Thomasson A, Barbon AR, Lopéz JF and Modrý D (2013) Treatment of atoxoplasmosis in the blue-crowned laughing thrush (*Dryonastes courtoisi*). *Avian Pathology* **42(6)**, 569–571

Tramadol
(Tramadol ER*, Ultracet*, Ultram*, Zamadol*)
POM CD SCHEDULE 3

Formulations: Oral: 50 mg tablets; 100 mg, 200 mg, 300 mg extended release tablets; smaller tablet sizes (10 mg, 25 mg) are available from some veterinary wholesalers; 5 mg/ml, 100 mg/ml oral liquid. **Injectable:** 50 mg/ml solution (may be difficult to source in the UK).

Action: Some metabolites of tramadol are agonists at all opioid receptors, particularly mu receptors. The parent compound also inhibits the re-uptake of noradrenaline and 5-HT, and stimulates presynaptic 5-HT release, which provides an alternative pathway for analgesia involving the descending inhibitory pathways within the spinal cord. In humans, good and poor metabolizers of tramadol are described, with good metabolizers developing more opioid-like effects following drug administration and improved analgesia. Whether similar individual differences in metabolism of tramadol occur in other species is currently unknown.

Use: Management of mild to moderate acute pain and as an adjunctive analgesic in the management of chronic pain resulting from osteoarthritis or neoplasia. The recommended dose range is currently largely empirical due to a lack of combined PK/PD studies. Perioperatively, injectable tramadol is used instead of opioids to provide analgesia for acute pain, although the injectable preparation can be difficult to obtain in the UK. Tramadol has similar actions to morphine but causes less respiratory depression, sedation and GI side effects. It is attractive as an adjunct to manage chronic pain because it can be given orally; however, a larger body of evidence to support dose recommendations is needed. In rabbits 4.4 mg/kg i.v. had no clinically significant impact on the MAC of isoflurane. Oral tramadol at 11 mg/kg in rabbits did not reach a plasma concentration of tramadol or O-desmethyltramadol that would provide sufficient analgesia in humans for clinically acceptable periods.

Safety and handling: Normal precautions should be observed.

Contraindications: No information available.

Adverse reactions: Contraindicated in humans with epilepsy. Owners should be informed that there may be a slightly increased risk of seizures in treated animals. Sedation can occur in some animals and dosages should be adjusted for the individual.

Drug interactions: Tramadol can be given in combination with other classes of analgesic drugs such as NSAIDs, amantadine and gabapentin. It has the potential to interact with drugs that inhibit central 5-HT and noradrenaline re-uptake such as tricyclic antidepressants (e.g. amitriptyline), monoamine oxidase inhibitors (e.g. selegiline), selective serotonin re-uptake inhibitors and some opioids (e.g. fentanyl, pethidine and buprenorphine), causing serotonin syndrome that can result in seizures and death. Should signs of serotonin syndrome develop (manifest in mild form as hyperthermia, elevated blood pressure and CNS disturbances such as hypervigilance and excitation) these must be managed symptomatically and contributing drug treatments stopped.

DOSES

Mammals: Ferrets: 5 mg/kg p.o., s.c. q12–24h; **Rabbits:** 3–10 mg/kg p.o. q8–12h (note: analgesic dose not determined) [a,b]; **Rats:** 10–20 mg/kg p.o., s.c. q8–12h; **Mice:** 10–40 mg/kg s.c. q12h; **Primates:** 3 mg/kg p.o. or 1.5 mg/kg i.v. q24h [c]; **Hedgehogs:** 2–4 mg/kg p.o. q12h.

Birds: Bald eagles: 5 mg/kg p.o. q12h; **Hispaniolan Amazon parrots:** 30 mg/kg p.o. q6h to achieve human therapeutic levels [d,e]. Reduced thermal withdrawal response for 6 hours post-dosing; **Red-tailed hawks:** 15 mg/kg p.o. q12h to achieve human therapeutic levels.

Reptiles: Chelonians: 5–10 mg/kg i.m., p.o. q24–48h [f]; **Bearded dragons:** 11 mg/kg p.o.

Amphibians, Fish: No information available.

References

[a] Kelly KR, Pypendop BH, Christe KL (2015) Pharmacokinetics of tramadol following intravenous and oral administration in male rhesus macaques (*Macaca mulatta*). *Journal of Veterinary Pharmacology and Therapeutics* **38**, 375–382

[b] Egger CM, Souza MJ, Greenacre CB, Cox SK and Rohrbach BW (2009) Effect of intravenous administration of tramadol hydrochloride on the minimum alveolar concentration of isoflurane in rabbits. *American Journal of Veterinary Research* **70(8)**, 945–949

[c] Souza MJ, Greenacre CB and Cox SK (2008) Pharmacokinetics of orally administered tramadol in domestic rabbits (*Oryctolagus cuniculus*). *American Journal of Veterinary Research* **69(8)**, 979–982

[d] Geelen S, Guzman DSM, Souza MJ *et al.* (2013) Antinociceptive effects of tramadol hydrochloride after intravenous administration to Hispaniolan Amazon parrots (*Amazona ventralis*). *American Journal of Veterinary Research* **74(2)**, 201–206

[e] Souza MJ, Gerhardt L and Cox S (2013) Pharmacokinetics of repeated oral administration of tramadol hydrochloride in Hispaniolan Amazon parrots (*Amazona ventralis*). *Americal Journal of Veterinary Research* **74(7)**, 957–962

[f] Baker BB, Sladky KK and Johnson SM (2011) Evaluation of the analgesic effects of oral and subcutaneous tramadol administration in red-eared slider turtles. *Journal of the American Veterinary Medical Association* **238(2)**, 220–227

Travoprost

(Travatan*) **POM**

Formulations: Ophthalmic: 40 µg/ml (0.004%) solution in 2.5 ml bottle.

Action: Agonist for receptors specific for prostaglandin F. It reduces intraocular pressure by increasing uveoscleral outflow.

Use: Its main indication is in the management of primary glaucoma and it is useful in the emergency management of acute primary glaucoma (superseding mannitol and acetazolamide). Often used in conjunction with other topical antiglaucoma drugs such as carbonic anhydrase inhibitors. It may be useful in the management of lens subluxation despite being contraindicated in anterior lens luxation. Travoprost has comparable activity to latanoprost.

Safety and handling: Normal precautions should be observed.

Contraindications: Uveitis and anterior lens luxation.

Adverse reactions: Miosis, conjunctival hyperaemia and mild irritation may develop. Increased iridial pigmentation has been noted in humans.

Drug interactions: Do not use in conjunction with thiomersal-containing preparations.

DOSES
Mammals: Rabbits: 1 drop/eye q12h.
Birds, Reptiles, Amphibians, Fish: No information available.

Tretinoin see **Vitamin A**
Triazinone see **Toltrazuril**

Tricaine mesilate (Metacaine, TMS, Tricaine mesylate, Tricaine methane sulponate)
(Finquel, MS 222, Nytox, Tricaine, **Tricaine PHARMAQ**) **POM-VPS**

Formulations: Immersion: 100% powder for dissolution in water.

Action: Tricaine is highly lipid soluble and rapidly absorbed across the gills, resulting in anaesthesia by impeding peripheral nerve signal transmission to the CNS.

Use: For the sedation, immobilization, anaesthesia and euthanasia of fish. Ideally, the drug should be dissolved in water from the tank or pond of origin to minimize problems due to changes in water chemistry. The dry powder is very soluble in both fresh and marine water, and may be added directly or made into a stock solution (e.g. 100 mg/ml) for more accurate dosing. Before use, the pH of the anaesthetic solution should be buffered with sodium bicarbonate to the same pH of the water of origin. The anaesthetic solution should be used on the day of preparation and be well aerated during use. Food should be withheld for 12–24 h before anaesthesia to reduce the risk of regurgitation. The stage of anaesthesia reached is determined by the concentration used and the duration of exposure, since absorption continues throughout the period of immersion. Potency and toxicity increases with increasing temperature. Salinity and water hardness reduce toxicity and increase the dose required. Small fish are more sensitive to the drug than large fish. Different species vary in their response and may require different concentrations. It is recommended to use the lower dose rates to test the selected drug concentration and exposure time with a small group before medicating large numbers. Anaesthetized fish should be returned to clean water from their normal environment to allow recovery. For euthanasia, 5–10 times the normal anaesthetic dose should be used and the fish kept in the solution for at least 60 minutes after respiration ceases.

Safety and handling: The powder should be stored dry and stock solutions stored in sealed dark bottles.

Contraindications: Should not be used in the following tropical fish species: *Apistogramma* (*Mikrogeophagus*) *ramirezi*, *Balantiocheilos melanopterus*, *Etroplus suratensis*, *Melanotaenia maccullochi*, *Monodactylus argenteus*, *Phenacogrammus interruptus* and *Scatophagus argus*.

Adverse reactions: No information available.

Drug interactions: No information available.

DOSES
Fish: 50–250 mg/l by immersion for induction of anaesthesia; 25–100 mg/l by immersion for maintenance of anaesthesia[1].
Mammals, Birds, Reptiles, Amphibians: No information available.

References
[1] Sneddon LU (2012) Clinical anesthesia and analgesia in fish. *Journal of Exotic Pet Medicine* **21**, 32–43

Trilostane
(Vetoryl) **POM-V**

Formulations: Oral: 10 mg, 30 mg, 60 mg, 120 mg capsules.

Action: Blocks adrenal synthesis of glucocorticoids. Effects on mineralocortioids are relatively minor.

Use: Treatment of pituitary- and adrenal-dependent hyperadrenocorticism. It is not considered to be useful in treating ferrets with hyperadrenocorticism. Perform ACTH stimulation tests (start test 3–5h post-dosing) at 10 days, 4 weeks, 12 weeks and then every 3 months. The aim is for a post-ACTH cortisol of 40–120 nmol/l. In cases where clinical signs persist or polydipsia appears within the 24-hour period, ACTH stimulation tests performed later in the day and/or sequential cortisol determinations may be needed for dose adjustment (either mg/kg or frequency). Dosage adjustments may be necessary even after prolonged periods of stability.

Safety and handling: Normal precautions should be observed.

Contraindications: Do not use in patients with renal or hepatic insufficiency.

Adverse reactions: In humans, idiosyncratic reactions include diarrhoea, colic, muscle pain, nausea, hypersalivation and rare cases of skin changes (rash or pigmentation). Clinical hypoadrenocorticism can be seen. Adrenal necrosis has been reported. Adrenal hyperplasia has been noted with prolonged treatment but the effects of this are unknown. Prolonged adrenal suppression after drug withdrawal has been noted in some cases.

Drug interactions: Trilostane should not be administered concurrently with other drugs that suppress adrenal function (e.g. mitotane, itraconazole).

DOSES
Mammals: Rodents: 2–4 mg/kg p.o. q24h.
Birds, Reptiles, Amphibians, Fish: No information available.

Trimethoprim/Sulphonamide
(Potentiated sulphonamides)
(Co-Trimazine, Duphatrim, Metaxol, Norodine, **Sulfatrim**, Tribrissen, Trimacare, Trimediazine, Trimedoxine, Trinacol, Septrin*) **POM-V**

Formulations: Trimethoprim and sulphonamide are formulated in a ratio of 1:5.
- Injectable: trimethoprim 40 mg/ml and sulfadiazine 200 mg/ml (240 mg/ml total) suspension.
- Oral: 16 mg/ml trimethoprim and 80 mg/ml sulfamethoxazole (Sulfatrim), 200 mg sulfamethoxazole and 40 mg trimethoprim per 5 ml = 48 mg/ml suspension (Septrin paediatric suspension). Trimethoprim and sulfadiazine are also available in a variety of tablet sizes designated by the amount of trimethoprim (e.g. 20 mg, 80 mg).

Action: Trimethoprim and sulphonamides block sequential steps in the synthesis of tetrahydrofolate, a cofactor required for the synthesis of many molecules, including nucleic acids. Sulphonamides block the synthesis of dihydropteroic acid by competing with para-aminobenzoic acid, and trimethoprim inhibits the enzyme dihydrofolate reductase, preventing the reduction of dihydrofolic acid to tetrahydrofolic acid. This two-step mechanism ensures that bacterial resistance develops more slowly than to either agent alone. In addition, the effect of the combination tends to be bactericidal as against a bacteriostatic effect of either agent alone.

Use: Licensed in rabbits, pigeons and bearded dragons for treatment of coccidiosis. Many organisms are susceptible, including *Nocardia*, *Brucella*, Gram-negative bacilli, some Gram-positive organisms (*Streptococcus*), plus *Pneumocystis carinii* and *Toxoplasma gondii*. *Pseudomonas* and *Leptospira* are usually resistant. Trimethoprim/sulphonamide is useful in the management of urinary, respiratory tract and prostatic infections, but ineffective in the presence of necrotic tissue. Trimethoprim alone may be used for urinary, prostatic, systemic salmonellosis and respiratory tract infections. Fewer adverse effects are seen with trimethoprim alone. Trimethoprim is a weak base which becomes ion-trapped in fluids that are more acidic than plasma (e.g. prostatic fluid and milk). Monitor tear production particularly during long-term use and in animals susceptible to keratoconjunctivitis sicca. Ensure patients receiving sulphonamides are well hydrated and are not receiving urinary acidifying agents. Used for the treatment of bacterial infections and intestinal coccidiosis in fish and reptiles.

Safety and handling: Normal precautions should be observed.

Contraindications: Avoid use in animals with keratoconjunctivitis sicca (KCS) or previous history of adverse reaction to sulphonamides (e.g. KCS or polyarthritis). Beware use in reptiles where renal disease is suspected.

Adverse reactions: Acute hypersensitivity reactions are possible with sulphonamide products; they may manifest as a type III hypersensitivity reaction. Sulphonamides may reversibly suppress thyroid function. Dermatological reactions (e.g. toxic epidermal necrolysis) have been associated with the use of sulphonamides in some animals. Sulphonamide crystal formation can occur in the urinary tract, particularly in animals producing very concentrated acidic urine.

Drug interactions: Antacids may decrease the bioavailability of sulphonamides if administered concomitantly. Urinary acidifying agents will increase the tendency for sulphonamide crystals to form within the urinary tract. Concomitant use of drugs containing procaine may inhibit the action of sulphonamides since procaine is a precursor for para-amino benzoic acid. When using the Jaffe alkaline picrate reaction assay for creatinine determination, trimethoprim/sulphonamide may cause an overestimation of approximately 10%.

DOSES

See Appendix for guidelines on responsible antibacterial use.
Doses (mg) of total product (trimethoprim + sulphonamide).

Mammals: Ferrets: 15–30 mg/kg p.o., s.c. q12h; **Rabbits:** 30 mg/kg p.o., s.c. q24h; **Guinea pigs, Chinchillas, Hamsters:** 15–30 mg/kg p.o., i.m., s.c. q12–24h; **Rats, Mice, Gerbils:** 50–100 mg/kg p.o., s.c. q24h; **Primates:** 15 mg/kg p.o. q12h or 30 mg/kg s.c. q24h; **Prosimians:** 25 mg/kg p.o. q12h; **Marsupials:** 10–20 mg/kg p.o., i.m. q12–24h; **Sugar gliders:** 10–20 mg/kg p.o. q12–24h; **Hedgehogs:** 30 mg/kg p.o., s.c., i.m. q12h.

Birds: 8–30 mg/kg i.m. q12h or 20–100 mg/kg p.o. q12h; **Pigeons:** 475–970 mg/l drinking water.

Reptiles: 25 mg/kg p.o. q24h for 7 days for coccidiosis.

Amphibians: 3 mg/kg p.o., s.c. q24h.

Fish: 30 mg/kg i.m. q48h for 10 days or 30 mg/kg in feed q24h for 10 days.

Tropicamide

(Mydriacyl*, Tropicamide*) **POM**

Formulations: Ophthalmic: 0.5%, 1% solution, single-use vials, 5 ml bottle.

Action: Inhibits acetylcholine at the iris sphincter and ciliary body muscles, causing mydriasis (pupil dilation) and cycloplegia (paralysis of the ciliary muscle). Ineffective in birds and reptiles because of the complex arrangement of musculature in the iris and ciliary body.

Use: Synthetic, short-acting antimuscarinic used for mydriasis and cycloplegia. It is the mydriatic of choice for intraocular examination due to its rapid onset (20–30 min) and short duration of action (4–12 h). Tropicamide is more effective as a mydriatic than as a cycloplegic and is therefore less effective than atropine in relieving ciliary body muscle spasm associated with uveitis. Use with care in patients with lens luxation.

Safety and handling: Normal precautions should be observed.

Contraindications: Avoid in glaucoma.

Adverse reactions: No information available.

Drug interactions: No information available.

DOSES
Mammals: Rabbits, Chinchillas, Hamsters, Rats: 1 drop per eye, repeat after 20–30 min if necessary.
Birds, Reptiles: Ineffective because of the complex arrangement of musculature in the iris and ciliary body.
Amphibians, Fish: No information available.

Tylosin

(Bilosin, Pharmasin, Tylan, Tyluvet) **POM-V**

Formulations: Injectable: 200 mg/ml solutions (Bilosin, Tylan, Tyluvet). Oral: 100 g/bottle soluble powder (Tylan).

Action: A bacteriostatic macrolide antibiotic that binds to the 50S ribosomal subunit, suppressing bacterial protein synthesis.

Use: Tylosin has good activity against mycoplasmas and has the same antibacterial spectrum of activity as erythromycin but is generally less active against bacteria.

Safety and handling: Normal precautions should be observed.

Contraindications: Do not give other than via nebulization to rabbits, guinea pigs, chinchillas, hamsters or degus.

Adverse reactions: GI disturbances. The activity of tylosin is enhanced in an alkaline pH. Tylosin can cause pain at the site of injection.

Drug interactions: Not well documented in small animals. It does not appear to inhibit the same hepatic enzymes as erythromycin.

DOSES
See Appendix for guidelines on responsible antibacterial use.

Mammals: Ferrets, Rats, Mice: 10 mg/kg p.o., i.m., s.c. q12h; Not recommended for rabbits, guinea pigs, chinchillas, hamsters or degus other than by nebulization, as for birds.

Birds: 20–40 mg/kg i.m. q8–12h (not chickens) or by nebulization of 100 mg diluted in 5 ml DMSO and 10 ml saline; **Pigeons:** 50 mg/kg p.o. q24h, 25 mg/kg i.m. q6–8h or 800 mg/l drinking water; **Passerines:** 1 g/l drinking water for 7–10 days.

Reptiles: 5 mg/kg i.m. q24h every 10–60 days.

Amphibians, Fish: No information available.

Ursodeoxycholic acid (UDCA)
(Destolit*, Ursodeoxycholic acid*, Ursofalk*,
Ursogal*) **POM**

Formulations: Oral: 150 mg, 300 mg, 500 mg tablets;
250 mg capsule; 50 mg/ml suspension.

Action: A relatively hydrophilic bile acid with cytoprotective effects
in the biliary system. It inhibits ileal absorption of hydrophobic bile
acids, thereby reducing their concentration in the body pool;
hydrophobic bile acids are toxic to hepatobiliary cell membranes
and may potentiate cholestasis. It also has an immunomodulatory
effect, and may modify apoptosis of hepatocytes.

Use: An adjunctive therapy for patients with liver disease,
particularly where cholestasis is present. Anecdotal use only in
ferrets.

Safety and handling: Normal precautions should be observed.

Contraindications: No information available.

Adverse reactions: Vomiting is a rare effect. Serious
hepatotoxicity has been recognized in rabbits and non-human
primates. Some human patients have an inability to sulphate
lithocholic acid (a naturally occurring metabolite of UDCA), which is
a known hepatotoxin; the veterinary significance of this is unclear.

Drug interactions: Aluminium-containing antacids may bind to
UDCA, thereby reducing its efficacy.

DOSES
Mammals: Ferrets: 10–15 mg/kg p.o. q12–24h.
Birds, Reptiles, Amphibians, Fish: No information available.

Vecuronium
(Norcuron*) **POM**

Formulations: Injectable: 10 mg powder for reconstitution.

Action: Inhibits the actions of acetylcholine at the neuromuscular junction by binding competitively to the alpha subunit of the nicotinic acetylcholine receptor on the post-junctional membrane.

Use: Used topically as a mydriatic in birds; ensure solution does not contain surface-penetrating agent. Provision of neuromuscular blockade during anaesthesia. This may be to improve surgical access through muscle relaxation, to facilitate positive pressure ventilation or for intraocular surgery. Intermediate dose-dependent duration of action of approximately 20 min. Has no cardiovascular effects and does not cause histamine release. Monitoring (using a nerve stimulator) and reversal of the neuromuscular blockade are recommended to ensure complete recovery before the end of anaesthesia. Hypothermia, acidosis and hypokalaemia will prolong the duration of neuromuscular blockade. In healthy animals repeated doses are relatively non-cumulative and it can be given by infusion i.v. to maintain neuromuscular blockade. It is metabolized by the liver; therefore in animals with liver dysfunction atracurium is advised rather than vecuronium.

Safety and handling: Unstable in solution and so is presented as a freeze-dried powder. The prepared solution can be diluted further if required.

Contraindications: Do not administer systemically unless the animal is adequately anaesthetized and facilities to provide positive pressure ventilation are available.

Adverse reactions: No information available.

Drug interactions: Neuromuscular blockade is more prolonged when vecuronium is given in combination with volatile anaesthetics, aminoglycosides, clindamycin and lincomycin.

DOSES
Birds: 1 drop of 0.8 mg/ml solution in 0.9% saline applied topically to eye; repeat after 2 minutes [a,b].
Mammals, Reptiles, Amphibians, Fish: No information available.

References
[a] Hendrix DV and Sims MH (2004) Electroretinography in the Hispaniolan Amazon parrot (*Amazona ventralis*). *Journal of Avian Medicine and Surgery* **18(2)**, 89–94
[b] Ramer JC, Paul-Murphy J, Brunson D and Murphy CJ (1996) Effects of mydriatic agents in cockatoos, African gray parrots and Blue-fronted Amazon parrots. *Journal of the American Veterinary Medical Association* **208(2)**, 227–230

Verapamil

(Cordilox*, Securon*, Verapamil*) **POM**

Formulations: Injectable: 2.5 mg/ml solution. **Oral:** 40 mg, 80 mg, 120 mg, 160 mg tablets.

Action: Inhibits inward movement of calcium ions through slow (L-type) calcium channels in myocardial cells, cardiac condution tissue and vascular smooth muscle. Verapamil causes a reduction in myocardial contractility (negative inotrope), depressed electrical activity (slows AV conduction) and vasodilation (cardiac vessels and peripheral arteries and arterioles).

Use: In rabbits may be used perioperatively to minimize formation of surgical adhesions. Patients with severe hepatic disease may have a reduced ability to metabolize the drug; reduce the dose by 70%.

Safety and handling: Normal precautions should be observed.

Contraindications: Do not use in patients with 2nd or 3rd degree AV block, hypotension, sick sinus syndrome, left ventricular dysfunction or heart failure.

Adverse reactions: Can cause hypotension, bradycardia, dizziness, precipitation or exacerbation of congestive heart failure, nausea, constipation and fatigue in humans. The likelihood of adverse reactions is decreased by dilution and slow administration of the product where given i.v.

Drug interactions: Do not use concurrently with beta-blockers. Both drugs have a negative inotropic and chronotropic effect and the combined effect can be profound. Co-administration with sodium channel blockers may also lead to cardiovascular depression and hypotension. Verapamil activity may be adversely affected by vitamin D or calcium salts. Cimetidine may increase the effects of verapamil. Verapamil may increase the blood levels of digoxin, digitoxin or theophylline, leading to potentially toxic effects from these drugs. Calcium-channel blockers may increase intracellular vincristine. The neuromuscular blocking effects of non-depolarizing muscle relaxants may be enhanced by verapamil.

DOSES

Mammals: Rabbits: 0.2 mg/kg very slow i.v., s.c., p.o. after surgery and repeated q8h for 9 doses or 2.5–25 µg (micrograms)/kg/h i.p., s.c.; rapid i.v. administration can cause cardiac failure and sudden death, and s.c. or p.o. routes are advised instead; Hamsters: 0.25–0.5 mg/kg s.c. q12h.

Birds, Reptiles, Amphibians, Fish: No information available.

Vincristine
(Oncovin*, Vincristine*) **POM**

Formulations: Injectable: 1 mg, 2 mg, 5 mg vials.

Action: Interferes with microtubule assembly, causing metaphase arrest and ultimately resulting in cell death.

Use: With other neoplastic agents in the treatment of ferret neoplastic diseases, particularly lymphoma. Has been used to treat lymphoma in a green iguana. Use with caution in patients with hepatic disease, leucopenia, infection, or pre-existing neuromuscular disease. Solution is locally irritant and must be administered i.v. through a carefully pre-placed catheter.

Safety and handling: Cytotoxic drug; see specialist texts for further advice on chemotherapeutic agents. Store under refrigeration.

Contraindications: No information available.

Adverse reactions: Include peripheral neuropathy, ileus, GI tract toxicity/constipation and severe local irritation if administered perivascularly. Potentially myelosuppressive.

Drug interactions: Concurrent administration of vincristine with drugs that inhibit cytochromes of the CYP3A family may result in decreased metabolism of vincristine and increased toxicity. If vincristine is used in combination with crisantaspase it should be given 12–24 hours before the enzyme. Administration of crisantaspase with or before vincristine may reduce clearance of vincristine and increase toxicity.

DOSES
See Appendix for chemotherapy protocols in ferrets

Mammals: Ferrets: 0.12–0.2 mg/kg i.v. as part of chemotherapy protocol for lymphoma[1].

Birds: 0.1 mg/kg i.v. q7–14d[2].

Reptiles: 0.008 mg/kg i.v. as part of chemotherapy protocol for lymphoma (one case report in the green iguana)[3].

Amphibians, Fish: No information available.

References
[1] Antinoff N and Hahn K (2004) Ferret oncology. *Veterinary Clinics of North America: Exotic Animal Practice* **7**, 579–626

[2] Rivera S, McClearen JR and Reavill DR (2009) Treatment of nonepitheliotropic cutaneous B-cell lymphoma in an umbrella cockatoo (*Cacatua alba*). *Journal of Avian Medicine and Surgery* **23(4)**, 294–303

[3] Folland DW, Johnston MS, Thamm DH and Reavill D (2011) Diagnosis and management of lymphoma in a green iguana (*Iguana iguana*). *Journal of the American Veterinary Medical Association* **239(7)**, 985–991

Virkon S
(Virkon S aquatic tablets*)

Formulations: Marketed as a water sanitizer and comprises a mixture of oxyzones, fruit acid salts and potassium monopersulphonate. **Immersion:** 5 g tablet for dissolution in water.

Action: No information available.

Use: For the reduction of viruses, bacteria and some parasites in koi carp ponds. This is a modified version of Virkon S with the amount of detergent reduced since this is toxic to aquatic animals, and the fragrance removed. Do not add directly to the pond: the tablets must be dissolved in water before adding slowly to the pond at the point where the water enters from the filtration system, to aid dispersal. An initial dose of 8 mg/l is recommended. If further weekly dosing at 2 mg/l is required, then 10% of the pond water should be changed prior to dosing. The product is deactivated by UV light. Repeated dosing can result in a build-up of the surfactant, resulting in some foaming, which can be reduced by partial water changes.

Safety and handling: Normal precautions should be observed.

Contraindications: No information available.

Adverse reactions: No information available.

Drug interactions: No information available.

DOSES
Fish: 2–8 mg/l by prolonged immersion initially, then 2 mg/l weekly as required.
Mammals, Birds, Reptiles, Amphibians: No information available.

Vitamin A (Retinol, Isotretinoin, Tretinoin)
(Retin-A*, Roaccutane*) POM

Formulations: Injectable: Vitamin A (retinol) 50,000 IU/ml (only available on special order from France and the USA at time of writing). Oral: 10 mg, 20 mg isotretinoin capsules (Roaccutane). Topical: 0.025% tretinoin cream; 0.01% tretinoin gel (Retin-A).

Action: Nutritional fat-soluble hormone that regulates gene expression. Tretinoin (all-trans retinoic acid) is the acid form of vitamin A and isotretinoin (13-cis retinoic acid) is an isomer of tretinoin.

Use: Treatment of hypovitaminosis A. Also used in conjunction with other appropriate therapies for sebaceous adenitis in rabbits. Animals receiving oral dosing should be monitored for vitamin A toxicity. Avoid concurrent use of oral and topical preparations because of toxicity. Avoid using formulations of vitamins A, D3 and E that are authorized for farm animals as they are too concentrated for small animal use.

Safety and handling: Vitamin A is teratogenic; gloves should be worn when applying topical preparations. Avoid contact with eyes, mouth or mucous membranes. Minimize exposure of the drug to sunlight.

Contraindications: Do not use in pregnant animals.

Adverse reactions: Many adverse effects are reported in humans following the use of oral isotretinoin, predominantly involving the skin, haematological parameters, hepatotoxicity, nervous system and bone changes. Depression, anorexia and skin sloughing are reported in reptiles following overdose. Teratogenic if administered in the first trimester or at high doses. Redness and skin pigmentation may be seen after several days. It changes the lipid content of tears, which can result in keratoconjunctivitis sicca (KCS). It may also cause hyperlipidaemia and can be hepatotoxic at high doses. Prolonged use of vitamin A can promote loss of calcium from bone and lead to hypercalcaemia. Do not use topical preparations simultaneously with other topical drugs.

Drug interactions: Numerous, depending on preparation and route given. Consult specialist tests before using with another drug. Oral vitamin A may alter ciclosporin levels, which should therefore be monitored closely.

DOSES
Mammals: Rabbits: 500–1000 IU/kg i.m. once; **Guinea pigs, Sugar gliders:** 50–500 IU/kg i.m. or 10 mg beta carotene/kg food; **Hamsters:** 50–500 IU/kg i.m. or 2 µg (micrograms) vitamin A palmitate/g food; **Hedgehogs:** 400 IU/kg p.o., i.m. q24–48h; only give parenterally for up to 2 doses, thereafter orally.
Birds: 1000–20,000 IU/animal i.m. once or p.o. q12h.
Reptiles: 1000–2000 IU/kg p.o. q7–14d.
Amphibians: 1000 IU/kg p.o. daily for 14 days, then q7d.
Fish: No information available.

Vitamin B complex
(Anivit 4BC, Duphafral Extravite, Dupharal, Multivitamin injection, Vitamin B tablets)
POM-VPS, general sale

Formulations: Various preparations containing varying quantities of vitamins are available, authorized for farm animals only. Most are for parenteral use and all those are POM-VPS.

Action: Cofactors for enzymes of intermediary metabolism and biosynthesis.

Use: Multiple deficiencies of B vitamins may occur in patients with renal or hepatic disease or significant anorexia. Dosages and routes vary with individual products. Check manufacturer's recommendations prior to use. Most products are intended for large animal use and some may contain vitamin C and other vitamins or minerals.

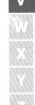

Safety and handling: All B vitamins are photosensitive and must be protected from light. Multidose vials require aseptic technique for repeated use.

Contraindications: No information available.

Adverse reactions: Anaphylaxis may be seen when used i.v. and products should be given slowly and/or diluted with i.v. fluids. Use of large animal products which also contain fat-soluble vitamins (A, D, E, K) may lead to toxicity.

Drug interactions: None reported.

DOSES
Mammals: **Rabbits:** 0.02–0.4 ml/animal s.c., i.m. q24h or as required; **Rodents:** 0.02–0.2 ml/kg s.c., i.m. q24h or as required; **Marsupials:** 0.01–0.02 ml/kg i.m. q24h or as required; **Sugar gliders:** 0.01–0.2 ml/kg s.c, i.m.; **Hedgehogs:** 1 ml/kg s.c., i.m. q24h or as required.

Birds: 1–3 mg/kg i.m. once. Should aim to achieve 10–30 mg/kg thiamine. Care must be taken not to exceed 3 mg/kg pyridoxine HCl (vitamin B6) as toxicity (acute death in 24–48 hours) recorded in raptors and pigeons [a].

Reptiles, Amphibians, Fish: No information available.

References
[a] Sarmour J (2013) Acute toxicity after administration of high doses of vitamin B6 (pyridoxine) in falcons. *Proceedings of the 1st International Conference on Avian, Herpetological and Exotic Mammal Medicine*, Weisbaden, Germany

Vitamin B1 (Thiamine)
(Vitamin B1) POM-V, general sale

Formulations: Injectable: 100 mg/ml solution (authorized for veterinary use, though only in farm animals). **Oral:** various.

Action: Cofactor for enzymes in carbohydrate metabolism, it forms a compound with ATP to form thiamine diphosphate/thiamine pyrophosphate employed in carbohydrate metabolism. It does not affect blood glucose.

Use: Thiamine supplementation is required in deficient animals. Although uncommon this may occur in animals fed raw fish diets (containing thiaminase) or uncooked soy products. Thiamine may be beneficial in alleviating signs of lead poisoning and ethylene glycol intoxication. It is used in birds, reptiles and amphibians for the treatment of cerebral cortical necrosis.

Safety and handling: Protect from air and light; multidose vials require aseptic technique for repeated use.

Contraindications: Do not use in pregnant animals unless absolutely necessary.

Adverse reactions: Anaphylaxis can be seen with i.v. use; dilute with fluids and/or give slowly if using i.v. Adverse effects in pregnant animals are documented.

Drug interactions: There are no specific clinical interactions reported, although thiamine may enhance the activity of neuromuscular blocking agents.

DOSES
Mammals: Ferrets, Rabbits: 1–2 mg/kg s.c., i.m. q12–24h for several days until signs resolve.
Birds: 10–30 mg/kg i.m. q24h [a].
Reptiles: Thiamine deficiency: 25–35 mg/kg p.o., i.m., s.c. q24h.
Amphibians: Thiamine deficiency: 25 mg/kg of feed fish.
Fish: No information available.

References
[a] Carnarius M, Hafez HM, Henning A, Henning HJ and Lierz M (2008) Clinical signs and diagnosis of thiamine deficiency in juvenile goshawks (*Accipiter gentilis*). *Veterinary Record* **163(7)**, 215–17

Vitamin B12 (Cyanocobalamin, Hydroxocobalamin)
(Anivit B12 250 and 1000, Neo-Cytamen (hydroxocobalamin) Vitbee 250 and 1000)
POM-VPS
Formulations: Injectable: 0.25 mg/ml, 1 mg/ml solutions.

Action: Essential cofactor for enzymes involved in DNA and RNA synthesis and in carbohydrate metabolism.

Use: Cyanocobalamin is used to treat vitamin B12 deficiency. Such a deficiency may develop in patients with significant disease of the distal ileum, small intestinal bacterial overgrowth and exocrine pancreatic insufficiency. In humans, hydroxocobalamin has almost completely replaced cyanocobalamin in the treatment of vitamin B12 deficiency.

Safety and handling: Must be protected from light.

Contraindications: Do not give i.v.

Adverse reactions: Hypersensitivity to the phenol preservative in the injectable solutions can occur; patients should be monitored after injections for rash, fever and urticaria.

Drug interactions: None reported.

DOSES
Mammals: Rabbits: 20–50 µg (micrograms)/kg monthly to continue as long as deficiency is present.
Birds: 0.25–5 mg/kg i.m. q7d.
Reptiles: 0.05 mg/kg i.m., s.c.
Amphibians, Fish: No information available.

Vitamin C (Ascorbic acid)
(Numerous trade names) **POM, general sale**

Formulations: Injectable: 100 mg/ml. **Oral:** Various strength tablets, capsules, powders and liquids.

Action: Water-soluble antioxidant, also critical for crosslinking collagen precursors (growth and repair of tissue) and is involved in protein, lipid and carbohydrate metabolism.

Use: Vitamin C is used to reduce methaemoglobinaemia associated with paracetamol toxicity. Supplemental vitamin C may be required in conditions of increased oxidative stress, in cachexic patients and in those requiring nutritional support. Vitamin C is not endogenously produced by guinea pigs, and must be present in the diet.

Safety and handling: Normal precautions should be observed.

Contraindications: Avoid use in patients with liver disease.

Adverse reactions: May cause anaphylaxis if given i.v. Vitamin C supplementation may increase liver damage by increasing iron accumulation. Prolonged use can increase the risk of urate, oxalate and cystine crystalluria and stone formation.

Drug interactions: Large doses (oral or injectable) will acidify the urine and may increase the renal excretion of some drugs (e.g. mexiletine) and reduce the effect of some antibacterial drugs in the genitourinary system (e.g. aminoglycosides).

DOSES
Mammals: Rabbits: 50–100 mg/kg p.o., s.c. q12h;
Guinea pigs: maintenance: 10–30 mg/kg/day p.o., s.c. or 200–400 mg/l drinking water; hypovitaminosis C: 100–200 mg/kg p.o. q24h;
Primates: 25 mg/kg p.o. q12h or 30–100 mg/kg p.o., s.c. q24h [a,b];
Hedgehogs: 50–200 mg/kg p.o., s.c. q24h.
Reptiles: 10–20 mg/kg i.m. q7d.
Birds, Amphibians, Fish: No information available.

References
[a] Eisele PH, Morgan JP, Line AS and Anderson JH (1992) Skeletal lesions and anemia associated with ascorbic acid deficiency in juvenile rhesus macaques. *Laboratory Animal Science* **42(3)**, 245–249
[b] Ratterree MS, Didier PJ, Blanchard JL, Clarke MR and Schaeffer D (1990) Vitamin C deficiency in captive non-human primates fed a commercial primate diet. *Laboratory Animal Science* **40(2)**, 165–168

Vitamin D (1,25-dihydroxycolecalciferol (active vitamin D3), colecalciferol (vitamin D3)) (Alfacalcidol*, AT 10*, Calcijex*, Calcitriol*, One-alpha*, Rocaltrol*) **POM-VPS, POM**

Formulations: Oral: Alfacalcidol 2 µg/ml solution (One-alpha), 0.25–1 µg capsules (Alfacalcidol; One-alpha), Calcitriol 0.25 µg capsules (Calcitriol; Rocaltrol), Dihydrotachysterol 0.25 µg/ml solution (AT 10). **Injectable:** Calcitriol 1 µg/ml solution (Calcijex).

Action: In conjunction with other hormones (calcitonin and parathormone) regulates calcium homeostasis through numerous complex mechanisms, including accretion of calcium to bone stores, absorption of calcium from dietary sources.

Vitamin D is a general term used to describe a range of hormones that influence calcium and phosphorus metabolism. They include vitamin D2 (ergocalciferol or calciferol), vitamin D3 (colecalciferol), dihydrotachysterol, alfacalcidol and calcitriol (1,25-dihydroxycole-calciferol, the active form of vitamin D3). These different drugs have differing rates of onset and durations of action.

Use: Chronic management of hypocalcaemia when associated with low parathyroid hormone concentrations which are most commonly associated with iatrogenic hypoparathyroidism following thyroidectomy and immune-mediated hypoparathyroidism. Calcitriol has also been used in the management of renal secondary hyperparathyroidism; in this circumstance it reduces serum parathyroid hormone concentrations. Dihydrotachysterol has an onset of action within 24 hours and raises serum calcium within 1–7 days, with a discontinuation time of 1–3 weeks for serum calcium levels to normalize. Calcitriol and alfacalcidol (1-alpha-hydroxycolecalciferol) have a rapid onset of action (1–2 days) and a short half-life (<1 day); they are the preferred forms for use. Vitamin D requires two hydroxylations (one in the liver and the other in the kidney) to become active. Thus, only the active form (calcitriol) should be used in patients with renal failure. Vitamin D3 is used in birds and reptiles for the treatment of nutritional secondary hyperparathyroidism in combination with calcium and ultraviolet light. Vitamin D has a very narrow therapeutic index and toxic doses are easily achieved resulting in soft tissue calcification. Serum calcium and preferably ionized calcium concentrations need to be monitored closely and frequently. Avoid using formulations of vitamins A, D3 and E that are authorized for farm animals as they are too concentrated for small animal use.

Safety and handling: Normal precautions should be observed.

Contraindications: Do not use in patients with hyperphosphataemia or malabsorption syndromes. Do not use in pregnant animals.

Adverse reactions: Hypercalcaemia and hyperphosphataemia.

Drug interactions: Corticosteroids may negate the effect of vitamin D preparations. Sucralfate decreases absorption of vitamin D. Drugs that induce hepatic enzyme systems (e.g. barbiturates) will increase the metabolism of vitamin D and lower its effective dose. Magnesium- or calcium-containing antacids may cause hypermagnesaemia or hypercalcaemia when used with vitamin D. Thiazide diuretics may also cause hypercalcaemia with concurrent use. Hypercalcaemia may potentiate the toxic effects of verapamil or digoxin; monitor carefully.

DOSES
Mammals: Primates: 110 IU/100 g p.o. q24h (marmosets).
Birds: Hypovitaminosis D: 3300–6600 IU/kg i.m. once (calcitriol)[1].
Reptiles: 200–1000 IU/kg p.o., i.m. q7d. Oral administration may be safer than i.m.
Amphibians: 2–3 IU/ml in a continuous bath with 2.3% calcium gluconate; 100–400 IU/kg p.o. q24h.
Fish: No information available.

References
[1] de Matos R (2008) Calcium metabolism in birds. *Veterinary Clinics of North America: Exotic Animal Practice* **11(1)**, 59–82

Vitamin E (Alpha tocopheryl acetate)
(Multivitamin injection, Vitamin E suspension)
POM-VPS

Formulations: Oral: 20 mg/ml, 100 mg/ml suspension. Injectable: component of multivitamin injectable preparations.

Action: Lipid-soluble antioxidant also regulates gene expression and is involved in cellular metabolism of sulphur compounds.

Use: Vitamin E supplementation is very rarely required in small animals. Patients with exocrine pancreatic insufficiency and other severe malabsorptive diseases may be at risk of developing deficiency. Its use has been suggested for numerous conditions, including discoid lupus, demodicosis and hepatic diseases including fibrosis. These are, however, only anecdotal suggestions and there may be some significant risks. Avoid using formulations of vitamins A, D3 and E that are authorized for farm animals as they are too concentrated for small animal use.

Safety and handling: Normal precautions should be observed.

Contraindications: Do not use in patients at high risk for thrombosis. Do not use in neonates.

Adverse reactions: Thrombosis. Anaphylactoid reactions have been reported.

Drug interactions: Vitamin E may enhance vitamin A absorption, utilization and storage. Vitamin E may alter ciclosporin pharmacokinetics and, if used concurrently, ciclosporin therapy should be monitored by checking levels.

DOSES

Mammals: Primates: 3.75 IU/kg i.m. q3d with selenium at 1.15 mg/kg i.m. for 30 days (myopathy); **Marsupials:** 25–100 IU/animal i.m. q24h or 400 IU/animal i.m. post-capture restraint (macropods).

Birds: 0.06 mg/kg i.m. q7d in psittacids for hypovitaminosis E; once only in raptors to prevent/treat capture myopathy[a].

Reptiles: 1 IU/kg i.m. q24h for 7–14 days.

Amphibians: 1 mg/kg p.o., i.m. q7d or 200 IU/kg of feed.

Fish: No information available.

References

[a] Schink B, Hafez HM and Lierz M (2008) Alpha-tocopherol in captive falcons: reference values and dietary impact. *Journal of Avian Medicine and Surgery* **22(2)**, 99–102

Vitamin K1 (Phytomenadione)
(Vitamin K1 Laboratoire TVM, Konakion*)
POM-V, NFA-VPS

Formulations: Injectable: 10 mg/ml. Oral: 50 mg tablets.

Action: Involved in the formation of active coagulation factors II, VII, IX and X by the liver.

Use: Toxicity due to coumarin and its derivatives. Before performing liver biopsy in patients with prolonged coagulation times. Deficient states may also occur in prolonged significant anorexia. Although vitamin K is a fat-soluble vitamin its biological behaviour is like that of a water-soluble vitamin; it has a relatively short half-life and there are no significant storage pools. It may still require 6–12 hours for effect. One-stage prothrombin time is the best method of monitoring therapy. Use a small gauge needle when injecting s.c. or i.m. in a patient with bleeding tendencies.

Safety and handling: Normal precautions should be observed.

Contraindications: Avoid giving i.v. if possible.

Adverse reactions: Anaphylactic reactions have been reported following i.v. administration. Safety not documented in pregnant animals.

Drug interactions: Many drugs will antagonize the effects of vitamin K, including aspirin, chloramphenicol, allopurinol, diazoxide, cimetidine, metronidazole, erythromycin, itraconazole, propranolol and thyroid drugs as well as coumarin-based anticoagulants. If the patient is on other long-term medications it is advisable to check specific literature. The absorption of oral vitamin K is reduced by mineral oil.

DOSES

Mammals:

- Ferrets:
    - Known 1st generation coumarin toxicity or vitamin K1 deficiency: Initially 2.5 mg/kg s.c. in several sites, then 1–2.5 mg/kg in divided doses p.o. q8–12h for 5–7 days.
    - Known 2nd generation coumarin (brodifacoum) toxicity: Initially 5 mg/kg s.c. in several sites, then 2.5 mg/kg p.o. q12h for 3 weeks, then re-evaluate coagulation status. The patient's activity should be restricted for 1 week following treatment. Evaluate the coagulation status 3 weeks after cessation of treatment.
    - Known inandione (diphacinone) or unknown anticoagulant toxicity: Initially 2.5–5 mg/kg s.c. over several sites, then 2.5 mg/kg p.o. divided q8–12h for 3–4 weeks. Re-evaluate coagulation status 2 days after stopping therapy. If the PT time is elevated, continue therapy for 2 additional weeks. If not elevated, repeat PT in 2 days. If normal, the animal should be rested for 1 week, if abnormal then continue therapy for an additional week and re-check PT times as above.
- **Rabbits, Rodents:** 1–10 mg/kg i.m. as needed depending upon clinical signs/clotting times.
- **Primates:** 1 mg/kg p.o., i.m. q8h.
- **Sugar gliders:** 2 mg/kg s.c. q24–72h.

Birds: 0.2–2.5 mg/kg i.m., p.o. q6–12h until stable, then q24h [a].

Reptiles: 0.5 mg/kg i.m. q24h.

Amphibians, Fish: No information available.

References

[a] Murray M and Tseng F (2008) Diagnosis and treatment of secondary anticoagulant rodenticide toxicosis in a red-tailed hawk (*Buteo jamaicensis*). *Journal of Avian Medicine and Surgery* **22(1)**, 41–46

Voriconazole
(Vfend, Voriconzole) **POM**

Formulations: Oral: 50 mg, 200 mg tablets; 40 mg/ml oral suspension. Injectable: 200 mg powder for reconstitution.

Action: Triazole antifungal agent that inhibits the cytochrome systems involved in the synthesis of ergosterol in fungal cell membranes, causing increased cell wall permeability and allowing leakage of cellular contents.

Use: Treatment of aspergillosis, candidiasis, blastomycosis, coccidioidomycosis, cryptococcosis, sporotrichosis, histoplasmosis, a variety of dermatomycoses and *Malassezia*. It is widely distributed in the body, although low concentrations are found in tissues with low protein contents (e.g. CSF, ocular fluid and saliva). Treatment of chytridiomycisis in amphibians.

Safety and handling: Normal precautions should be observed.

Contraindications: Pregnancy. Avoid use if liver disease is present.

Adverse reactions: Vomiting, diarrhoea, anorexia, salivation, depression and apathy, abdominal pain, hepatic toxicosis, drug eruption, ulcerative dermatitis and limb oedema could potentially occur.

Drug interactions: In humans, antifungal imidazoles and triazoles inhibit the metabolism of antihistamines (particularly terfenadine), oral hypoglycaemics, and antiepileptics and glucocorticoids. Plasma concentrations of ciclosporin, benzodiazepines and vincristine may be increased by voriconazole.

DOSES
Mammals: Rabbits: 1% solution applied topically for fungal keratitis.
Birds: Raptors: 12.5 mg/kg p.o. q12h (some recommend 12.5 mg/kg q12h, then q24h after 3 days)[a]; **Grey Parrots:** 12–18 mg/kg p.o. q12h[b]; **Amazon Parrots:** 18 mg/kg p.o. q8h[c]; Similar dose rates may be used intravenously in urgent cases or in spinal cases.
Reptiles: Bearded dragons: 10 mg/kg p.o. q24h[d].
Amphibians: Poison dart frogs: 1.25 µg (micrograms)/ml q24h topically *via* spray for 7 days[e].
Fish: No information available.

References
[a] Di Somma A, Bailey T, Silvanose C and Garcia-Martinez C (2007) The use of voriconazole for the treatment of aspergillosis in falcons (*Falco* species). *Journal of Avian Medicine and Surgery* **21(4)**, 307–317

[b] Flammer K, Nettifee Osborne JA, Webb DJ *et al.* (2008) Pharmacokinetics of voriconazole after oral administration of single and multiple doses in African grey parrots (*Psittacus erithacus timneh*). *American Journal of Veterinary Research* **69(1)**, 114–121

[c] Sanchez-Migallon Guzman D, Flammer K, Papich MG *et al.* (2010) Pharmacokinetics of voriconazole after oral administration of single and multiple doses in Hispaniolan Amazon parrots (*Amazona ventralis*). *American Journal of Veterinary Research* **71(4)**, 460–467

[d] Van Waeyenberghe L, Baert K, Pasmans F *et al.* (2010) Voriconazole, a safe alternative for treating infections caused by the Chrysosporium anamorph of Nannizziopsis vriesii in bearded dragons (*Pogona vitticeps*). *Medical Mycology* **48(6)**, 880–885

[e] Martel A, Van Rooij P, Vercauteren G *et al.* (2011) Developing a safe antifungal treatment protocol to eliminate *Batrachochytrium dendrobatidis* from amphibians. *Medical Mycology* **49(2)**, 143–149

Xylazine

(Chanazine, Nerfasin, Rompun, Sedaxylan, Virbaxyl, Xylacare, Xylapan) **POM-V**

Formulations: Injectable: 20 mg/ml solution.

Action: Agonist at peripheral and central alpha-2 adrenoreceptors, producing dose-dependent sedation, muscle relaxation and analgesia.

Use: Has been largely superseded by medetomidine or dexmedetomidine and is no longer recommended. Used to provide sedation and premedication when used alone or in combination with opioid analgesics. Xylazine combined with ketamine is used to provide a short duration (20–30 minutes) of surgical anaesthesia. Xylazine is less specific for the alpha-2 adrenoreceptor than are medetomidine and dexmedetomidine and causes significant alpha-1 adrenoreceptor effects. This lack of specificity is likely to be associated with the poorer safety profile of xylazine compared with medetomidine and dexmedetomidine. Xylazine also sensitizes the myocardium to catecholamine arrhythmias, which increases the risk of cardiovascular complications. Xylazine is a potent drug that causes marked changes in the cardiovascular system. It should not be used in animals with cardiovascular or systemic disease affecting cardiovascular performance. Atipamezole is not licensed as a reversal agent for xylazine, but it is effective and can be used to reverse the effects of xylazine if an overdose is given. Spontaneous arousal from deep sedation following stimulation can occur with all alpha-2 agonists; aggressive animals sedated with xylazine must still be managed with caution. Xylazine stimulates growth hormone production and may be used to assess the pituitary gland's ability to produce this hormone (xylazine stimulation test).

Safety and handling: Normal precautions should be observed.

Contraindications: Do not use in animals with cardiovascular or other systemic disease. Use of xylazine in geriatric patients is also not advisable. It causes increased uterine motility and should not be used in pregnant animals, nor in animals likely to require or receiving sympathomimetic amines. Due to effects on blood glucose, use in diabetic animals is not recommended. Avoid when vomiting is contraindicated (e.g. foreign body, raised intraocular pressure).

Adverse reactions: Xylazine has diverse effects on many organ systems as well as the cardiovascular system. It causes a diuresis by suppressing ADH secretion, a transient increase in blood glucose by decreasing endogenous insulin secretion, mydriasis and decreased intraocular pressure.

Drug interactions: When used for premedication, xylazine will significantly reduce the dose of all other anaesthetic agents required to maintain anaesthesia.

DOSES

When used for sedation is generally given as part of a combination. See Appendix for sedation protocols in all species.

Mammals: Primates: 0.5–2.2 mg/kg i.m. for sedation or 0.5–3 mg/kg in combination with ketamine at 10–20 mg/kg for anaesthesia; **Marsupials:** 5 mg/kg in combination with ketamine at 10–25 mg/kg; **Hedgehogs:** 0.5–1.0 mg/kg i.m.

Birds: Do not use.

Reptiles: No longer recommended as superseded by medetomidine and dexmedetomidine.

Amphibians: 10 mg/kg intracoelomic q12–24h appears to have an analgesic effect in laboratory studies in Xenopus frogs[a].

Fish: No information available.

References

[a] Terril-Robb L, Suckow M and Grigdesby C (1996) Evaluation of the analgesic effects of butorphanol tartarate, xylazine hydrochloride and flunixin meglumine in leopard frogs (*Rana pipiens*). *Contemporary Topics in Laboratory Animal Science* **35**, 54–56

Zinc salts
(Numerous trade names) **GSL**

Formulations: Oral: various zinc sulphate, zinc gluconate, zinc acetate and chelated zinc preparations.

Action: Primarily involved in DNA and RNA synthesis, although also involved in essential fatty acid synthesis, WBC function and numerous reactions in intermediary metabolism. When administered orally can reduce GI absorption and hepatic uptake of copper.

Use: Zinc-responsive dermatoses. Proposed benefits also exist in chronic liver disease and hepatic encephalopathy. Bioavailability of elemental zinc varies depending on formulation: zinc acetate and chelated forms: highest; gluconate: intermediate; sulphate: lowest. Higher bioavailability is also associated with improved tolerance.

Safety and handling: Normal precautions should be observed.

Contraindications: Patients with copper deficiency.

Adverse reactions: Nausea, vomiting and occasional diarrhoea. Haemolysis may occur with large doses or serum levels >10 mg/ml particularly if a coexistent copper deficiency exists.

Drug interactions: Significant interactions with other divalent heavy metals such as iron and copper can occur and long-term administration of zinc may lead to decreased hepatic copper or iron stores and functional deficiency. Penicillamine and ursodeoxycholic acid may potentially inhibit zinc absorption; the clinical significance is unclear. Zinc salts may chelate oral tetracycline and reduce its absorption; separate doses by at least 2 hours. Zinc salts may reduce the absorption of fluoroquinolone antibiotics.

DOSES
Mammals: Primates: 2.5 μg (micrograms)/animal p.o. q24h for 3 days.
Birds, Reptiles, Amphibians, Fish: No information available.

Appendix I: general information

Abbreviations

In general abbreviations should not be used in prescription writing. However, it is recognized that at present some Latin abbreviations are used when prescribing. These should be limited to those listed here.

Abbreviations used in prescription writing

a.c.	Before meals
ad. lib.	At pleasure
amp.	Ampoule
b.i.d.	Twice a day
cap.	Capsule
g	Gram
h	Hour
i.c.	Intracoelomic
i.m.	Intramuscular
i.p.	Intraperitoneal
i.v.	Intravenous
m^2	Square metre
mg	Milligram
ml	Millilitre
o.m.	In the morning
o.n.	At night
p.c.	After meals
prn	As required
q	Every, e.g. q8h = every 8 hours
q.i.d./q.d.s	Four times a day
q.s.	A sufficient quantity
s.c.	Subcutaneous
s.i.d.	Once a day
Sig:	Directions/label
stat	Immediately
susp.	Suspension
tab	Tablet
t.i.d./t.d.s.	Three times a day

Other abbreviations used in this Formulary

ACE	Angiotensin converting enzyme
ACTH	Adrenocorticotropic hormone
AV	Atrioventricular
CBC	Complete blood count
CHF	Congestive heart failure
CNS	Central nervous system
COX	Cyclo-oxygenase
CRI	Continuous rate infusion
CSF	Cerebrospinal fluid
d	Day(s)
DIC	Disseminated intravascular coagulation
ECG	Electrocardiogram
GI	Gastrointestinal
h	Hour(s)
Hb	Haemoglobin
MAOI	Monoamine oxidase inhibitor
min	Minute
p.o.	By mouth, orally
PU/PD	Polyuria/polydipsia
RBC	Red blood cell
SSRI	Selective serotonin re-uptake inhibitor
STC	Special Treatment Certificate
VPC	Ventricular premature contraction
WBC	White blood cell
wk	Week(s)

Writing a prescription

A 'veterinary prescription' is defined by EU law as 'any prescription for a veterinary medicinal product issued by a professional person qualified to do so in accordance with applicable national law'. The word 'veterinary' takes its normal meaning 'of or for animals'. In the UK there are two classes of medicines available only on veterinary prescription, POM-V and POM-VPS, described in the Introduction. Only in the case of POM-V medicines does the veterinary prescription have to be issued by a veterinary surgeon. The act of prescribing is taken to mean the decision made by the prescriber as to which product should be supplied, taking account of the circumstances of the animals being treated, the available authorized veterinary medicinal products and the need for responsible use of medicines. Good prescription principles include the following. Only 1, 8, 10 and 12 are legal requirements; the remainder are good practice.

1   Print or write legibly in ink or otherwise so as to be indelible. Sign in ink with your normal signature. Include the date on which the prescription was signed.
2   Use product or approved generic name for drugs in capital letters – do not abbreviate. Ensure the full name is stated, to include the pharmaceutical form and strength.
3   State duration of treatment where known and the total quantity to be supplied.
4   Write out microgram/nanogram – do not abbreviate.
5   Always put a 0 before an initial decimal point (e.g. 0.5 mg), but avoid the unnecessary use of a decimal point (e.g. 3 mg not 3.0 mg).
6   Give precise instructions concerning route/dose/formulation. Directions should preferably be in English without abbreviation. It is recognized that some Latin abbreviations are used (p.311).
7   Any alterations invalidate the prescription – rewrite.
8   Prescriptions for Schedule 2 and most Schedule 3 Controlled Drugs must be entirely handwritten and include the total quantity in both words and figures, the form and strength of the drug.
9   The prescription should not be repeated more than three times without re-checking the patient.
10 Include both the prescriber's and the client's names and addresses.
11 Include the directions that the prescriber wishes to appear on the labelled product. It is good practice to include the words 'For animal treatment only'.
12 Include a declaration that 'This prescription is for an animal under my care' or words to that effect.
13 If drugs that are not authorized for veterinary use are going to be used when there is an alternative that is 'higher' in the prescribing cascade, there should be a clear clinical justification made on an individual basis and recorded in the clinical notes or on the prescription.

The following is a standard form of prescription used:

From: *Address of practice*   *Date*

Telephone No.

Animal's name and identification   *Owner's name*
(species, breed, age and sex)   *Owner's address*

Rx
- *Print name, strength and formulation of drug*
- *Total quantity to be supplied*
- *Amount to be administered*
- *Frequency of administration*
- *Duration of treatment*
- *Any warnings*
- *If not a POM-V and prescribed under the 'Cascade',*
  this must be stated
- For animal treatment only
- For an animal under my care

Non-repeat/repeat X *1, 2 or 3*

Name, qualifications and signature of veterinary surgeon

Guidelines for responsible antibacterial use

Following these guidelines will help to maximize therapeutic success of antibacterial agents whilst at the same time minimizing the development of antibacterial resistance, thereby safeguarding antimicrobials for future veterinary and human use. These guidelines should be read in conjunction with the updated *BSAVA Guide to the Use of Veterinary Medicines*, the PROTECT ME guidance and individual drug monographs (www.bsavalibrary.com). It is important that the veterinary profession uses antibacterials prudently in order to: minimize the selection of resistant veterinary pathogens (and therefore safeguard animal health); minimize possible resistance transfer to human pathogens; and retain the right to prescribe certain antibacterials.

It is important to remember that antibacterials do not make organisms resistant, but they do create selective pressure on populations of organisms. Resistance may be inherent, evolved (by chromosomal DNA changes) or acquired (by plasmid transfer). Resistance is reduced by the following:

1 **Reducing the expectation of antibacterial prescriptions.**
   Educate clients not to expect antibacterials when they are not appropriate; e.g. viral infections.
2 **Minimizing and ideally avoiding prophylactic use.**
   - Prophylactic antibacterial use may be appropriate in certain medical situations; for example, when an animal is considered to be at increased risk due to concurrent disease or immunosuppressant therapy and is in contact with other infected animals.

- Prophylactic antibacterial use may be appropriate in the perioperative period, although it should not be a substitute for good asepsis. Examples of appropriate criteria for perioperative antibacterial use include:
  - Prolonged surgical procedures (>1.5 hours)
  - Introduction of an implant into the body
  - Procedures where introduction of infection would be catastrophic (e.g. CNS surgery)
  - Where there is an obvious identified break in asepsis
  - Bowel surgery with a risk of leakage
  - Dentistry with associated periodontal disease
  - Contaminated wounds.
- In exotic pets, the choice of an appropriate antibiotic will be highly dependent on the species or group of species and the likely spectrum of bacterial involvement, and great care must be taken to avoid any known adverse effects (e.g. on gut microflora in rabbits and rodents).

3 **Culturing appropriate material for sensitivity testing.**
- The results from culture and sensitivity tests considerably assist the choice of which antibacterial to use.
- Culture is not required in every case, but when prolonged courses of antibacterials are likely to be needed (e.g. pyodermas, otitis externa, deep or surgical wound infections) then culture will improve the animal's treatment.

4 **Knowing the features of antibacterials.** There are three key areas that veterinary surgeons must have a working knowledge of.
- **Spectrum of activity.** Many of the antibacterials in routine veterinary use are broad-spectrum; however, to minimize resistance the narrowest spectrum agent should be chosen. Some specific examples of spectra covered are:
  - Anaerobes – metronidazole, clindamycin, many of the penicillins (especially the narrow spectrum penicillins such as Penicillin G) and cephalosporins
  - Gram-positive bacteria – penicillins, cephalosporins, lincosamides and macrolides
  - Gram-negative bacteria – aminoglycosides and fluoroquinolones.
- **Distribution.** Many of the antibacterial classes are well distributed around the body, and it is important to be aware of some of the specifics of distribution. Key examples (in mammals) include:
  - Aminoglycosides are poorly distributed. They are not absorbed from the GI tract and even if given systemically distribution can be quite restricted. Conversely, it means that they are very appropriate for local delivery
  - Beta-lactams attain high concentrations in the urinary tract due to filtration and secretion into the renal tubule. Levels attained may be many times higher than plasma concentrations. Fluoroquinolones also attain extremely high levels in the urinary tract
  - Lipid-soluble basic antibacterials such as the

    macrolides and lincosamides become ion-trapped (concentrate) in sites such as the prostate gland and the mammary gland.

- **Adverse effects/toxicity.** These must be considered in the context of the individual animal and in relation to concurrent treatment or pre-existing conditions.

5 **Use the antibacterial you have chosen appropriately**.
- Consider the practicalities and owner compliance.
- Give the appropriate **dose**, for the appropriate **frequency** and the appropriate **duration**. Too little or too much antibacterial will contribute to resistance and inappropriate use will lead to treatment failure.
- Is the antibacterial **time-** or **concentration-dependent**? (Refer to the *BSAVA Guide to the Use of Veterinary Medicines* (www.bsavalibrary.com) for an explanation of these terms.)

6 **Assess the response.** Part of this may be carrying out repeated culture and sensitivity testing, where appropriate, and amending treatment if indicated from the results. If you are using an antibacterial which your clinical experience, or the results of culture and sensitivity, suggests should be effective in a particular situation and treatment fails, then this should be reported through the Suspected Adverse Reaction Surveillance Scheme (SARSS) organized by the Veterinary Medicines Directorate (VMD), as this is important in monitoring resistance development.

7 **Certain antibacterials should be used judiciously.** This means that their use as first line agents should be avoided, and they should only be used when other agents are ineffective (ideally determined by culture and sensitivity testing). These include:
- Fluoroquinolones
- Third and fourth generation cephalosporins
- Amikacin.

The VMD has published guidelines for responsible antibiotic use under the cascade which state that 'it is justified, on a case-by-case basis, to prescribe an antibiotic on the cascade in the interests of minimizing the development of restance'. Consequently, use of an alternative antibiotic may be justified, rather than first-line use of a licensed fluoroquinolone in an exotic animal, if the veterinary surgeon feels that this is appropriate for the individual case.

8 **Certain antibacterials should probably NOT be used in veterinary species.** These are agents of last resort in human patients and include:
- Vancomycin
- Carbapenams such as imipenam.

In addition to written guidelines on which antibacterials should be used and the appropriate dosing regimens, there should be a practice policy in terms of appropriate criteria warranting antibacterials. For example, it is feasible to work out appropriate first option antibacterials for uncomplicated urinary tract infections and surgical prophylaxis, which should then be used by all practice members.

Antibacterials in small mammals

Antibacterial therapy in several small mammal species poses a greater risk when compared with other species due to the suppression of normal bacterial flora, resulting in overgrowth of other species, notably *Clostridium*, resulting in enterotoxaemia and death. Mice, rats, ferrets and usually gerbils are fairly resistant, whereas hamsters, guinea pigs, chinchillas, degus and rabbits are more susceptible. The risk of enterotoxaemia is related to several factors, including the drug selected, the dose, the route of administration and the animal's nutritional status and general health. Antibiotics that have been associated with this problem when given orally include penicillins, lincosamides, aminoglycosides (possibly), cephalosporins and erythromycin. Some species appear more sensitive to certain drugs than others, while some medications actually appear well-tolerated by alternative routes (for example, injectable benzylpenicillin in rabbits). See individual monographs for more details.

Dosing small and exotic animals

Veterinary surgeons who are unfamiliar with the actions of a particular drug in a given exotic species are advised to consult the drug monograph and more complete references.

The size of some species of exotic pets makes dosing difficult and care must be taken when calculating small doses. Some points to bear in mind when dosing are:

- Where powders are to be dissolved in water, sterile water for injection should be used
- Most solutions may be diluted with water for injection or 0.9% saline
- Dilution will be necessary when volumes <0.1 ml are to be administered
- Suspensions cannot be diluted
- Use 1 ml syringes for greatest accuracy
- Specialist laboratories with a Veterinary Specials Authorization should be contacted to reformulate drugs.

Doses provided in this Formulary are intended for exotic pet species. They should not be used for commercial production species of fish or poultry, or large mammals. Established poultry texts should be consulted for treating individual chickens.

Composition of intravenous fluids

Fluid	Na$^+$ (mmol/l)	K$^+$ (mmol/l)	Ca^{2+} (mmol/l)	Cl$^-$ (mmol/l)	HCO$_3^-$ (mmol/l)	Dext. (g/l)	Osmol. (mosl/l)
0.45% NaCl	77			77			155
0.9% NaCl	154			154			308
5% NaCl	856			856			1722
Ringer's	147	4	2	155			310
Lactated Ringer's (Hartmann's)	131	5	2	111	29 *		280
Darrow's	121	35		103	53 *		312
0.9% NaCl + 5.5% Dext.	154			154		50	560
0.18% NaCl + 4% Dext.	31			31		40	264
Duphalyte **		2.6	1.0	3.6		454	Unknown

Dext. = Dextrose; Osmol. = Osmolality. * Bicarbonate is present as lactate.
** Also contains a mixture of vitamins and small quantities of amino acids and 1.2 mmol/l of MgSO$_4$

Safety and handling of chemotherapeutic agents

Most drugs used in veterinary practice do not pose a major hazard to the person handling them or handling an animal treated with them (or its waste). Chemotherapeutic agents are the exception. People who are exposed to these drugs during their use in animals risk serious side effects. In addition, chemotherapeutic agents pose a serious risk to patient welfare if not used correctly. They should only be used when absolutely indicated (i.e. histologically-confirmed diseases that are known to be responsive to them). Investigational use should be confined to controlled clinical trials.

Personnel

- The preparation and administration of cytotoxic drugs should only be undertaken by trained staff.
- Owners and staff (including cleaners, animal caretakers, veterinary surgeons) involved in the care of animals being treated with cytotoxic drugs must be informed (and proof available that they have been informed) of:
  - The risks of working with cytotoxic agents
  - The potential methods for preventing aerosol formation and the spread of contamination
  - The proper working practices for a safety cabinet
  - The instructions in case of contamination
  - The principles of good personal protection and hygiene practice.
- As a general rule, pregnant women and immunocompromised personnel should not be involved in the process of preparing and/or administering cytotoxic agents, caring for animals that

have been treated with cytotoxic drugs, or cleaning of the areas these animals have come into contact with. It is the responsibility of the employee to warn their supervisors if they are pregnant, likely to become pregnant or are immunocompromised.

Equipment and facilities

- All areas where cytotoxic agents are prepared and/or administered, or where animals who have received cytotoxic drugs are being cared for, should be identified by a clear warning sign. Access to these areas should be restricted.
- Ideally a negative pressure pharmaceutical isolator with externally ducted exhaust filters, which has been properly serviced and checked, should be used. If such an isolator is not available then a suitably modified Class 2B Biological Safety Cabinet (BSC) may be used.
- There must be adequate materials for cleaning of spilled cytotoxic agents (cytotoxic spill kit).
- Closed or semi-closed systems should be used to prevent aerosol formation and control exposure to carcinogenic compounds. Special spike systems (e.g. Codan and Braun) can be used. Other systems specifically developed for the use of cytotoxic agents are recommended (e.g. Spiros, Tevadaptor, Oncovial and PhaSeal). If such systems are not available, then at the very least infusion sets and syringes with Luer-lock fittings should be used.

Preparation of cytotoxic drugs

- Manipulation of oral or topical medicines containing cytotoxic drugs should be avoided. If a drug concentration is required that is not readily available, then a specialist laboratory with a Veterinary Specials Authorization should be contacted to reformulate the drug to the desired concentration. This may be useful for drugs such as piroxicam, hydroxycarbamide and lomustine. Tablets should never be crushed or split. If reformulation is not possible then using smaller sized tablets or adjusting the dosage regimen is often sufficient.
- When drug preparation is complete, the final product should be sealed in a plastic bag or other container for transport before it is taken out of the ventilated cabinet. It should be clearly labelled as containing cytotoxic drugs.
- All potentially contaminated materials should be discarded in special waste disposal containers, which can be opened without direct contact with hands/gloves (e.g. a foot pedal). Local regulations as to the disposal of this waste should be followed.
- There should be a clear procedure regarding how to handle cytotoxic drugs following an injection accident.
- During the preparation and administration of cytotoxic drugs, personal protection should be worn, including special disposable chemoprotective gloves, disposable protective clothing, and eye and face protection.

- After the preparation and/or administration of cytotoxic drugs, or after nursing a treated animal, the area used should be properly cleaned using a specific protocol before other activities commence.

Administration of cytotoxic drugs

- All necessary measures should be taken to ensure that the animal being treated is calm and cooperative. If the temperament of the animal is such that a safe administration is not to be expected, then the veterinary surgeon has the right (and is obliged) not to treat these animals.
- Many cytotoxic drugs are irritant and must be administered via a preplaced i.v. catheter. Administration of bolus injections should be done through a catheter system, which should be flushed with 0.9% NaCl before, during and after the injection.
- Heparinized saline should be avoided as it can interact with some chemotherapeutic drugs (e.g. doxorubicin).
- Drugs should be administered safely using protective medical devices (such as needleless and closed systems) and techniques (such as priming of i.v. tubing by pharmacy personnel inside a ventilated cabinet or priming in line with non-drug solutions).
- The tubing should never be removed from a fluid bag containing a hazardous drug, nor should it be disconnected at other points in the system until the tubing has been thoroughly flushed. The i.v. catheter, tubing and bag should be removed intact when possible.
- Hands should be washed with soap and water before leaving the drug administration area.
- Procedures should be in place for dealing with any spillages that occur and for the safe disposal of waste. In the event of contact with skin or eyes, the affected area should be washed with copious amounts of water or normal saline. Medical advice should be sought if the eyes are affected.

Procedures for nursing patients receiving chemotherapy

- Special wards or designated kennels with clear identification that the patients are being treated with cytotoxic agents are required.
- Excreta (saliva, urine, vomit, faeces) are all potentially hazardous after the animal has been treated with cytotoxic drugs, and should be handled and disposed of accordingly.
- During the period of risk, personal protective equipment (such as disposable gloves and protective clothing) should be worn when carrying out nursing procedures.
- All materials that have come into contact with the animal during the period of risk should be considered as potentially contaminated.
- After the animal has left the ward, the cage should be cleaned according to the cleaning protocol.

Guidelines for owners

- All owners should be given written information on the potential hazards of the cytotoxic drugs. Written information on how to deal with the patient's excreta (saliva, urine, vomit, faeces) must also be provided.

- If owners are to administer tablets themselves, then written information on how to do this must also be provided. Drug containers should be clearly labelled with 'cytotoxic contents' warning tape.

Further information

For further information readers are advised to consult specialist texts and the guidelines issued by the European College of Veterinary Medicine – Companion Animals (ECVIM-CA) on 'Preventing occupational and environmental exposure to cytotoxic drugs in veterinary medicine'.

Percentage solutions

The concentration of a solution may be expressed on the basis of weight per unit volume (w/v) or volume per unit volume (v/v).

% w/v = number of grams of a substance in 100 ml of a liquid
% v/v = number of ml of a substance in 100 ml of liquid

% Solution	g or ml/100 ml	mg/ml	Solution strength
100	100	1000	1:1
10	10	100	1:10
1	1	10	1:100
0.1	0.1	1	1:1000
0.01	0.01	0.1	1:10,000

Drugs usage in renal and hepatic insufficiency

With failure of liver or kidney, the excretion of some drugs may be impaired, leading to increased serum concentrations. Note: this information is based on mammals and may not be directly applicable to birds, reptiles, amphibians and fish.

Renal failure

a. Double the dosing interval or halve the dosage in patients with severe renal insufficiency. Use for drugs that are relatively non-toxic.

b. Increase dosing interval 2-fold when creatinine clearance (Ccr) is 0.5–1.0 ml/min/kg, 3-fold when Ccr is 0.3–0.5 ml/min/kg and 4-fold when Ccr is <0.3 ml/min/kg.

c. Precise dose modification is required for some toxic drugs that are excreted solely by glomerular filtration, e.g. aminoglycosides. This is determined by using the dose fraction K_f to amend the drug dose or dosing interval according to the following equations:

Modified dose reduction = normal dose $\times K_f$
Modified dose interval = normal dose interval/K_f
where K_f = patient Ccr/normal Ccr

Where Ccr is unavailable, Ccr may be estimated at 88.4/serum creatinine (µmol/l) (where serum creatinine is <350 µmol/l). K_f may be estimated at 0.33 if urine is isosthenuric or 0.25 if the patient is azotaemic.

Drug	Nephrotoxic	Dose adjustment in renal failure
Amikacin	Yes	c
Amoxicillin	No	a
Amphotericin B	Yes	c
Ampicillin	No	a
Cefalexin	No	b
Chloramphenicol	No	N, A
Digoxin	No	c
Gentamicin	Yes	c
Oxytetracycline	Yes	CI
Penicillin	No	a
Streptomycin	Yes	b
Tobramycin	Yes	c
Trimethoprim/ sulphonamide	Yes	b, A

a, b, c = Refer to section above on dose adjustment; A = Avoid in severe renal failure; CI = Contraindicated; N = normal dose.

APPENDIX I: GENERAL INFORMATION

APPENDIX II: PROTOCOLS

INDEX: THERAPEUTIC CLASS

INDEX: GENERIC AND TRADE NAMES

Hepatic insufficiency

Drug clearance by the liver is affected by many factors and thus it is not possible to apply a simple formula to drug dosing. The table below is adapted from information in the human literature.

Drug	DI	CI
Aspirin		✓
Azathioprine		✓
Cefotaxime	✓	
Chloramphenicol		✓
Clindamycin		✓
Cyclophosphamide	✓	
Diazepam		✓
Doxorubicin	✓	
Doxycycline	✓	
Furosemide	✓	
Hydralazine	✓	
Lidocaine	✓	
Metronidazole	✓	
Morphine	✓	
NSAIDs	✓	
Oxytetracycline		✓
Pentobarbital	✓	
Phenobarbital	✓	
Propranolol	✓	
Theophylline	✓	
Vincristine	✓	

CI = Contraindicated; avoid use if at all possible. DI = A change in dose or dosing interval may be required.

Suspected Adverse Reaction Surveillance Scheme (SARSS)

The Veterinary Medicines Directorate (VMD) has a website (www.gov.uk/government/organisations/veterinary-medicines-directorate) to report any and all suspected adverse reactions in an animal or a human to a veterinary medicinal product, or in an animal treated with a human medicine. Anyone can report a suspected adverse reaction in this way. An 'adverse reaction' includes lack of efficacy and known side effects. It is only by completing such forms that the changes in the prevalence of problems can be documented.

The online report form is preferred; however, if you would prefer to use a paper copy you can download and print an Animal Form to report an adverse reaction in an animal to a veterinary medicine or to a human product. Alternatively, download and print a Human Form to report an adverse reaction in a human to a veterinary medicinal product. Post the forms to the address at the top of the reports.

If you have any questions please call the VMD pharmacovigilance team on **01932 336911**.

Further reading

British National Formulary No. 78 (2019) British Medical Association and the Royal Pharmaceutical Society of Great Britain

Carpenter JW (2018) *Exotic Animal Formulary, 5th edn.* Elsevier, St Louis

Compendium of Data Sheets for Animal Medicines (2020) National Office of Animal Health, Enfield, Middlesex

Giguére S, Prescott JF, Baggot JD and Walker RD (2013) *Antimicrobial Therapy in Veterinary Medicine, 5th edn.* Wiley Blackwell, Iowa

Monthly Index of Medical Specialties (2019) Haymarket Medical Publications, London

Papich MG (2015) *Saunders Handbook of Veterinary Drugs, 4th edn.* Elsevier, St Louis

Plumb DC (2018) *Plumb's Veterinary Drug Handbook, 9th edn.* Wiley Blackwell, New Jersey (also available from www.plumbsveterinarydrugs.com)

Useful websites

www.bnf.org
British National Formulary – registration required through academic institutions to use BNF online but can order paper copy of BNF from this site.

www.bsavalibrary.com
British Small Animal Veterinary Association online Library – links to *Journal of Small Animal Practice,* and contains the *BSAVA Guide to the Use of Veterinary Medicines* and searchable online Formularies (free access for BSAVA members).

www.bva.co.uk/News-campaigns-and-policy/Policy/medicines/veterinary-medicines/
British Veterinary Association. Information on the Prescribing Cascade.

www.bvzs.org/images/uploads/BVZS_dispensing_guidelines.pdf
British Veterinary Zoological Society. Information on the Prescribing Cascade.

www.chemopet.co.uk
Chemopet – company that will reformulate a wide range of injectable and oral chemotherapy drugs.

www.emea.europa.eu/ema/
European Medicines Agency.

www.gov.uk/government/organisations/veterinary-medicines-directorate
Veterinary Medicines Directorate – in particular is useful for repeat applications for special import certificates (SICs) and special treatment certificates (STCs) and the electronic Summary of Product Characteristics (eSPCs).

www.medicines.org.uk/emc
Electronic Medicines Compendium.

www.ncbi.nlm.nih.gov/pubmed
PubMed is a widely used free service of the U.S. National Library of Medicine and the National Institutes of Health that allows users to search abstracts in the medical literature. All major veterinary publications covered.

www.noahcompendium.co.uk
NOAH compendium site.

www.novalabs.co.uk/
Site for a company that will reformulate many drugs into conveniently sized tablets.

www.rcvs.org.uk/setting-standards/advice-and-guidance/code-of-professional-conduct-for-veterinary-surgeons/supporting-guidance/veterinary-medicines/
Royal College of Veterinary Surgeons. Information on the Prescribing Cascade.

www.specialslab.co.uk
Site for a company that will reformulate many drugs into conveniently sized tablets.

www.wiley.com
Journal of Small Animal Practice – free for BSAVA members, free abstracts and pay per article for others.

Appendix II: protocols

Chemotherapy protocols

The metabolism of small mammals, birds and reptiles is markedly different from dogs, cats and humans. Therefore, extrapolation of doses is risky to the patient and extrapolation of safety data (such as the length of time that an animal may excrete a cytotoxic drug) is risky to the owners and staff handling the animals. The lack of any proper evidence base for the use of cytotoxic agents in these species means that any attempt to use them cannot be shown to be safe, either to the animal or to the people who come into contact with that animal. For this reason doses of these agents are generally not provided in the Formulary, other than for ferrets where established protocols have been published[a] (see below), and the use of these agents in such species is strongly discouraged until such time as better monitoring facilities are available in veterinary practice and there are sufficient cases to undertake effective clinical trials.

References
[a] Webb JK, Graham JE, Burgess KE and Antinoff N (2019) Presentation and survival time of domestic ferrets (*Mustela putorius furo*) with lymphoma treated with single-and multi-agent protocols: 44 cases (1998–2016). *Journal of Exotic Pet Medicine* **31**, 64–67

Chemotherapy protocols for lymphoma: ferrets

Note: the suggested protocols are based on clinical application and case studies and extrapolated from other species; there are no primary controlled trials in ferrets. A CBC should be performed prior to the administration of any chemotherapeutic agents.

Option 1

Week	Day	Drug	Dose and route
1	1	Prednisolone	1–2 mg/kg p.o. q12h continued throughout course of therapy
		Vincristine	0.025 mg/kg i.v.
	3	Cyclophosphamide	10 mg/kg p.o., s.c.
2	8	Vincristine	0.025 mg/kg i.v.
3	15	Vincristine	0.025 mg/kg i.v.
4	22	Vincristine	0.025 mg/kg i.v.
	24	Cyclophosphamide	10 mg/kg p.o., s.c.
7	46	Cyclophosphamide	10 mg/kg p.o., s.c.
9	63	Prednisolone	Taper dose down gradually to 0 over the next 4 wks

Option 2

Week	Drug	Dose and route
1	Vincristine	0.025 mg/kg i.v.
	L-Asparginase[a]	400 IU/kg intraperitoneal
	Prednisolone	1 mg/kg p.o. q24h continued throughout course of therapy
2	Cyclophosphamide	10 mg/kg p.o., s.c.
3	Doxorubicin	1 mg/kg i.v.
4	Vincristine	0.025 mg/kg i.v.
5	Cyclophosphamide	10 mg/kg p.o., s.c.
6	Doxorubicin	1 mg/kg i.v.
8	Vincristine	0.025 mg/kg i.v.
10	Cyclophosphamide	10 mg/kg p.o., s.c.
12	Vincristine	0.025 mg/kg i.v.
14	Methotrexate	0.5 mg/kg i.v.

[a] Premedicate with diphenhydramine at 1–2 mg/kg i.m. 30 minutes prior to administration to prevent an anaphylactic response.

Option 3 [a]

Week	Drug	Dose and route
−3	L-Asparginase[b]	400 IU/kg s.c.
1	Vincristine	0.12 mg/kg i.v.
	Prednisolone	1 mg/kg p.o. q24h continued throughout course of therapy
	Cyclophosphamide	10 mg/kg p.o.
2	Vincristine	0.12 mg/kg i.v.
3	Vincristine	0.12 mg/kg i.v.
4, 7, 10, 13, etc. (q3wks)	Vincristine	0.12 mg/kg i.v.
	Cyclophosphamide	10 mg/kg p.o.
Rescue	Doxorubicin[b]	1–2 mg/kg i.v. slow infusion

[a] Antinoff N and Hahn K (2004) Ferret oncology: diseases, diagnostics and therapeutics. *Veterinary Clinics of North America: Exotic Animal Practice* **7**, 579–625
[b] Premedicate with diphenhydramine at 1–2 mg/kg i.m., s.c. 30 minutes prior to administration to prevent an anaphylactic response.

Option 4 (avoiding i.v. route) [1]

Week	Drug	Dose and route
1	L-Asparginase [a]	10,000 IU/m^2 s.c.
	Cyclophosphamide	250 mg/m^2 p.o., s.c. (in 50 ml/kg NaCl s.c.)
	Prednisolone	2 mg/kg p.o. q24h for 7 days then q48h throughout course of therapy
2	L-Asparginase [a]	10,000 IU/m^2 s.c.
3	L-Asparginase [a]	10,000 IU/m^2 s.c.
	Cytosine arabinoside	300 mg/m^2 s.c. q24h for 2 days (dilute 100 mg in 1 ml sterile water)
4	L-Asparginase [a]	10,000 IU/m^2 s.c.
5	Cyclophosphamide	250 mg/m^2 p.o., s.c. (in 50 ml/kg NaCl)
7	Methotrexate	0.8 mg/kg i.m.
9	Cyclophosphamide	250 mg/m^2 p.o., s.c. (in 50 ml/kg NaCl)
11	Cytosine arabinoside	300 mg/m^2 s.c. q24h for 2 days (dilute 100 mg in 1 ml sterile water)
	Chlorambucil	1 tablet/ferret p.o.
13	Cyclophosphamide	250 mg/m^2 p.o., s.c. (in 50 ml/kg NaCl)
15	Procarbazine	50 mg/m^2 p.o. q24h for 14 days
18	Cyclophosphamide	250 mg/m^2 p.o., s.c. (in 50 ml/kg NaCl)
20	Cytosine arabinoside	300 mg/m^2 s.c. q24h for 2 days (dilute 100 mg in 1 ml sterile water)
23	Cyclophosphamide	250 mg/m^2 p.o., s.c. (in 50 ml/kg NaCl)
26	Procarbazine	50 mg/m^2 p.o. q24h for 14 days
28	Repeat weeks 20–26 if not in remission for 3 cycles	

Note: perform a CBC at weeks 2, 4, 7, 8, 12, 16, 17 and 27; if severe myelosuppression, reduce dose by 25% for subsequent treatments of the previously used drug.
[a] Premedicate with diphenhydramine at 1–2 mg/kg i.m., s.c. 30 minutes prior to administration to prevent an anaphylactic response.
[1] Antinoff N and Williams BH (2012) Neoplasia. In: *Ferrets, Rabbits and Rodents*, ed. KE Quesenberry and JW Carpenter, pp. 103–121. Elsevier Saunders, Missouri

Sedation/immobilization protocols

Sedative combinations for ferrets

- Ketamine (5–8 mg/kg i.m.) plus medetomidine (80–100 μg (micrograms)/kg i.m.) or dexmedetomidine (40–50 μg (micrograms)/kg i.m.) to which can be added butorphanol (0.1–0.2 mg/kg i.m.) or buprenorphine (0.02 mg/kg i.m.) [a,b].
- Ketamine (5–20 mg/kg i.m.) plus midazolam (0.25–0.5 mg/kg i.m.) or diazepam (0.25–0.5 mg/kg i.m.) will provide immobilization or, at the higher doses, a short period of anaesthesia.
- Ketamine (7–10 mg/kg i.m., s.c.) plus medetomidine (20 μg (micrograms)/kg i.m., s.c.) plus midazolam (0.5 mg/kg i.m., s.c.) will provide anaesthesia; concurrent oxygenation is recommended.

References

[a] Ko JC, Heaton-Jones TG and Nicklin CF (1997) Evaluation of the sedative and cardiorespiratory effects of medetomidine, medetomidine-butorphanol, medetomidine-ketamine and medetomidine-butorphanol-ketamine in ferrets. *Journal of the American Animal Hospital Association* **33(5)**, 438–448

[b] Scherntjamer A, Lendl CE, Hartmann K et al. (2011) Medetomidine/midazolam/ ketamine anaesthesia in ferrets: effects on cardiorespiratory parameters and evaluation of plasma drug concentrations. *Veterinary Anaesthesia and Analgesia* **38(5)**, 439–450

Sedative combinations for rabbits

- Ketamine (3–5 mg/kg i.v. or 5–10 mg/kg i.m., s.c.) in combination with medetomidine (0.05–0.1 mg/kg i.v. or 0.1–0.3 mg/kg s.c., i.m.) or dexmedetomidine (0.025–0.05 mg/kg i.v. or 0.05–0.15 mg/kg s.c., i.m.) and butorphanol (0.05–0.1 mg/kg i.m., i.v., s.c.) or buprenorphine (0.02–0.05 mg/kg i.m., i.v., s.c.).
- Fentanyl/fluanisone (0.1–0.3 ml/kg i.m.) plus diazepam (0.5–1 mg/kg i.v., i.m. or 2.5–5.0 mg/kg intraperitoneal) or midazolam (0.25–1.0 mg/kg i.v., i.m., intraperitoneal).
- The combinations above will provide immobilization/light anaesthesia, usually sufficient to allow intubation for maintenance with a volatile agent.
- Ketamine (15 mg/kg i.m.) in combination with medetomidine (0.25 mg/kg i.m.) and buprenorphine (0.03 mg/kg i.m.) will provide general anaesthesia [a,b,c], but use of lower doses of medetomidine and ketamine followed by intubation and use of a volatile agent is recommended in practice.

References

[a] Grint NJ and Murison PJ (2008) A comparison of ketamine-midazolam and ketamine-medetomidine combinations for induction of anaesthesia in rabbits. *Veterinary Anaesthesia and Analgesia* **35(2)**, 113–121

[b] Murphy KL, Roughan JV, Baxter MG and Flecknell PA (2010) Anaesthesia with a combination of ketamine and medetomidine in the rabbit: effect of premedication with buprenorphine. *Veterinary Anaesthesia and Analgesia* **37(3)**, 222–229

[c] Orr HE, Roughan JV and Flecknell PA (2005) Assessment of ketamine and medetomidine anaesthesia in the domestic rabbit. *Veterinary Anaesthesia and Analgesia* **32(5)**, 271–279

Sedative combinations for other small mammals

- Medetomidine (50 μg (micrograms)/kg i.m.) or dexmedetomidine (25 μg (micrograms)/kg i.m.) plus, if needed, ketamine (2–4 mg/kg i.m.) [a,b,c,d,e,f].
- Other combinations as for rabbits. Combinations can also be administered intraperitoneal in small rodents.

References

[a] Bakker J, Uilenreef JJ, Pelt ER et al. (2013) Comparison of three different sedative-anaesthetic protocols (ketamine, ketamine-medetomidine and alphaxalone) in common marmosets (Callithrix jacchus). BMC Veterinary Research **9(1)**, 113

[b] Buchanan KC, Burge RR and Ruble GR (1998) Evaluation of injectable anaesthetics for major surgical procedures in guinea pigs. Contemporary Topics in Laboratory Animal Science **37(4)**, 58–63

[c] Dang V, Bao S, Ault A et al. (2008) Efficacy and safety of five injectable anesthetic regimens for chronic blood collection from the anterior vena cava of guinea pigs. Journal of American Association of Laboratory Animal Science **47(6)**, 56–60

[d] Hedenqvist P, Roughan JV and Flecknell PA (2000) Effects of repeated anaesthesia with ketamine/medetomidine and of pre-anaesthetic administration of buprenorphine in rats. Laboratory Animals **34(2)**, 207–211

[e] Jang HS, Choi HS, Lee SH, Jang KH and Lee MG (2009) Evaluation of the anaesthetic effects of medetomidine and ketamine in rats and their reversal with atipamezole. Veterinary Anaesthesia and Analgesia **36(4)**, 319–327

[f] Nevalainen T, Pyhälä L, Voipio HM and Virtanen R (1989) Evaluation of anaesthetic potency of medetomidine-ketamine combination in rats, guinea pigs and rabbits. Acta Veterinaria Scandinavica **85**, 139–143

Note: Reduce doses if animal is debilitated. For all small mammals, for deeper anaesthesia, intubation (if possible) and use of a volatile agent is recommended, rather than using higher doses of injectable agents.

Sedative combinations for birds

Injectable anaesthesia is best avoided unless in field situations (i.e. no gaseous anaesthesia available) or for the induction of large (e.g. swans/ratites), diving (e.g. ducks) or high-altitude birds. Even in these species, gaseous induction and maintenance (e.g. with isoflurane/sevoflurane) would still be the normal recommendation wherever possible. Sedation and premedicants are rarely used, as extra handling will add to the general stress of the situation. On occasions, diazepam (0.2–0.5 mg/kg i.m.) or midazolam (0.1–0.5 mg/kg i.m.) may be used; alternatively, either drug may be used at 0.05–0.15 mg/kg i.v. Parasympatholytic agents (such as atropine) are rarely used as their effect is to make respiratory excretions more viscous, thus increasing the risk of tube blockage.

- Propofol: 10 mg i.v. by slow infusion to effect; supplemental doses up to 3 mg/kg [a,b].
- Alfaxalone (2–4 mg/kg i.v.) is an alternative to propofol for the induction of anaesthesia in large birds or those with a dive response.
- Ketamine/diazepam combinations can be used for induction and muscle relaxation. Ketamine (30–40 mg/kg) plus diazepam (1.0–1.5 mg/kg) are given slowly i.v. to effect. May also be given i.m. but this produces different effects in different species and specific literature or specialist advice should be consulted. Ketamine (10 mg/kg i.m.) and diazepam (0.2–0.5 mg/kg i.m.) can be used as premedication/sedation (pigeons, Amazon parrots) prior to the administration of sevoflurane/isoflurane [c,d].
- **Raptors:** Ketamine (2–5 mg/kg i.m.) plus medetomidine (25–100 µg (micrograms)/kg) (lower dose rate i.v.; higher rate i.m.). This combination can be reversed with atipamezole at 65 µg (micrograms)/kg i.m. Ketamine should be avoided in vultures.

References

[a] Fitzgerald G and Cooper JE (1990) Preliminary studies on the use of propofol in the domestic pigeon (Columba livia). Research in Veterinary Science **49(3)**, 334–338

[b] Hawkins MG, Wright BD, Pascoe PJ *et al.* (2003) Pharmacokinetics and anesthetic and cardiopulmonary effects of propofol in red-tailed hawks (*Buteo virginianus*) and great horned owls (Bubo virginianus). *American Journal of Veterinary Research* **64(6)**, 677–683

[c] Azizpour and Hassani Y (2012) Clinical evaluation of general anaesthesia in pigeons using a combination of ketamine and diazepam. *Journal of the South African Veterinary Association* **83(1)**, 12

[d] Paula VV, Otsuki DA, Auler Júnior JO *et al.* (2013) The effect of premedication with ketamine, alone or with diazepam, on anaesthesia with sevoflurane in parrots (*Amazona aestival*). *BMC Veterinary Research* **9**, 142

Sedative combinations for reptiles

- Alfaxalone provides deep sedation/anaesthesia in chelonians (preferable to perform intermittent positive pressure ventilation with 100% oxygen after administration to prevent hypoxia). Can be used at 2–4 mg/kg i.v. or intraosseously for induction but effects are dependent on species and temperature.
  - **Chelonians: Red-eared sliders, Horsfield tortoises:** 10 mg/kg i.m. (light sedation) up to 20 mg/kg i.m. for surgical anaesthesia [a,b]; **Macquarie river turtles:** 9 mg/kg i.v. [c]
  - **Lizards, Snakes:** <9 mg/kg i.v. [d]; **Green iguanas:** 10 mg/kg i.m. (light sedation) up to 30 mg/kg i.m. for surgical anaesthesia [e] or 5 mg/kg i.v. [f] (for sufficient sedation to allow intubation); **Veiled chameleons:** 5 mg/kg i.v. (for sufficient sedation to allow intubation) [g]
- Propofol (5–10 mg/kg i.v. or intraosseously) will give 10–15 minutes of sedation/light anaesthesia (preferable to perform intermittent positive pressure ventilation with 100% oxygen after administration to prevent hypoxia).
  - **Red-eared sliders:** 10–20 mg/kg i.v. (higher doses required for successful intubation).
  - **Green iguanas:** 5–10 mg/kg iv., intraosseous.
  - **Brown tree snakes:** 5 mg/kg i.v.
- Ketamine as sole agent: Ketamine alone may result in variable sedation, poor muscle relaxation and prolonged recovery at higher dose rates. Usually combined with alpha-2 agonists and/or opioids/midazolam to provide deep sedation/light anaesthesia (see below).
- Alpha-2 agonists as sole agents: Although single agent use has been reported, it is generally preferable to use medetomidine or dexmedetomidine in combination with opioids and/or ketamine and/or midazolam for more reliable sedation (see below).
- Benzodiazepines as sole agents: Although single agent used has been reported, it is generally preferable to use midazolam in combination with opioids and/or ketamine and/or alpha-2 agonists for more reliable sedation (see below).
- Ketamine/alpha-2 agonist mixtures:
  - Ketamine (5–10 mg/kg i.m., i.v.) plus medetomidine (100–200 μg (micrograms)/kg i.m., i.v.) (deep sedation to light anaesthesia in gopher tortoises [h] and red-eared sliders [i]); may reverse medetomidine with atipamezole at 5 times the medetomidine dose (i.e. 0.5–1.0 mg/kg atipamezole)
  - Ketamine (2 mg/kg s.c.) plus dexmedetomidine (100 μg (micrograms)/kg s.c.) and midazolam (1 mg/kg s.c.) (moderate sedation in red-eared sliders [j])

- The addition of an opioid (e.g. morphine) to the mixture should be considered for potentially painful procedures (see monograph).
- Ketamine/benzodiazepine mixtures:
  - **Chelonians, Snakes:** Sedation to light anaesthesia: Ketamine (20–60 mg/kg i.m.) plus midazolam (1–2 mg/kg i.m.) or diazepam (**Chelonians:** 0.2–1 mg/kg i.m.; **Snakes:** 0.2–0.8 mg/kg i.m.) has been recommended for sedation.
- Ketamine/opioid mixtures:
  - Ketamine (10–30 mg/kg i.m.) plus butorphanol (0.5–1 mg/kg i.m.) has been recommended for sedation.
- Opioid/midazolam mixtures:
  - Butorphanol (0.4 mg/kg i.m.) plus midazolam (2 mg/kg i.m.) may be administered for pre-anaesthetic sedation.

References

[a] Hansen LL and Bertelsen MF (2013) Assessment of the effects of intramuscular administration of alfaxalone with and without medetomidine in Horsfield's tortoises (*Agrionemys horsfieldii*). *Veterinary Anaesthesia and Analgesia* **40(6)**, 68–75

[b] Kischinovsky M, Duse A, Wang T and Bertelsen MF (2013) Intramuscular administration of alfaxalone in red-eared sliders (*Trachemys scripta elegans*) – effect of dose and body temperature. *Veterinary Anaesthesia and Analgesia* **40(1)**, 13–20

[c] Scheelings TF (2013) Use of intravenous and intramuscular alfaxalone in Macquarie river turtles (*Emydura macquarii*). *Proceedings of the Association of Reptilian and Amphibian Veterinarians*, p. 71

[d] Scheelings TF, Baker RT, Hammersley G *et al.* (2011) A preliminary investigation into the chemical restraint with alfaxalone of selected Australian squamate species. *Journal of Herpetological Medicine and Surgery* **21**, 63–67

[e] Bertelsen MF and Sauer CD (2011) Alfaxalone anaesthesia in the green iguana (*Iguana iguana*). *Veterinary Anaesthesia and Analgesia* **38(5)**, 461–466

[f] Knotek Z, Hrda A, Knotkova Z, Barazorda Romero S and Habich A (2013) Alfaxalone anaesthesia in birds. *Acta Veterinaria Brno* **82**, 109–114

[g] Knotek Z, Hrda A, Kley N and Knotkova Z (2011) Alfaxalone anesthesia in veiled chameleon (*Chamaeleo calyptratus*). *Proceedings of the Association of Reptilian and Amphibian Veterinarians*, pp. 179–181

[h] Dennis C and Heard DJ (2002) Cardiopulmonary effects of a medetomidine-ketamine combination administered intravenously in gopher tortoises. *Journal of the American Veterinary Medical Association* **220(10)**, 1516–1519

[i] Greer LL, Jenne KJ and Diggs HE (2001) Medetomidine-ketamine anesthesia in red-eared slider turtles (*Trachemys scripta elegans*). *Journal of the American Association for Laboratory Animal Science* **40(3)**, 8–11

[j] Mans C, Drees R, Sladky KK, Hatt JM and Kircher PR (2013) Effects of body position and extension of the neck and extremities on lung volume measure via computed tomography in red-eared slider turtles (*Trachemys scripta elegans*). *Journal of the American Veterinary Medical Association* **243(8)**, 1190–1196

Sedative combinations for fish

All anaesthetics are administered by immersion and the stage of anaesthesia reached is determined by the concentration used and the duration of exposure, since absorption continues throughout the period of immersion. There are significant species differences in their response to the drugs and it is advised that the lower dose rates are used for unfamiliar species, marine and tropical fish. Many products and stock solutions should be kept in a dark bottle and protected from light. Ideally, the anaesthetic solution should be made up using water from the tank or pond of origin to minimize problems due to changes in water chemistry. It should be used on the day of preparation and well aerated during use. Food should be withheld for 12–24 hours before anaesthesia to reduce the risk of regurgitation, which may cause damage to gill tissues. Monitoring heart rate during prolonged procedures using a Doppler probe or ultrasound scanner is advisable since this is a direct reflection of the level of anaesthesia. Following the procedure, anaesthetized fish should be returned to clean water from their normal environment to allow recovery.

- Tricaine mesilate (MS-222) (50–250 mg/l by immersion) produces an acidic solution and should be buffered with sodium bicarbonate to maintain the same pH as the original environmental water conditions. The dry powder is very soluble in water and can be added directly or a stock solution can be made up to facilitate accurate dosing.
- Benzocaine (25–200 mg/l by immersion) is insoluble in water and must be dissolved in acetone or ethanol. For example, a stock solution of 100 g benzocaine/l of ethanol produces 100 mg/ml to facilitate accurate dosing.
- 2-Phenoxyethanol (0.1–0.5 ml/l by immersion) must be whisked vigorously into the water to improve solubility.

Anaesthetics, analgesics and NSAIDs

Adrenoreceptor antagonists
Atipamezole 27
Antiarthritis drugs
Polysulphated
glycosaminoglycan 243
Inhalational anaesthetics
Isoflurane 166
Nitrous oxide 215
Sevoflurane 266
Injectable anaesthetics
Alfaxalone 8
Fentanyl/Fluanisone 131
Ketamine 171
Propofol 254
(see also Sedation/immobilization protocols in the Appendix)
Local anaesthetics
Benzocaine 36
Bupivacaine 42
Eugenol 124
Lidocaine 180
Mepivacaine 195
Phenoxyethanol 236
Tricaine mesilate 288
Muscle relaxants
Atracurium 28
Rocuronium 263
Vecuronium 295
Mydriatics
Atracurium 28
Non-opioid analgesics
Amantadine 13
Tramadol 286

Non-steroidal anti-inflammatory drugs
Aspirin 25
Carprofen 54
Celecoxib 65
Dimethylsulfoxide 105
Ketoprofen 173
Meloxicam 194
Paracetamol 225
Piroxicam 242
Tolfenamic acid 284
Opioid analgesics
Alfentanil 10
Buprenorphine 43
Butorphanol 46
Fentanyl 129
Methadone 196
Morphine 209
Pethidine 232
Naloxone 212
Parasympatholytics
Atropine 29
Glycopyrronium 151
Sedatives
Acepromazine 1
Dexmedetomidine 96
Diazepam 98
Medetomidine 191
Midazolam 204
Xylazine 308
(see also Sedation/immobilization protocols in the Appendix)
Sympathomimetics
Adrenaline 6

Anti-infectives

(see also Guidelines for responsible antibacterial use in the Appendix)

Anthelmintics
Emodepside 117
Fenbendazole 127
Levamisole 177
Mebendazole/Closantel 190
Oxfendazole 219
Piperazine 241
Praziquantel 248
Pyrantel 258

Antibacterials
Aminoglycosides
Amikacin 13
Framycetin 141
Gentamicin 147
Neomycin 213
Streptomycin 273
Tobramycin 283
Beta-lactams
Amoxicillin 19
Ampicillin 22
Aztreonam 33
Cloxacillin 83
Co-amoxiclav 84

Anti-neoplastic

(see also Safety and handling of chemotherapeutic agents and Chemotherapy protocols in the Appendix)

Behaviour modifiers

Amitriptyline 18
Clomipramine 82
Diphenhydramine 107
Doxepin 112
Fluoxetine 138

Haloperidol 154
Mirtazapine 206
Paroxetine 226
Propentofylline 253

Blood and immune system

Anticoagulants
Aspirin 25
Heparin (low molecular weight) 154
Heparin (unfractionated) 155
Blood and substitutes
Haemoglobin glutamer 153

Colony-stimulating growth factors
Erythropoietin 123
Immunosuppressives
Azathioprine 30
Ciclosporin 74

Cardiovascular

Alpha blockers
Phenoxybenzamine 235
Antiarrhythmics
Digoxin 102
Verapamil 296
Antiplatelet aggregators
Aspirin 25
Beta blockers
Atenolol 25
Carvedilol 56
Propranolol 255
Diuretics
Furosemide 143
Hydrochlorothiazide 158

Positive inotropes
Dopamine 108
Pimobendan 239
Vasodilators
Benazepril 34
Diltiazem 103
Enalapril 118
Glyceryl trinitrate 151
Hydralazine 157
Imidapril 162
Prazosin 249

Dermatological

Antifungals
Terbinafine 278
Antihistamines
Chlorphenamine 72
Cyproheptadine 90
Diphenhydramine 107
Hydroxyzine 159
Cleansers and sebolytics
Chlorhexidine 70
Ecto- and endoparasiticides
Ivermectin 169
Milbemycin 206
Selamectin 265
Ectoparasiticides
Acetic acid 3
Acriflavine 5
Amitraz 17
Chloramine-T 68
Chloroquine 72

Cypermethrin 89
Cyromazine 90
Diflubenzuron 101
Emamectin benzoate 116
Fipronil 132
Formaldehyde 140
Fresh water 142
Imidacloprid 161
Lufenuron 184
Methoprene 198
Moxidectin 210
Nitenpyram 214
Potassium permanganate 245
Pyriproxyfen 259
Hormone replacements
see Endocrine
Immunosuppressives
Ciclosporin 74

APPENDIX I: GENERAL INFORMATION
APPENDIX II: PROTOCOLS
INDEX: THERAPEUTIC CLASS
INDEX: GENERIC AND TRADE NAMES

Genito-urinary tract

Antifibrotics
Colchicine 85
Diuretics
Furosemide 143
Phosphate binders
Chitosan 66
Urethral relaxants
Diazepam 98
Phenoxybenzamine 235

Urinary alkalinizers
Potassium citrate 245
Urinary incontinence
Phenylpropanolamine 237
Urinary retention
Bethanecol 38
Urolithiasis
Allopurinol 11
Penicillamine 227
Potassium citrate 245

Metabolic

Antidotes
Acetylcysteine 3
Charcoal 65
Colestyramine 86
Deferoxamine 92

Dimercaprol 104
Edetate calcium disodium 116
Methylthioninium chloride 200
Penicillamine 227
Pralidoxime 247

Neuromuscular system

Antiepileptics
Diazepam 98
Gabapentin 146
Imepitoin 161
Levetiracetam 178
Midazolam 204
Phenobarbital 233

Phenytoin 238
Potassium bromide 244
Euthanasia
Pentobarbital 230
Osmotic diuretics
Mannitol 186

Nutritional/fluids

(see also table of composition of intravenous fluids in the Appendix)

Crystalloids
Sodium chloride 271
Glucose supplements
Glucose 149
Mineral and electrolyte supplements
Iron salts 164
Sodium bicarbonate 270
Zinc salts 310

Nutritional supplements
Acetic acid 3
Amino acid solutions 15
Glutamine 150
Vitamin supplements
Vitamin A 298
Vitamin B complex 299
Vitamin B1 300
Vitamin B12 301
Vitamin C 302
Vitamin D 303
Vitamin E 304
Vitamin K1 305

APPENDIX I: GENERAL INFORMATION
APPENDIX II: PROTOCOLS
INDEX: THERAPEUTIC CLASS
INDEX: GENERIC AND TRADE NAMES

Ophthalmic

Antibacterials
Ciprofloxacin 77
Moxifloxacin 211
Antivirals
Aciclovir 4
Glaucoma therapy
Dorzolamide 110
Latanoprost 176
Timolol maleate 282
Travoprost 287
Immunosuppressives
Ciclosporin 74
Mydriatics
Phenylephrine 236
Tropicamide 292

Non-steroidal anti-inflammatory drugs
Diclofenac 100
Flurbiprofen 139
Ketorolac 175
Tear substitutes
Carbomer 980 52
Hyaluronate 156
Hypromellose 160
Paraffin 226
Polyvinyl alcohol 243
Topical anaesthetics
Proxymetacaine 257
Tetracaine 279

Respiratory system

Anti-inflammatory steroids
Fluticasone 140
Bronchodilators
Acetylcysteine 3
Aminophylline 16
Propentofylline 253
Salbutamol 264
Terbutaline 278
Theophylline 280

Mucolytics
Bromhexine 39
Nasal decongestants
Phenylpropanolamine 237
Respiratory stimulants
Doxapram 110